Vaccine Design

The Role of Cytokine Networks

NATO ASI Series

Advanced Science Institutes Series

A series presenting the results of activities sponsored by the NATO Science Committee, which aims at the dissemination of advanced scientific and technological knowledge, with a view to strengthening links between scientific communities.

The series is published by an international board of publishers in conjunction with the NATO Scientific Affairs Division

A Life Sciences **B Physics**	Plenum Publishing Corporation New York and London
C Mathematical and Physical Sciences **D Behavioral and Social Sciences** **E Applied Sciences**	Kluwer Academic Publishers Dordrecht, Boston, and London
F Computer and Systems Sciences **G Ecological Sciences** **H Cell Biology** **I Global Environmental Change**	Springer-Verlag Berlin, Heidelberg, New York, London, Paris, Tokyo, Hong Kong, and Barcelona

PARTNERSHIP SUB-SERIES

1. Disarmament Technologies	Kluwer Academic Publishers
2. Environment	Springer-Verlag
3. High Technology	Kluwer Academic Publishers
4. Science and Technology Policy	Kluwer Academic Publishers
5. Computer Networking	Kluwer Academic Publishers

The Partnership Sub-Series incorporates activities undertaken in collaboration with NATO's Cooperation Partners, the countries of the CIS and Central and Eastern Europe, in Priority Areas of concern to those countries.

Recent Volumes in this Series:

Volume 293—Vaccine Design: The Role of Cytokine Networks
edited by Gregory Gregoriadis, Brenda McCormack, and Anthony C. Allison

Volume 294—Vascular Endothelium: Pharmacologic and Genetic Manipulations
edited by John D. Catravas, Allan D. Callow, and Una S. Ryan

Volume 295—Prions and Brain Diseases in Animals and Humans
edited by Douglas R. O. Morrison

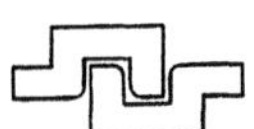

Series A: Life Sciences

Vaccine Design

The Role of Cytokine Networks

Edited by

Gregory Gregoriadis and
Brenda McCormack

School of Pharmacy
University of London
London, England

and

Anthony C. Allison

Dawa Corporation
Belmont, California

Plenum Press
New York and London
Published in cooperation with NATO Scientific Affairs Division

Proceedings of a NATO Advanced Study Institute on
Vaccine Design: The Role of Cytokine Networks,
held June 24 – July 5, 1996,
in Cape Sounion, Greece

NATO-PCO-DATA BASE

The electronic index to the NATO ASI Series provides full bibliographical references (with keywords and/or abstracts) to about 50,000 contributions from international scientists published in all sections of the NATO ASI Series. Access to the NATO-PCO-DATA BASE is possible via a CD-ROM "NATO Science and Technology Disk" with user-friendly retrieval software in English, French, and German (©WTV GmbH and DATAWARE Technologies, Inc. 1989). The CD-ROM contains the AGARD Aerospace Database.

The CD-ROM can be ordered through any member of the Board of Publishers or through NATO-PCO, Overijse, Belgium.

Library of Congress Cataloging-in-Publication Data

On file

ISBN 0-306-45818-7

A Division of Plenum Publishing Corporation
233 Spring Street, New York, N.Y. 10013

http://www.plenum.com

10 9 8 7 6 5 4 3 2 1

Printed in the United States of America

PREFACE

During the last decade or so vaccine development has been facilitated by rapid advances in the molecular and cell biology of the immune system. This has laid the foundations of a new generation of vaccines exemplified by subunit vaccines produced through gene cloning and by synthetic peptides mimicking small regions of proteins on the outer coat of viruses. However, as subunit and peptide vaccines are only weakly or non-immunogenic, there is a real need for strategies to improve their potency.

This book contains the proceedings of the 5th NATO Advanced Studies Institute (ASI), "Vaccine Design: The Role of Cytokine Networks," held at Cape Sounion Beach, Greece, during 24 June–5 July 1996 and deals in depth with the role of basic immunology in the regulation of immunity and vaccine design. Special emphasis is given to the use of cytokines in conjuction with vaccines with the aim of improving their potency or the use of vaccines designed to improve cytokine production. We express our appreciation to Dr. J.-L. Virelizier and Dr. G. Kollias for their cooperation in planning the ASI and to Mrs. Concha Perring for her excellent production of the manuscripts. The ASI was held under the sponsorship of NATO Scientific Affairs Division and generously co-sponsored by SmithKline Beecham Pharmaceuticals (Philadelphia). Financial assistance was also provided by Connaught Laboratories Ltd. (Ontario), Pasteur Merieux (Marcy l'Étoile), Biochine (Siena), Help SA (Athens), and Avanti Polar Lipids Inc. (Birmingham, USA).

Gregory Gregoriadis
Brenda McCormack
Anthony C. Allison

CONTENTS

Vaccine Design

The Role of Cytokine Networks

THE ROLE OF CYTOKINES IN THE ACTION OF IMMUNOLOGICAL ADJUVANTS

Anthony C. Allison

Dawa Corporation
Belmont, CA 94002 U.S.A.

INTRODUCTION

Three classes of adjuvants - mineral oil emulsions, aluminium salts, and saponin - have long been used to augment immune responses in vaccination. Each has its own advantages and limitations, and during the last decade new adjuvants have been developed. These complement a new group of antigens, including proteins produced by recombinant technology and synthetic peptides, which require adjuvants to elicit protective immune responses. Some of the recently developed adjuvant formulations are already approved for use in human and veterinary vaccines. This paper describes immunomodulating bacterial products and synthetic derivatives, as well as two-phase (lipid in water) vehicles for antigens. It also reviews briefly what adjuvants are required to do and what is known of their mode of action, with special reference to the role of cytokines.

DEFINITIONS

An adjuvant is a substance or procedure which augments specific immune responses to antigens. A carrier is an immunogenic molecule which, when bound to a second molecule, augments immune responses to the latter. Examples of carriers are the protein components of glycoconjugates that increase antibody responses to bacterial capsular polysaccharides and proteins bound to peptides which increase anti-peptide responses. A carrier is thus distinguished from a vehicle, which is a two-phase system that facilitates uptake of antigens by antigen-presenting cells and transports antigens from injection sites to lymphoid tissues. Examples of vehicles are liposomes, ISCOMs and microfluidized squalene emulsions. Adjuvants frequently contain immunomodulators, which induce the production of cytokines and augment immune responses. Examples are muramyl peptides, lipopolysaccharides and derivatives, and certain cationic detergents. The combination of an immunomodulator with a vehicle, to optimize activity, is an adjuvant formulation.

Vaccine Design: The Role of Cytokine Networks
Edited by Gregoriadis *et al.*, Plenum Press, New York, 1997

AFFINITIES AND ISOTYPES OF ANTIBODIES

Traditionally the efficacy of adjuvants has been judged by the levels of antibodies elicited (using a convenient test, such as ELISA or haemagglutination). While these assays have provided useful information, they should now be supplemented by other measures of the quantity and quality of antibodies elicited. Preferably, antibody levels should be quantified by tests relevant to function, such as neutralization of bacterial toxins or viruses, killing of tumor cells or induced cytostasis. Because of potential problems with solid-phase assays, at least some measurements of antibody levels using fluid-phase assays should be made. In addition to the quantities of antibodies elicited by a vaccine, two properties of the antibodies are likely to be important for protection: their affinity for antigen and their isotype. To neutralize a virus or bacterial toxin, antibodies should bind them with sufficiently high affinity. If the complexes are not removed by phagocytic cells, antibodies must bind to a virus or toxin with an affinity of at least the same order as the natural receptor. Measurements of affinities by dissociation from antigen bound to a surface, using low pH or chaotropic agents, have limitations. In the author's laboratory methods have been developed to measure the quantities and affinities of antibodies in the fluid phase (Kenney et al., 1990).

Another important property of antibodies is their isotype. Antibodies of the immunoglobulin G (IgG) class pass from the vascular to the extravascular compartment more easily than those of the IgM class, only the former are transferred across the placenta or by milk to fetuses and newborn animals. Antibodies of some isotypes efficiently activate complement, bind to high-affinity receptors on monocytes, and act synergistically with antibody-dependent effector cells (ADCC), to produce cytotoxicity. Examples are IgG2a antibodies in mice and IgG1 antibodies in humans, both of which bind to high affinity FcγI receptors. Studies with isotype-switch variants of murine monoclonal antibodies (which have the same Fab regions, so binding to antigen is comparable) show that IgG2a antibodies confer better protection against tumors than those of other isotypes (Kaminski et al., 1986). Studies with "reshaped" human antibodies, genetically constructed to have antigen-binding hypervariable regions like those of rodent monoclonals, confirm the superiority of the human IgG1 isotype in ADCC-mediated lysis (Reichmann et al., 1988). The desirability of developing an adjuvant formulation that preferentially elicits high-affinity antibodies of the IgG2a isotype in mice and IgG1 in humans is apparent.

Antibodies elicited should be directed to determinants exposed in native antigens; modern adjuvants augment the formation of such antibodies, whereas Freund's adjuvant can denature antigens and elicit antibodies against internal determinants (Kenney et al., 1989).

CELL-MEDIATED IMMUNITY

Helper T-lymphocytes are required for the formation of antibodies against most antigens. Activation of helper T-cells is one important function of adjuvants. Effector T-lymphocytes, able to lyse target cells in a genetically restricted fashion, and to produce mediators such as IFN-γ and lymphotoxin, contribute to host resistance aganist some viruses, bacteria, parasites and tumours (Schulz et al., 1991; Doherty et al., 1992). The importance of antigen presentation in eliciting protective immune responses can be illustrated by studies with peptide antigens of tumours (Toes et al., 1996). Under some conditions cytotoxic T-lymphocytes (CTL) are elicited, and this is correlated with protection against tumour cell outgrowth. Under other conditions peptide vaccination leads to functional deletion of tumour-specific CTL and inability to reject tumours.

It is likely, therefore, that for optimal protection against tumours and some infectious agents, eg, herpesviruses, the elicitation of cell-mediated immunity is desirable. Tests for cell-mediated immunity should include not only delayed hypersensitivity but also proliferative responses to the antigen and the release of IL-2, IFN-γ and lymphotoxin. Cytotoxicity for autologous or syngeneic infected target cells should also be studied. If mice or rats are used, syngeneic target cells are readily available. With outbred species, such as humans and subhuman primates, B-cells transformed by Epstein-Barr virus, transfected with a vaccinia virus or other vector expressing the antigen under consideration (eg, HIV antigens - Walker et al., 1988), can provide autologous target cells for studies of genetically-restricted cell-mediated cytotoxicity.

IMMUNOMODULATORS

Muramyl Dipeptides (MDP)

Ellouz et al. (1974) showed that the minimal component of bacterial cell walls with adjuvant activity is N-acetylmuramyl-L-alanyl-D-isoglutamine (muramyl dipeptide or MDP). When MDP is added to Freund's incomplete adjuvant (FIA) the isotype of antibodies changes and cell-mediated immunity is elicited. MDP itself is pyrogenic, and produces in experimental animals changes similar to Reiter's syndrome observed in humans with some bacterial infections: arthritis and anterior uveitis. MDP in mineral oil emulsions injected into rats induces adjuvant arthritis, and in rabbits MDP produces uveitis: increased vascular permeability and a leukocytic infiltrate of the uveal tract of the eye (Waters et al., 1986).

In several laboratories analogues of MDP were synthesized to identify components with better separation of adjuvant activity from undesirable side effects. An analogue in which L-threonine replaces L-alanine in MDP gives good separation (Allison and Byars, 1986); the hydroxyl group of threonine allows the formation of an additional internal hydrogen bond, thereby stabilizing the molecule in a preferred configuration. The threonyl analogue of MDP is a potent adjuvant, does not induce adjuvant arthritis in rats and induces uveitis in rabbits only when used in very high concentrations (Waters et al., 1986).

Monophosphoryl Lipid A (MPL)

The adjuvant-active component of lipopolysaccharide endotoxins of Gram-negative bacteria (LPS) is lipid A, as confirmed by total synthesis. Lipid A is pyrogenic, and elicits systemic responses similar to those produced by MDP. Efforts have been made to separate adjuvant activity of lipid A derivatives from side effects. Lipid A is a disaccharide of glucosamine with two phosphate groups (at the 1′and 4′ positions of the disaccharide) and five or six fatty acid chains, usually C_{12} or C_{16} in length. Under mildly acid conditions, one phosphate group can be removed, leaving 4′-monophosphoryl lipid A (MPL). This retains adjuvant activity, but is much less toxic than lipid A (Ribi et al., 1993). MPL, suitably formulated, is being used in human vaccines.

ANTIGEN-CARRYING VEHICLES

Oil-in Water Emulsions

Water-in-oil emulsions, such as Freund's adjuvants, form depots at injection sites, which become infiltrated by leukocytes. There is inevitably some inflammation. Excision of injection sites after an interval does not impair immune responses, which suggests either that cells carry the antigen to depots in lymphoid tissues, or that emulsified antigen migrates to lymphoid tissues. To facilitate uptake of antigens by antigen-presenting cells and transport into lymph, and to use a more acceptable lipid, Allison and Byars (1986) developed squalene or squalane emulsions in an aqueous phase. Squalene is a naturally occurring, abundant precursor of cholesterol; squalane is saturated and more stable than squalene, which is convenient in a formulation. Squalane occurs naturally in sebaceous secretions. The squalene/squalane emulsions in buffered saline are prepared by microfluidization in the presence of an emulsifying agent or agents. The combination of threonyl-MDP with such an emulsion is designated SAF.

Liposomes

Another lipid-in-water system which can transport antigens to lymphoid tissues is liposomes. These single or concentric phospholipid bilayers are versatile vehicles for antigens and immunomodulators such as lipid A. Water-soluble antigens can be entrapped within liposomes or bound to their surface, while lipophilic peptides or other antigens can be solubilized in the phospholipid bilayers. Allison and Gregoriadis (1974) showed that diphtheria toxoid in liposomes elicits higher antibody responses than free toxoid, and since then liposomes have been used in many experimental vaccines (Gregoriadis, 1990).

A liposome-based human vaccine is now marketed in Switzerland (Glück, 1995). It is named immunopotentiating reconstituted influenza virosomes (IRIV), small unilamellar vesicles bearing influenza virus haemagglutinin (HA) and hepatitis A virus. The HA is believed to function as a fusogen favouring processing in antigen-presenting cells as well as a carrier augmenting the formation of antibodies against hepatitis A virus (Glück, 1995). When peptides are presented in liposomes carrier effects can occur without covalent linkage of hapten to carrier (Gregoriadis et al., 1993). IRIV elicit good antibody responses to both influenza HA and hepatitis A determinants, and open the way for other liposomally based human vaccines.

ANTIGEN-PRESENTING CELLS

We performed the first analyses of the cell types responding to antigens and adjuvants using cell transfer (Unanue et al., 1969; Spitznagel et al., 1970). These experiments showed that adjuvants such as LPS or Bordetella pertussis initially interact with antigen-presenting cells and not lymphocytes. Moreover, adjuvants could not bypass the requirement for helper T-lymphocytes (Allison and Davies, 1971). For many years macrophages were thought to be the predominant antigen-presenting cells. However, macrophages in lymph nodes and the spleen can be efficiently depleted using a bisphosphonate in liposomes, and such depletion augments immune responses to soluble and viral antigens (Van Rooijen and Sanders, 1994). This suggests that while macrophages partially digest large organisms for presentation of antigens, in a human or domestic animal responding to subunit vaccines other antigen-presenting cells play a major role. Three such cell types have been defined.

Dendritic Cells (DC)

Cells of this lineage originate in the bone marrow, migrate through the blood to the skin and interstitial tissues and then migrate through afferent lymphatics to the T-dependent areas of lymph nodes, where they are termed interdigitating cells. DC isolated from the spleen (Steinman, 1991) have similar properties and are probably of the same lineage. DC efficiently present antigens associated with their surfaces to T-lymphocytes, initiating T-dependent immune responses (Macatonia et al., 1995).

The initiation of an immune response in the skin, for example to a contact sensitizer, is associated with a migration of DC from the skin to lymph nodes of the drainage chain

(Cumberpatch and Kimber, 1995). The DC which arrive in lymph nodes show markers of maturation manifested by higher expression of MHC class II antigens and of intercellular adhesion molecule-1 than in skin DC. Injection of a small dose of LPS into muscle results in migration of DC to draining lymph nodes.

Information has accumulated about the cytokines that promote the generation of DC from human $CD34^+$ precursor cells in the bone marrow or peripheral blood, as well as the migration of DC from tissues such as skin to the lymph nodes of the drainage chain. The combination of TGF-β1, TNF-α, GM-CSF and stem cell factor (SCF) provides optimal generation of functional DC from $CD34^+$ precursors (Strobl et al., 1996). GM-CSF increases expression of MHC class II molecules and ICAM-1 on DC and their efficiency of antigen presentation (Heufler et al., 1988). The cytokine principally responsible for induced migration of DC from tissues to lymph nodes is TNF-α (Cumberpatch and Kimber, 1995). An early effect of adjuvants is likely to be inducing the migration of DC from sites of injection of antigen to lymph nodes, as well as promoting the maturation of these cells, thereby increasing the efficiency of antigen presentation to T-cells.

Follicular Dendritic Cells (FDC)

Follicular dendritic cells are found in lymphoid follicles in lymph nodes, spleen and other sites (Szakal et al., 1989). Their branching cytoplasmic extensions are closely associated with B-lymphocytes. FDC express CD4 and high-affinity complement (CR2) receptors (CD21). Immune complexes binding FDC become localized on beaded cell-membrane extensions, and can remain there for a long time (months). Some antigen is endocytosed by CD21-bearing follicular B-lymphocytes expressing class II major histocompatibility antigens. The antigen can be demonstrated for at least one week by immunocytochemistry in endocytic vacuoles within B-cells; in such a compartment they may be partially digested for presentation to T-lymphocytes.

B-Lymphocytes

Evidence has accumulated that B-lymphocytes efficiently present antigens to T-lymphocytes (Ron and Sprent, 1987). In fact, depletion of B-cells by repeated injections of antibody against the μ-chain of immunoglobulin markedly decreases responses to antigens of T-lymphocytes in peripheral lymphoid tissues (Ron and Sprent, 1987). A major role of surface-membrane immunoglobulin receptors for antigens on B-cells may be to bind the antigen for subsequent T-cell presentation, especially in secondary T-cell responses. The so-called "original antigenic sin" recall phenomenon is explicable in these terms.

TARGETING ANTIGENS TO ANTIGEN-PRESENTING CELLS

It has long been known that activation of complement facilitates the localization of antigens on FDC and the induction of B memory (MacLennan, 1994). The underlying mechanism has recently been clarified. Two fragments of activated C3 are C3dg and C3d, which bind to CR2 (CD21) on FDC and B-lymphocytes (Dempsey et al., 1996); C3d binds CD21, a B-cell membrane protein that associates with CD19 and amplifies proliferative responses of these cells. Hen egg lysozyme (HEL) fused to murine C3d, to produce a recombinant model targeted antigen, was found to elicit antibodies in mice much more efficiently than HEL itself (Dempsey et al., 1996). Adjuvants such as LPS activate complement by the alternative pathway. Squalene emulsions have the same effect, and liposomes of compositions that activate complement are more efficient adjuvants than other liposomes

(Allison and Byars, 1992). Thus targeting antigens to FDC, through binding of C3d to CD21, may be an important requirement for eliciting antigen-specific B-cell proliferation and thereby establishing immunological memory. We are currently exploring the hypothesis that targeting antigens to dendritic cells augments T-cell responses.

SELECTION BY ADJUVANTS FOR THE PRODUCTION OF ANTIBODIES OF HIGH AFFINITY AND PROTECTIVE ISOTYPES

For reasons discussed above, it frequently is desirable to elicit antibodies of high affinities and protective isotypes, e.g. IgG2a in the mouse. It has long been known that the use of particular adjuvants can influence the isotypes of antibodies. An example is the use of low doses of antigen with alum, B. pertussis or saponin to produce IgE antibodies in the mouse (Hamaoka et al., 1973) and rat (Vijay et al., 1979). Antigens administered to guinea pigs in FIA mainly elicit antibodies of the γ_1 isotype whereas with the complete adjuvant γ_2 antibodies are formed (White, 1976). In the author's laboratory comparisons have been made of antibodies elicited by human serum albumin and recombinant human interleukin-1α administered to mice in different adjuvants by the intraperitoneal and subcutaneous routes (Kenney et al., 1989). Considerable differences were observed: FCA elicited high levels of antibodies (these were not of high affinity, with many directed to epitopes not exposed on the native molecule); SAF elicited the highest proportion of antibodies of the IgG2a isotype; antibodies against IL-1 were potent in neutralizing biological activity of the molecule (with cells from the mice used to produce monoclonal antibodies); and aluminum hydroxide elicited mainly IgG1 antibodies (Kenney et al., 1989). Thus, adjuvants can select for the isotype of antibodies formed.

ROLE OF CYTOKINES IN ISOTYPE SELECTION

Evidence is accumulating that cytokines play a role in isotype selection in the mouse and in cultured human cells (Finkelman et al., 1990). IFN-γ augments the production of IgG2a antibodies in mice, whereas IL-4 augments IgG1 and IgE antibodies, explaining why adjuvants that are designed to increase cell-mediated immunity - such as FCA and SAF - concurrently select for antibodies of the IgG2a isotype. Potent T-cell-mediated responses to antigenic stimulation release IFN-γ (from both the helper and cytotoxic subset of T-cells) which augments the formation of IgG2a antibodies. Adjuvants which less consistently stimulate T-cell responses, such as aluminum hydroxide, favour production of IgG1 and IgE antibodies by stimulating release of more IL-4 than IFN-γ. This interpretation was proposed by Allison and Byars (1992) and discussed in the context of stimulating the Th1 subset of T-lymphocytes by Audibert and Lise (1993). We found that SAF increases the number of cells producing IL-2 and IFN-γ, but not those producing IL-4, in the lymph nodes draining sites of antigen injection. Dendritic cells can produce IL-12, a dominant cytokine involved in the development of $CD4^+$ T-lymphocytes which produce IFN-γ (Macatonia et al., 1995). Production of IL-12 by DC appears to be an early and crucial event in the cascade of cytokines formed in lymphoid tissues responding to antigens in the presence of adjuvants. The importance of IFN-γ in this cascade is illustrated by observations on IFN-γ receptor-deficient mice (Schijns et al., 1994). In these mice antiviral Th1-type responses occur, but the generation of protective antiviral antibodies is profoundly impaired.

PRIMARY AND SECONDARY CYTOKINE CASCADES

When an infectious agent invades the connective tissue of the skin or another site, early innate humoral and cellular defense mechanisms are followed by acquired immune responses. In the innate response cytokines such as TNF-α and GM-CSF recruit leukocytes and activate them for microbial killing. Complement activation enhances chemotaxis of leukocytes and phagocytosis of invading organisms. TNF-α also promotes the migration of DC to lymph nodes, while GM-CSF and other cytokines, acting together, increase the efficacy of DC as antigen-presenting cells. Microbial antigens associated with C3d are efficiently presented by FDC to B-cells. Thus innate immunity is reinforced by acquired immunity: the two are closely linked.

To improve vaccination it is necessary to mimic these events. For example, two-phase systems can be used to increase the efficiency of antigen uptake by DC and the transport of antigens to lymphoid tissue, with activated complement targeting antigens to FDC. Immunomodulators induce a primary cytokine cascade at injection sites: the production of small amounts of TNF-α, TGF-β1 and GM-CSF. These cytokines promote the migration and maturation of DC, thereby increasing the probability that antigen will be associated with DC as well as the efficiency of antigen presentation to T-cells. During a secondary cytokine cascade in draining lymph nodes DC produce IL-12, which augments the production of IFN-γ in T-cells, thereby favouring a Th1-pattern of response. IFN-γ selects for the production of antibody isotypes that are most efficient in host protection. Adjuvant formulations already developed induce these cascades of cytokines, but there is room for improvement of efficacy without toxicity. Developing adjuvant formulations that induce preferentially cell-mediated immunity or antibody formation would also be helpful for new vaccines, e.g. against cancer. Perhaps targeting antigens to DC or FDC will achieve that goal as well as selective cytokine induction.

PROTECTING MUCOSAL SURFACES

A great deal of effort is currently being made to immunize by mucosal routes to stimulate mucosal IgA production. While useful progress has been made, limitations in this strategy have become apparent, in particular the induction of good memory responses. Hence it is worth noting that systemic immunization can, in some situations, protect mucosal surfaces. According to current dogma, lymphocytes isolated from lymph or lymph nodes preferentially return to mucosal sites whereas lymphocytes from peripheral tissues preferentially migrate to peripheral tissues or lymphoid organs. However, Meeusen et al. (1996) have recently presented evidence that site-directed migration of lymphocytes can be determined by the functional phenotype of the lymphocyte, independent of their site of induction. Following either subcutaneous or mucosal immunization of sheep, antigen-specific proliferating T-cells were concentrated in peripheral lymph nodes and were virtually absent from intestinal lymph nodes. The authors propose that in peripheral lymphoid tissue, predominantly Th1 type of responses occur whereas in mucosal lymphoid tissue the response is predominantly of Th2-type.

Following subcutaneous immunizations of sheep with a recombinant protein from *Taenia ovis*, Rothel et al. (1996) found in efferent lymphatics large numbers of antigen-specific IgA-secreting cells. Injected IgA-secreting cells migrate preferentially to gut-associated lymphoid tissue. Thus induction of a mucosal IgA response may be achieved by peripheral vaccination.

Two examples of the use of our adjuvant formulation illustrate that subcutaneous immunization can protect mucosal surfaces. Guinea pigs vaccinated with recombinant gD-2t of herpes simplex virus in SAF were found to be protected against vaginal mucosal challenge with the virus (Byars et al., 1994). In the immunized animals lesions at challenge sites were markedly reduced and spread of virus to dorsal root ganglia, as well as systemically, was prevented. Prevention of nerve ganglion infection is correlated with reduced recurrence, which in a population could decrease viral transmission.

Another study was on a primate model of periodontitis, a common disorder in which the attachment tissues of the teeth and their alveolar bone housing are destroyed, resulting in tooth loss. The Gram-negative anaerobic bacterium Porphyromonas gingivalis has been closely linked to severe forms of periodontitis. Persson et al. (1994) showed that immunization of Macaca fascicularis with killed P. gingivalis in SAF inhibits progression of periodontal tissue destruction.

These remarks are not intended to imply that systemic immunization can substitute for mucosal immunization in all situations. Clearly that is not the case. However, when protective mucosal immunization is not easily elicited, it is worth investigating whether systemic vaccination is useful.

REFERENCES

Allison, A.C. and Davies, A.J.S. 1971. Requirement of thymus-dependent lymphocytes for potentiation by adjuvants of antibody formation. Nature, 233:330.

Allison, A.C. and Gregoriadis, G. 1974. Liposomes as immunological adjuvants. Nature, 252:252.

Allison, A.C. and Byars, N.E. 1986. An adjuvant formulation that selectively elicits the formation of antibodies of protective isotypes and cell-mediated immunity. J. Immun. Methods, 2:369.

Allison, A.C. and Byars, N.E. 1992. Adjuvants for a new generation of vaccines. Can. J. Infect. Dis., 3:84B.

Audibert, F.M. and Lise, L.D. 1993. Adjuvants: current status, clinical perspectives and future prospects. Immunol. Today, 14:281.

Byars, N.E., Fraser-Smith, E.B., Pecyk, R.A. et al. 1994. Vaccinating guinea pigs with recombinant glycoprotein D of herpes simplex virus in an efficacious adjuvant formulation elicits protection against vaginal infection. Vaccine, 12:200.

Cumberpatch, M. and Kimber, I. 1995. Tumour necrosis factor-α is required for accumulation of dendritic cells in draining lymph nodes and for optimal contact sensitization. Immunology, 84:31.

Dempsey, P.W., Allison, M.E.D., Akkaraju, S., Goodnow, C.C. and Fearon, D.T. 1996. C3d of complement as a molecular adjuvant: bridging innate and acquired immunity. Science, 271:348.

Doherty, P.C., Allen, W., Eichelberger, M. and Carding, S.R. 1992. Roles of ab and gd T-cell subsets in viral immunity. Annu. Rev. Immunol., 10:123.

Ellouz, F., Adam, A., Ciorbaru, R. and Lederer, E. 1974. Minimal structural requirements for adjuvant activity of bacterial peptidoglycans. Biochem. Biophys. Res. Comm., 59:1317.

Finkelman, F.D., Holmes, J., Katona, I.M. et al. 1990. Lymphokine control of in vivo immunoglobulin isotype selection. Annu. Rev. Immunol., 8:303.

Glück, R. 1995. Liposomal presentation of antigens for human vaccines, in: Powell, M.F., Newman, M.F. (eds.). Vaccine Design: The Subunit and Adjuvant Approach. Plenum Press, New York 1995; pp 325.

Gregoriadis, G. 1990. Immunological adjuvants: A role for liposomes. Immunol. Today, 11:89.

Gregoriadis, G., Wang, Z., Barenholz, Y. and Francis, M.J. 1993. Liposome-entrapped T-cell peptide provides help for a co-entrapped B-cell peptide to overcome genetic restriction in mice and induce immunological memory. Immunology, 80:535.

Hamaoka, T., Katz, D.H., Benacerraf, B. 1973. Hapten-specific antibody responses in mice. II. Cooperative interactions between adoptively transferred T- and B-lymphocytes in the development of an IgE response. J. Exp. Med., 138:538.

Heufler, C., Koch, F. and Schuler, G. 1988. Granulocyte/macrophage colony-stimulating factor and interleukin-1 mediate the maturation of epidermal Langerhans cells into potent immunostimulatory dendritic cells. J. Exp. Med., 167:700.

Kaminski, M.S., Kitamura, K. and Maloney, D.G. 1986. Importance of antibody isotype in monoclonal anti-idiotype therapy of murine B-cell lymphoma. A study of hybridoma class switch variants. J. Immunol., 136:1123.

Kenney, J.S., Hughes B.M. and Allison, A.C. 1989. Determination of antibody affinity and concentration by solution-phase microradioimmunoassay, in: Zola, H. (ed.) Laboratory Methods in Immunology. CRC Press, Boca Raton; pp 209.

Kenney, J.S., Hughes, B.W., Masada, M.P. and Allison, A.C. 1989. Influence of adjuvants on the quantity, affinity, isotype and epitope specificity of murine antibodies. J. Immunol. Methods, 21:157.

Macatonia, S.E., Hosken, N.A., Litton, M., Vieira, P., Hsieh, C.-S., culpepper, J.A., Wysocka, M., Trinchieri, G., Murphy, K.M. and O'Garra, A. 1995. Dendritic cells produce IL-12 and direct the development of Th1 cells from naive $CD4^+$ T-cells. J. Immunol., 154:5071.

MacLennan, I.C.M. 1994. Germinal centers. Annu. Rev. Immunol., 12:117.

Meeusen, E.N.T., Premier, R.R. and Brandon, M.R. 1996. Tissue-specific migration of lymphocytes: a key role for Th1 and Th2 cells? Immunol. Today, 17:421.

Persson, G.R., Engel, D., Whitney, C., Darueau, R., Weinberg, A., Brunsvold, M. and Page, R.C. 1994. Immunization against Porphyromonas gingivalis inhibits progression of experimental periodontitis in nonhuman primates. Infect. Immun., 62:1026.

Reichmann, L., Clark, M., Waldmann, H. and Winter, G. 1988. Reshaping human antibodies for therapy. Nature, 332:323.

Ribi, E., Ulrich, J.T. and Masihi, K.N. 1993. Immunopotentiating activities of monophosphoryl lipid A, in: Majde, J.A. (ed.) Immunopharmacology of Infectious Diseases: Vaccine Adjuvants and Modulation of Non-specific Resistance. Alan R. Liss, New York; pp 101.

Ron, Y. and Sprent, J. 1987. T-cell priming in vitro: A major role for B-cells in presenting antigen to T-cells in lymph nodes. J. Immunol., 138:2848.

Rothel, J.S., Corner, L.A., Seaw, H.-F., Wood, P.R. and Lightowlers, M.W. 1996. Antigen-specific IgA secreting cells induced by peripheral vaccination. Immunol. Cell. Biol., 74:278.

Schijns, V.E.C.J., Haagmans, B., Rijke, E.O., Huang, S., Aguet, M. and Horzunek, M.C. 1994. IFN-γ receptor-deficient mice generate antiviral Th1-characteristic cytokine profiles but altered antibody responses. J. Immunol., 153:2029.

Schulz, M., Zinkernagel, R.M. and Hengartner, H. 1991. Peptide-induced protection by cytotoxic T-cells. Proc. Natl. Acad. Sci. USA, 88:991.

Spitznagel, J.K. and Allison, A.C. 1970. Mode of action of adjuvants: effects on antibody responses to macrophages-associated bovine serum albumin. J. Immunol., 104:128.

Steinman, R.M. 1991. The dendritic cell system and its role in immunogenicity. Annu. Rev. Immunol., 9:271.

Strobl, H., Riedl, E., Scheinecker, C., Bello-Fernandez, C., Pickl, W.F., Rappersberger, K., Majdic, O. and Knapp., W. 1996. TGF-β1 promotes in vitro development of dendritic cells from $CD34^+$ hemopoietic progenitors. J. Immunol., 157:1499.

Szakal, A.K., Kosco, M.H. and Tew, J.G. 1989. Microanatomy of lymphoid tissue during humoral immune responses: Structure-function relationships. Annu. Rev. Immunol., 7:91.

Toes, R.E.M., Blom, R.J.J., Offringa, R., Kast, W.M. and Melief, C.J.M. 1996. Enhanced tumor outgrowth after peptide vaccination. J. Immunol., 156:3911.

Unanue, E.R., Askonas, B.A. and Allison, A.C. 1969. A role of macrophages in the stimulation of immune responses by adjuvants. J. Immunol., 103:71.

Van Rooijen, N. and Sanders, A. 1994. Liposome mediated depletion of macrophages: mechanism of action, preparation of liposomes and applications. J. Immunol. Methods, 174:83.

Vijay, H.M., Lavregne, G., Huang, H. and Bernstein, I.L. 1979. Preferential synthesis of IgE reaginic antibodies in rats immunized with alum adsorbed antigens. Int. Arch. Allergy Appl. Immunol., 59:227.

Walker, B.D., Flexner, C. and Paradis, T.J. 1988. HIV-1 reverse transcriptase is a target for cytotoxic T-lymphocytes in infected individuals. Science, 240:64.

Waters, R.V., Terrell, T.G. and Jones, G.H. 1986. Uveitis induction in the rabbit by muramyl dipeptides. Infect. Immun., 51:816.

White, R.G. 1976. The adjuvant effect of microbial products on the immune response. Rev. Microbiol., 30:579.

THE ROLE OF TUMOUR NECROSIS FACTOR IN LYMPHOID TISSUE FORMATION AND FUNCTION

Manolis Pasparakis, Eleni Douni, Lena Alexopoulou, and George Kollias

Department of Molecular Genetics, Hellenic Pasteur Institute, 127 Vas. Sophias Avenue, 115 21 Athens, Hellas

INTRODUCTION

Tumour necrosis factor and lymphotoxin-α (TNF and LTα) are multipotent cytokines showing a wide range of activities that extend beyond their well characterised pleiotropic proinflammatory properties to include diverse signals for cellular differentiation, proliferation and death. TNF is produced in response to various stimuli mainly by macrophages and T cells and is shown to be bioactive both as a transmembrane protein and as a homotrimeric secreted molecule (Vasali, 1992; Kriegler et al, 1988). LTα, originally identified as a major product of lymphocytes, exists as a secreted molecule only in a homotrimeric form (Paul and Ruddle, 1988), but it may also accumulate on the cellular membrane of lymphocytes when complexed with LTβ, a type II transmembrane protein that is another member of the TNF ligand family (Browning et al, 1993). LTα1β2 trimers signal exclusively through the LTα receptor(s) (Crowe et al, 1994), while TNFα and LTα share the same cell surface receptors, designated p55 and p75 TNF-R, which show common but also differential activities depending on the cell type in which they operate (Vandenabeele et al, 1995). p75 TNF-R signalling has been mainly implicated in lymphocyte proliferation (Espevik et al, 1990; Tartaglia et al, 1991) while the p55 TNF-R is generally known to mediate apoptosis (Tartaglia et al, 1993), a process in which the p75 TNF-R may also be involved (Grell et al, 1995; Zheng et al, 1995).

Our attempts to define a role for TNFα and its receptors in disease pathogenesis by overexpression of these proteins in transgenic systems (Douni et al, 1996), have led to the development and consequent characterisation of specific disease models which demonstrated the important role of this cytokine in the development of rheumatoid arthritis (Keffer et al, 1991; Probert et al, 1995b;Georgopoulos et al, 1996), systemic inflammation (Probert et al, 1993), and CNS inflammatory and demyelinating diseases (Probert et al, 1995a; Akassoglou et al, 1997). More recently, the generation of mice deficient in TNF (Pasparakis et al, 1996), LTα (De Togni et al, 1994; Matsumoto et al, 1996a; Matsumoto et al, 1996b), or their receptors (Matsumoto et al, 1996a; Rothe et al, 1993; Pfeffer et al, 1993; Le Hir et al, 1996) provided new insights into the physiological role played by these molecules in the development of secondary lymphoid tissues and in the organisation of the humoral immune response.

ROLE OF TNF IN LPS-INDUCED TOXICITY, ANTI-BACTERIAL HOST DEFENCE AND CONTACT HYPERSENSITIVITY RESPONSES

The prominent role of the TNF/ p55 TNF-R system in mediating the lethal toxicity of low dose LPS after sensitisation with D-galactosamine, was recently demonstrated in mice with a targeted deletion of either TNF or the p55TNF-R. These mice showed complete resistance to the effects of high dose LPS/D-Gal treatment (Pasparakis et al, 1996, Rothe et al, 1993; Pfeffer et al, 1993) a phenomenon in which the p75 TNF-R does not appear to contribute (Erickson et al, 1994). Interestingly, however, neither TNFα nor p55 or p75 TNF-R deficient mice are resistant to high doses of LPS alone, suggesting that in the absence of sensitisation to the lethal effects of LPS, other yet unidentified factors produced independently of TNF contribute to the observed toxicity.

Infection of mice with Listeria monocytogenes has served as a model system to assess the role of cytokines in promoting immune responses to microbial pathogens. Recent studies in cytokine knockout mice demonstrated an important role for both IFNγ (Dalton et al, 1993) and TNF (Pasparakis et al, 1996) in these processes. For example, both TNF and IFNγ knockout mice show severely impaired resistance to listeria and readily succumb to even low doses of this pathogen. However, although production of IFNγ seems necessary for the orchestration of the innate phase of the immune response to listeria, its presence is not required for the development of acquired immune responses to the bacteria (Harty and Bevan, 1995). The role of TNF in this latter phenomenon is not yet defined and TNF knockout mice should prove very useful to study this important question.

The role of TNF in regulating contact hypersensitivity (CH) responses has been controversial and studies in mice using neutralising anti-TNF antibodies have suggested either an enhancing (Cumberbatch and Kimber, 1992; Piguet et al, 1991; Bromberg et al, 1992) or an immunosuppressive (Kurimoto and Streilen, 1992; Kondo et al, 1995) role. In addition to the antibody studies, it has recently been reported that mice deficient for the p55TNF-R show enhanced CH responses suggesting an overall immunosuppressive role for this receptor (Kondo et al, 1995). In contrast, we have observed that TNF knockout mice develop decreased CH responses and have suggested an overall enhancing role for TNF in these processes (Pasparakis, 1996). To explain this apparent discrepancy a differential role for the p55 and the p75TNF-Rs during the different phases of the contact hypersensitivity reaction may be suggested. Our hypothesis is that TNF utilises the p75TNF-R to enhance the migration of allergen bearing Langerhan's cells to the draining lymph nodes serving a crucial immunostimulatory role in this phase of response. Consistent with this hypothesis is the finding that LC migration is not affected in mice lacking the p55 TNF-R (Wang et al, 1996). At a later stage, during the DTH response, TNF signalling through the p55TNF-R may have an immunosupressive role which may serve the restoration of homeostasis in the affected area.

ROLE OF TNF IN THE DEVELOPMENT AND ORGANISATION OF SPLENIC LYMPHOID FOLLICLES

One of the most interesting recent observations in the TNF field is the involvement of TNF and LT in the development and organisation of lymphoid tissue. A first surprising observation was that LTα knockout mice were lacking lymph nodes and Peyer's patches and

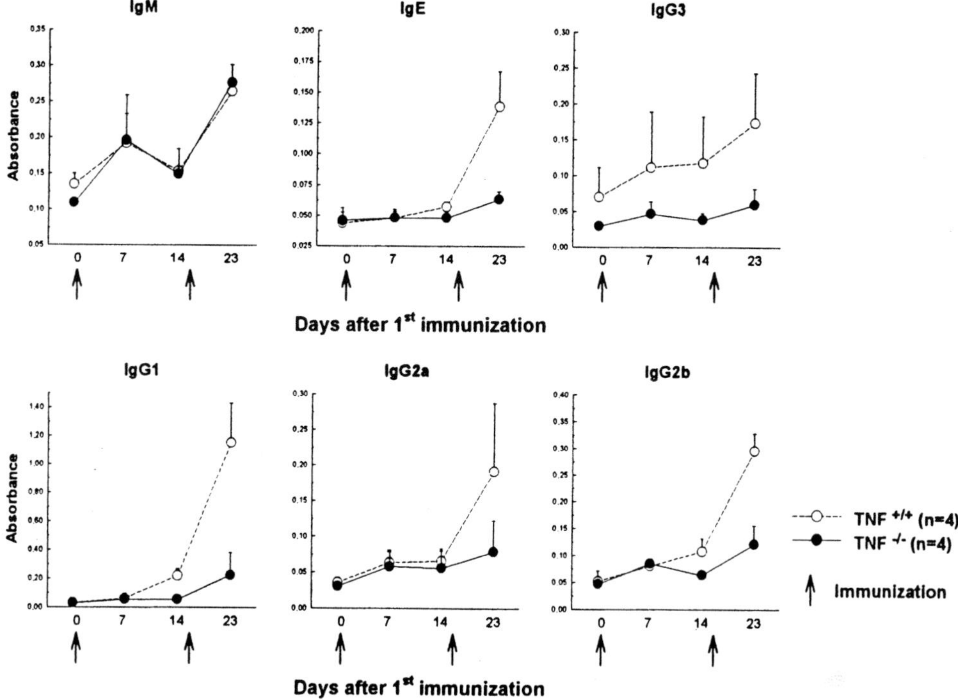

Figure 1. Measurement of serum antibody responses to the T-cell dependent antigen SRBC in wild type and TNF knockout mice. Mice were immunised intraperitoneally with 100 il of a 10% suspension of sheep red blood cells in sterile PBS on days 0 and 15, and were bled on days 0, 7 and 23. SRBC-specific serum antibodies were measured using isotype specific ELISAs.

that they were defective in the formation of distinct B and T cell areas in the spleen (De Togni et al, 1994). On the other hand, TNF or p55 TNF-R knockout mice show distinct B and T cell areas in all their lymphoid organs (i.e. spleen, lymph nodes and Peyer's patches), but fail to form structured B cell follicles, FDC networks and germinal centres (Pasparakis et al, 1996; Matsumoto et al, 1996a; Pasparakis et al, 1996b; Pasparakis et al, 1997). This activity of TNFα is most probably signalled exclusively through the p55 TNF-R, since no such defects can be observed in the p75 TNF-R knockout mice (Matsumoto et al, 1996a; Le Hir et al, 1996). The responsible mechanism for the TNF/p55TNF-R effect remains elusive, however, currently existing evidence suggests that it may lie in defective cell trafficking due to defective adhesion molecule expression, as was recently exemplified in p55 TNF-R knockout mice lacking expression of the adhesion molecule MAdCAM-1 in their splenic marginal zone (Neumann et al, 1996). Trafficking or differentiation defects may also explain the absence of organised FDC networks which may in turn explain the impaired formation of primary B cell follicles. Alternatively, an early and decisive developmental defect in the localisation of the FDC network may also be suggested. Further, exhaustive analysis of the cellular and molecular composition of lymphoid tissues in the TNF/LT and related receptor knockout mice, should identify interesting details on the specific role played by these molecules in the development and organisation of a functional lymphoid tissue.

Despite the absence of germinal centres, isotype switch to IgG1 and IgG2b in response to T cell dependent antigens (SRBC) was found operative in mice lacking either TNF (Pasparakis et al, 1996) or the p55 TNF-R (Le Hir et al, 1996). We have studied this

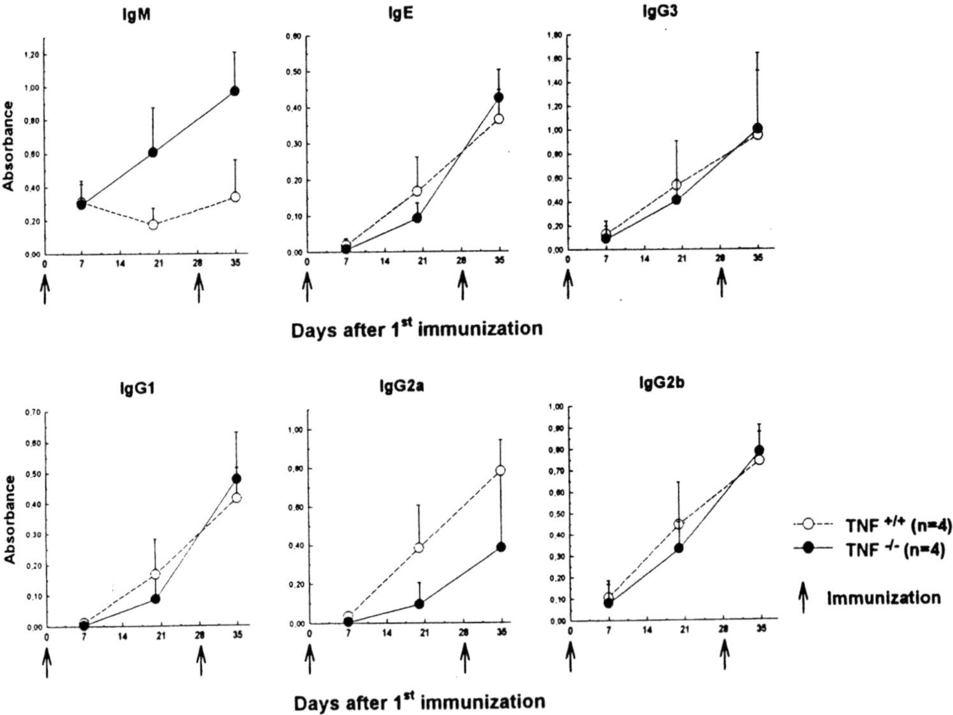

Figure 2. Measurement of anti-TNP serum antibodies in wild-type and TNF deficient mice upon immunisation with TNP-KLH. Mice were immunised intraperitoneally with 50 ìg TNP-KLH in complete Freund's adjuvant on day 0, and were boosted with an intraperitoneal injection of 5 ìg TNP-KLH in PBS on day 28. Blood samples were collected 7, 20 and 35 days after first immunisation, and anti-TNP antibodies were measured using isotype specific ELISAs.

phenomenon in further detail in TNF knockout mice and have observed a diminished response in several IgG classes following secondary immunisation with the SRBC antigen (Fig 1). Interestingly, when TNFα knockout mice where immunised with TNP-KLH in the presence of complete Freund's adjuvant, IgG1, IgG2b, IgG3 and IgE responses at day 35 following a primary (day 0) and a secondary (day 28) immunisation where found increased similarly to wild-type controls (Fig 2). This was not the case in IgG2a responses which were still found increased but severely compromised in comparison to the normal controls suggesting a role for TNFα in directing this specific recombination. It may therefore be suggested that although isotype switching can still occur in the absence of germinal centres and FDCs, prolonged antibody responses are generally impaired in TNFα or p55TNF-R knockout mice. This may be due to a defect in sustained antigen presentation which may be explained by the lack of organised FDC networks in these systems. On the other hand, adjuvant-induced immunisation (e.g in the TNP-KLH immunisation protocol) seems to overcome this defect probably by making the antigen available for longer periods of time.

IS THERE A ROLE FOR TNF IN "TERTIARY" LYMPHOID TISSUE DEVELOPMENT AT SITES OF INFLAMMATION?

In view of the proinflammatory (Keffer et al, 1991; Probert et al, 1995b; Georgopoulos et al, 1996; Probert et al, 1003; Probert et al, 1995a; Akassoglou et al, 1997) and lymphoid developmental activities (Pasparakis et al, 1996; Pasparakis et al, 1997) of TNF, we have hypothesised that overexpression of TNF, for example as it occurs at inflammatory sites, may trigger local development of tertiary lymphoid structures resembling those of secondary lymphoid organs. Confirmation that LTα-induced inflammation may show characteristics of organised lymphoid tissue, was recently provided in rat insulin promoter driven LTα transgenic mice which develop chronic inflammatory lesions in kidney and pancreas, and form lymph node-like structures in these areas (Kratz et al, 1996). To examine whether TNF, being a natural mediator of inflammation, could be inducing such processes, we have made use of previously described transgenic mouse lines engineered to overexpress human TNF in their T cells. These mice (CD2 huTNF-globin) develop systemic inflammation in peripheral organs such as the liver and lung and severe structural perturbations in the thymus (Probert et al, 1993). Immunohistochemical characterisation of these sites for several typical markers of secondary lymphoid tissue such as B220 (B cells), IgM (B cells), CD3 (T cells), FDCs (follicular dendritic cells) and IDCs (interdigitating dendritic cells), revealed the presense of organised lymphoid-like structures (manuscript in preparation). Flow cytometric analysis of such thymic follicles showed a lymph node-like B and T cell constitution and confirmed the presence of a high percentage of B220+ / IgM+ cells. It may therefore be suggested that in addition to its pro-inflammatory activities, TNF signalling through the p55 TNF receptor may direct local maturation of the immune response by orchestrating the appearance of structured lymphoid follicles within inflammatory sites. Elucidation of the mechanisms involved in these phenomena could provide useful applications for the treatment of chronic inflammatory and autoimmune diseases, including rheumatoid arthritis and myasthenia gravis, in which local antigen presentation and consequent epitope spreading may be dependent in the functioning of such newly formed lymphoid structures. Indeed, in the case of Myasthenia Gravis surgical removal of thymus, a tissue where most of these lymphoid structures have been reported, showed beneficial effects to the progression of disease (Leprince et al, 1990).

These phenomena highlight a role for cytokines such as TNFα and LTα in the induction of local lymphoid organogenesis, implicating them also as key determinants in processes such as local antigen presentation and consequent epitope spreading which are central to the pathogenesis of many autoimmune or chronic inflammatory diseases. It remains unclear, however, whether either or both cytokines are necessary for the induction of these phenomena and whether similar or divergent signalling pathways are used. Building up on this knowledge may provide useful applications for the therapeutic manipulation of related diseases or the design of more effective immunisation protocols as for example in efforts to build more effective vaccines.

Acknowledgements

This work was supported in part by the Greek Secretariat for Research and Technology and European Commission Grants BIO-CT96-0174 and BIO-CT96-0077.

REFERENCES

Akassoglou, K., Probert, L., Kontogeorgos, G. and Kollias, G., 1997, Astrocyte-specific but not neuron-specific transmembrane TNF triggers inflammation and degeneration in the central nervous system of transgenic mice. J.Immunol., 158: 438.

Bromberg, J.S., Chavin, K.D. and Kunkel, S.L., 1992, Anti-tumour necrosis factor antibodies suppress cell-mediated immunity in vivo. J.Immunol., 148:3412.

Browning, J.L., Ngam ek, A., Lawton, P., DeMarinis, J., Tizard, R., Chow, E.P., Hession, C., O'Brine Greco, B., Foley, S.F. and Ware, C.F., 1993, Lymphotoxin beta, a novel member of the TNF family that forms a heteromeric complex with lymphotoxin on the cell surface. Cell, 72:847.

Crowe, P.D., VanArsdale, T.L., Walter, B.N., Ware, C.F., Hession, C., Ehrenfels, B., Browning, J.L., Din, W.S., Goodwin, R.G. and Smith, C.A., 1994, A lymphotoxin-beta-specific receptor. Science, 264:707.

Cumberbatch, M., and Kimber, I., 1992. Dermal tumour necrosis factor-alpha induces dendritic cell migration to draining lymph nodes, and possibly provides one stimulus for Langerhan's cell migration. Immunology, 75:257.

Dalton, D.K., Pitts-Meek, S., Keshav, S., Figari, I.S., Bradley, A. and Stewart, T.A., 1993, Multiple defects of immune cell function in mice with disrupted interferon-gamma genes. Science, 259:1739.

Douni, E., Akassoglou, K., Alexopoulou, L., Georgopoulos, S., Haralambous, S., Hill, S., Kassiotis, G., Kontoyiannis, D., Pasparakis, M., Plows, D., Probert, L. and Kollias, G. 1996, Transgenic and knockout analyses of the role of TNF in immune regulation and disease pathogenesis. J. Inflamm., 47:27.

Erickson, S.L., de Sauvage, F.J., Kikly, K., Carver-Moore, K., Pitts-Meek, S., Gillett, N., Sheehan, K.C., Schreiber, R.D., Goeddel, D.V. and Moore, M.W., 1994, Decreased sensitivity to tumour-necrosis factor but normal T-cell development in TNF receptor-2-deficient mice. Nature, 372:560.

Espevik, T., Brockhaus, M., Loetscher, H., Nonstad, U. and Shalaby, R., 1990, Characterization of binding and biological effects of monoclonal antibodies against a human tumour necrosis factor receptor. J.Exp.Med., 171:415.

Georgopoulos, S., Plows, D. and Kollias, G., 1996, Transmembrane TNF is sufficient to induce localized tissue toxicity and chronic inflammatory arthritis in transgenic mice. J. Inflamm., 46:86.

Grell, M., Douni, E., Wajant, H., Lohden, M., Clauss, M., Maxeiner, B., Georgopoulos, S., Lesslauer, W., Kollias, G., Pfizenmaier, K. and Scheurich, P., 1995, The trans-membrane form of tumor necrosis factor is the prime activating ligand of the 80 kDa tumor necrosis factor receptor. Cell, 83:793.

Harty, J.T. and Bevan, M.J., 1995, Specific immunity to Listeria monocytogenes in the absence of IFN gamma. Immunity., 3:109.

Le Hir, M., Bluethmann, H., Kosco Vilbois, M.H., Muller, M., di Padova, F., Moore, M., Ryffel, B. and Eugster, H.P., 1996, Differentiation of follicular dendritic cells and full antibody responses require tumor necrosis factor receptor-1 signaling. J.Exp.Med., 183:2367.

Keffer, J., Probert, L., Cazlaris, H., Georgopoulos, S., Kaslaris, E., Kioussis, D. and Kollias, G., 1991, Transgenic mice expressing human tumour necrosis factor: a predictive genetic model of arthritis. EMBO J., 10: 4025.

Kondo, S., Wang, B., Fujisawa, H., Shivji, G.M., Echtenacher, B., Mak, T.W., and Sauder, D.N., 1995, Effect of gene-targeted mutation in TNF receptor (p55) on contact hypersensitivity and ultraviolet B-induced immunosuppression. J.Immunol., 155: 3801.

Kratz, A., Campos-Neto, A., Hanson, M.S. and Ruddle, N.H., 1996, Chronic inflammation caused by lymphotoxin is lymphoid neogenesis. J.Exp.Med., 183:1461.

Kriegler, M., Perez, C., DeFay, K., Albert, I. and Lu, S.D., 1988, A novel form of TNF/cachectin is a cell surface cytotoxic transmembrane protein: ramifications for the complex physiology of TNF. Cell, 53:45.

Kurimoto, I. and Streilein, J.W., 1992, *cis*-urocanic supression of contact hypersensitivity induction is mediated via tumour necrosis factor-á. J.Immunol., 148:3072.

Leprince, C., Cohen-Kaminsky, S., Berrih-Aknin, S., Vernet-Der Garabedian, B., Treton, D., Galanaud, P., and Richard, Y., 1990, Thymic B cells from myasthenia gravis patients are activated B cells. Phenotypic and functional analysis. J.Immunol., 145:2115.

Matsumoto, M., Mariathasan, S., Nahm, M.H., Baranyay, F., Peschon, J.J. and Chaplin, D.D., 1996a, Role of lymphotoxin and the type I TNF receptor in the formation of germinal centers. Science, 271:1289.

Matsumoto, M., Lo, S.F., Carruthers, C.J., Min, J., Mariathasan, S., Huang, G., Plas, D.R., Martin, S.M., Geha, R.S., Nahm, M.H. and Chaplin, D.D. (1996b). Affinity maturation without germinal centres in lymphotoxin-alpha-deficient mice. Nature, 382:462.

Neumann, B., Machleidt, T., Lifka, A., Pfeffer, K., Vestweber, D., Mak, T.W., Holzmann, B. and Kronke, M., 1996, Crucial role of 55-kilodalton TNF receptor in TNF-induced adhesion molecule expression and leukocyte organ infiltration. J.Immunol., 156:1587.

Pasparakis, M., Alexopoulou, L., Episkopou, V. and Kollias, G., 1996, Immune and inflammatory responses in TNF alpha-deficient mice: a critical requirement for TNF alpha in the formation of primary B cell follicles, follicular dendritic cell networks and germinal centers, and in the maturation of the humoral immune response. J.Exp.Med., 184:1397.

Pasparakis, M., Alexopoulou, L., Douni, E. and Kollias, G., 1996b, Tumour necrosis factors in immune regulation : everything that's interesting is ... new ! Cytokine and Growth Factor Review , 7:223.

Pasparakis, M., Alexopoulou, L., Grell, M., Pfizenmaier, K., Bluethmann, H. and Kollias, G., 1997, Intact Peyer's patch organogenesis yet defective formation of B lymphocyte follicles in peripheral lymphoid organs of mice deficient for tumour necrosis factor and its 55 kDa receptor. (Submitted for publication)

Paul, N.L., and Ruddle, N.H., 1988, Lymphotoxin. Annu.Rev.Immunol., 6:407.
Pfeffer, K., Matsuyama, T., Kundig, T.M., Wakeham, A., Kishihara, K., Shahinian, A., Wiegmann, K., Ohashi, P.S., Kronke, M. and Mak, T.W., 1993, Mice deficient for the 55 kd tumor necrosis factor receptor are resistant to endotoxic shock, yet succumb to L. monocytogenes infection. Cell, 73:457.
Piguet, P.F., Grau, G.E., Hauser, C. and Vassalli, P., 1991, Tumour necrosis factor is a critical mediator in hapten induced irritant and contact hypersensitivity reactions. J.Exp.Med., 173:673.
Probert, L., Plows, D., Kontogeorgos, G. and Kollias, G., 1995b, The type I interleukin-1 receptor acts in series with tumor necrosis factor (TNF) to induce arthritis in TNF-transgenic mice. Eur.J.Immunol., 25:1794.
Probert, L., Keffer, J., Corbella, P., Cazlaris, H., Patsavoudi, E., Stephens, S., Kaslaris, E., Kioussis, D. and Kollias, G., 1993, Wasting, ischemia, and lymphoid abnormalities in mice expressing T cell- targeted human tumor necrosis factor transgenes. J.Immunol., 151:1894.
Probert, L., Akassoglou, K., Pasparakis, M., Kontogeorgos, G. and Kollias, G., 1995a, Spontaneous inflammatory demyelinating disease in transgenic mice showing central nervous system-specific expression of tumor necrosis factor alpha. Proc.Natl.Acad. Sci. USA, 92:11294.
Rothe, J., Lesslauer, W., Lotscher, H., Lang, Y., Koebel, P., Kontgen, F., Althage, A., Zinkernagel, R., Steinmetz, M. and Bluethmann, H., 1993, Mice lacking the tumour necrosis factor receptor 1 are resistant to TNF-mediated toxicity but highly susceptible to infection by Listeria monocytogenes. Nature, 364:798.
Tartaglia, L.A., Weber, R.F., Figari, I.S., Reynolds, C., Palladino, M.A. and Goeddel D.V., 1991, The two different receptors for tumour necrosis factor mediate distinct cellular responses. Proc.Natl.Acad.Sci. USA, 88:9292.
Tartaglia, L.A., Ayres, T.M., Wong, G.H. and Goeddel, D.V., 1993, A novel domain within the 55 kd TNF receptor signals cell death. Cell, 74:845.
De Togni, P., Goellner, J., Ruddle, N.H., Streeter, P.R., Fick, A., Mariathasan, S., Smith, S.C., Carlson, R., Shornick, L.P., Strauss Schoenberger, J. and Chaplin, D., 1994, Abnormal development of peripheral lymphoid organs in mice deficient in lymphotoxin. Science, 264:703.
Vandenabeele, P. Declercq, W., Beyaert, R. and Fiers, W., 1995, Two tumour necrosis factor receptors: structure and function. Trends Cell Biol., 5:392.
Vassali, P., 1992, The pathophysiology of tumour necrosis factor. Annu.Rev.Immunol., 10:411.
Wang, B., Kondo, S., Shivji, G.M., Fujisawa, H., Mak, T.W. and Sauder, D.N., 1996, Tumour necrosis factor receptor II (p75) signalling is required for the migration of Langerhans' cells. Immunology, 88:284.
Zheng, L., Fisher, G., Miller, R.E., Peschon, J., Lynch, D.H. and Lenardo, M.J., 1995, Induction of apoptosis in mature T cells by tumour necrosis factor. Nature, 377:348.

DENDRITIC CELLS AND CYTOKINES

Jonathan M. Austyn

Nuffield Department of Surgery, University of Oxford,
John Radcliffe Hospital, Headington, Oxford OX3 9DU, UK

INTRODUCTION

Dendritic cells (DC) initiate T- and T-dependent immune responses (Austyn et al, in press; Austyn, 1992; Steinman, 1991). Different stages of the lineage are distributed within different anatomical compartments and have specialized functions that are designed to achieve this overall result. At least three specializations are apparent. First, DC progenitors that are produced within bone marrow of adult mammals travel in blood to seed the tissues. Second, within non-lymphoid tissues DC develop into an immature or "processing" stage with optimal capacities to internalize and process foreign antigens, synthesize MHC class II molecules, and assemble peptide-MHC class II complexes that can be expressed at the cell surface. Third, DC commence a maturation process within non-lymphoid tissues and migrate to secondary lymphoid tissues where, at the mature or "costimulatory" stage, the cells have optimal capacities to present foreign-peptide MHC class II complexes to resting T cells and to deliver specialized costimulatory signals for initiation of T cell activation.

DC presentation of exogenous antigens as peptide-MHC class II complexes favours the activation of CD4+ T cells, many of which are helper (and, in fact, one form of suppressor) T cells. Presentation of endogenous antigens as peptide-class I complexes favours the activation of CD8+ T cells, many of which are cytotoxic T cells. Once these T cells have been activated they can respond to other types of antigen-presenting cells (APC). The activated helper T cells can then secrete cytokines that act on the APC and induce or up-regulate cellular functions to facilitate elimination of antigens within the cell; an example is activation of macrophages that have internalized microorganisms. In contrast, activated cytotoxic T cells (CTL) can secrete cytolysins that kill the APC or "target cell"; an example is elimination of a cell that has been infected by a virus. It is therefore convenient to distinguish between the afferent phase of adaptive immune responses, when T cells are activated by DC, and the efferent phase when the activated T cells respond to other types of APC and generate a concerted response that is designed to eliminate the foreign antigen.

When antigen is first encountered, for example when a microorganism enters through a wound, an innate immune response ensues. This involves activation of plasma enzyme systems and the response of inflammatory cells. The complement, coagulation, fibrinolysis and kinin systems are closely interrelated, and activation of these components of innate immunity leads to recruitment of inflammatory cells such a polymorphonuclear leukocytes (e.g. neutrophils) and monocyte / macrophages which produce a wide variety of additional soluble mediators. An important consequence is the inflammatory response. It now seems likely that inflammation provides a central link between the innate and adaptive (lymphocyte-mediated) arms of the immune system. In particular, inflammatory mediators such as cytokines can act on DC and stimulate their maturation, migration and function. The purpose of this short article is to outline some of the ways that cytokines and other mediators can influence and control the behaviour of DC. Its relevance to the overall theme is that manipulation of these pathways may lead to strategies for the design and production of new or more effective vaccines.

DENDRITIC CELL PROGENITORS

As for other leukocytes, DC ultimately derive from haemopoietic stem cells but their precise branch point from other lineages is not yet clear. At least in vitro, an important cytokine for generation of DC is GM-CSF. DC can be grown from mouse bone marrow progenitors in the presence of this cytokine, and from human CD34+ bone marrow and cord blood progenitors that are cultured in GM-CSF plus TNF-alpha. Using these approaches, mixed colonies of DC, macrophages and neutrophils have been generated from mouse bone marrow (Inaba et al, 1993), and pure colonies of DC have been produced from human bone marrow progenitors that can be expanded in the presence of stem cell factor (c-kit ligand) (Young et al, 1995). In the mouse, administration of flt-3 ligand considerably increases the number of DC that can be isolated from lymphoid tissues, presumably by expanding the population of DC progenitors. Subsets of human CD34+ bone marrow cells and mouse thymic lymphoid precursor cells have also been identified that can give rise to DC and lymphoid, but not myeloid, cells (Galy et al, 1995). Hence at least two distinct committed stem cells that can give rise to DC of myeloid and lymphoid origin may exist. An additional complication is that DC-like cells can also be obtained by culture of human blood monocytes in GM-CSF plus IL-4, giving rise to cells at the immature or processing stage, and further maturation can be induced by addition of LPS, TNF-alpha, IL-1, or CD40 ligand (Sallusto and Lanzavecchia, 1994). These agents also have important effects on DC in tissues (see below).

NON-LYMPHOID DENDRITIC CELLS

DC progenitors enter non-lymphoid tissues but the lack of available markers precludes detailed estimates of their abundance. Both GM-CSF and LPS have been implicated in recruitment of DC progenitors to these sites. For example, increased numbers of DC are present in human skin after intradermal adminstration of GM-CSF, and local production of this cytokine increases the numbers in human lung and some lung cancers (Kaplan et al, 1992; Tazi et al, 1993). Systemic administration of LPS to mice has been shown to recruit MHC class II-negative DC progenitors to heart and kidney (Roake et al, 1995), and LPS delivered in aerosol form increases the number of DC in rat lung (McWilliam et al, 1994). From studies of the effects of GM-CSF on DC progenitors in vitro (see above) it seems possible that this cytokine both recruits the cells to non-lymphoid tissues and commits them to undergo further development to the immature "processing" stage, although definitive evidence for this is lacking at present.

MHC class II-positive DC are widely distributed throughout non-lymphoid tissues (Steinman, 1991) with the exception of the central nervous system and some "immunologically-privileged" sites such as testis. Cells such as Langerhans cells are situated in the epidermis of skin and related cells are present in all other epithelial sites such as the gastrointestinal, urogenital, and respiratory tracts. DC are also present within the interstitial spaces of solid organs such as heart and kidney. Isolation and characterization of these cells from a variety of sites has revealed that non-lymphoid DC are, in general, at the immature "processing" stage (Austyn et al, 1994). Their localization and function therefore allows them to perform a "sentinel" function in acquiring and processing antigens that gain access to these sites. However, before they can activate T cells, at least two essential steps are required: DC need to undergo a maturation process to the "costimulatory" stage, and they need to migrate to secondary lymphoid tissues where T cells are localized.

During maturation, DC undergo profound changes in phenotype and function (Austyn, 1992; Steinman, 1991). These events have been particularly well studied in the case of Langerhans cells, but generally consistent findings have been made during studies of other populations of DC isolated from non-lymphoid tissues. Important features of freshly-isolated Langerhans cells at the immature stage include: the capacity to internalize antigens by pinocytosis, macropinocytosis, phagocytosis and receptor-mediated endocytosis; a well developed endosomal / lysosomal system that includes specialized compartments for peptide loading (CIIV / MIIC); and high rate of biosynthesis of MHC class II molecules for loading with antigenic peptides. These features are essentially lost during maturation of LC, and the cells come to resemble DC that can be cultured from secondary lymphoid tissues. Important features of mature DC include: stable expression of foreign peptide-MHC complexes at the cell surface and new or increased expression of costimulatory molecules such as CD40, CD80 and CD86.

Maturation of Langerhans cells can be induced by culture in GM-CSF which is produced by keratinocytes in epidermal cell suspensions for example, and augmented by IL-1. Langerhans cells can themselves produce GM-CSF and IL-1-beta as well as chemokines such as MIP-1-alpha and MIP-2. During maturation they express higher levels of IL1 beta but decreased MIP-1 and MIP2. Importantly, mature Langerhans cells, like lymphoid DC, can produce IL-12 (see below). In vivo, maturation is initiated in non-lymphoid tissues and seems to continue as the cells migrate into secondary lymphoid tissues.

Migration of DC from non-lymphoid tissues can be induced by inflammatory cytokines and other agents such as LPS. For example, intradermal administration of IL-1 or TNF-alpha promotes the loss of Langerhans cells from mouse skin, and systemic administration of these cytokines (particularly the latter) can induce migration from mouse heart and kidney (Kimber et al, 1992; Roake et al, 1995). The same cytokines are produced in skin following topical application of agents such as contact sensitizers which have been shown to stimulate migration of Langerhans cells from the epidermis to regional lymph nodes. Systemic administration of LPS has also been shown to increase the flux of DC ("veiled cells") draining from the lamina propria of rat intestine, and to deplete DC from mouse heart and kidney (Roake et al, 1995; MacPherson et al, 1995). Whether or not these are direct effects of LPS on DC or responses of DC to LPS-induced cytokines such as TNF-alpha is not yet clear. Whatever the case it is important to note that during the response to LPS, the DC that migrate from non-lymphoid tissues (presumably into lymphoid tissues) are replaced by DC progenitors, presumably to repeat the cycle. This could be an important role of adjuvants in general in that they may facilitate uptake of antigens by immature DC, the maturation and migration of these cells into secondary lymphoid tissues, and recruitment of further waves of DC progenitors into the site of vaccination.

Migration of DC into secondary lymphoid tissues occurs by three pathways (Austyn, 1996). Firstly, DC from epithelial sites migrate via afferent lymph into regional lymph nodes. Secondly, DC from interstitial sites migrate both by this route and via blood to spleen. Third, DC in liver sinusoids can undergo a blood-lymph translocation and migrate via hepatic lymph to celiac nodes (Matsuno et al, 1996). These three routes apparently permit immune responses to be generated against antigens that gain access to three different anatomical compartments: epithelia, interstitial spaces, and blood.

LYMPHOID DENDRITIC CELLS

At least four features contribute to the potency and largely unique capacity of lymphoid DC to initiate T- and T-dependent responses: homing to T cell-rich areas of secondary lymphoid tissues, the ability to cluster with resting T cells in an antigen-independent manner, high level surface expression of foreign peptide-MHC complexes, and expression of costimulatory molecules for T cell activation. Lymphoid DC are relatively short-lived, end-stage cells. Their ultimate fate is unclear, but they almost certainly do not leave the lymphoid tissues. It seems likely that they undergo apoptosis in these sites, either as part of a regulated differentiation process or following interaction with activated T cells for example via Fas-Fas ligand interactions.

The initial interaction between DC and antigen-specific T cells may generate activated T cells that secrete IL-2. Subsequently, the activated CD4+ T cells (and probably CD8+ T cells) can develop into cells that secrete polarized patterns of cytokines. TH1 cells preferentially secrete IFN-gamma and IL-2, whereas TH2 cells secrete IL-4, IL-5, IL-10 and, in mice, IL-13; TH0 cells secreting intermediate spectra of cytokines have also been identified, and a subset of TH3 cells that preferentially secretes TGF-beta has been proposed. The decision as to which pathway predominates is controlled in large part by the cytokine milieu in which T cell activation occurs: TH1 cells are generated in the presence of IL-12 whereas TH2 cells require IL-4. Mature DC can secrete IL-12 and the default pathway for these cells may be the generation of TH1-type responses (Macatonia et al, 1995; Koch et al, 1996).

IL-12 is a heterodimeric cytokine composed of p35 and p40 subunits which assemble to form the bioactive p70 molecule. It can be produced by cells such as macrophages in response to LPS, phagocytosis of bacteria, and intracellular pathogens. This is likely to be important in early (predominantly innate) defence against viral, bacterial and parasitic infections. For example, IL-12 produced by macrophages can stimulate NK cells to secrete IFN-gamma which is a potent macrophage activating cytokine. However, production of IL-12 by DC is likely to be important in late (predominantly adaptive) defence against bacterial, parasitic and perhaps fungal infections. IL-12 primes CD4+ T cells for high IFN-gamma production, and contributes to the secretion of optimal levels of IFN-gamma and proliferation of TH1 cells. Production of high levels of IL-12 by mature DC is stimulated during their interaction with activated T cells. In vitro, this can be triggered by ligation of either CD40 or class II molecules on DC for example, suggesting that interactions with the CD40 ligand or T cell receptor of T cells may normally be important for production (Koch et al, 1996). In contrast, IL-4 and IL-10, which favour generation and function of TH2 cells, downregulate DC production of IL-12. Hence, lymphoid DC are not only responsible for T cell activation but contribute to control of the direction of the subsequent immune response.

REFERENCES

Austyn, J.M., Liddington, M.I. and MacPherson, G.G., Dendritic cells: migration in vivo. In: Weir, DM, Herzenberg LA, Blackwell C, Herzenberg LA (eds). Handbook of Experimental Immunology, 5th edition. In press.

Austyn, J.M.., 1992, : Antigen uptake and presentation by dendritic leukocytes. Seminars Immunol. 4:227.

Austyn, J.M., Hankins, D.F., Larsen, C.P., Morris, P.J., Rao, A.S. and Roake, J.A., 1994, Isolation and characterization of dendritic cells from mouse heart and kidney. J Immunol. 152:2401.

Austyn, J.M., 1996, New insights into the mobilization and phagocytic activity of dendritic cells [commentary]. J Exp Med. 183:1287.

Galy, A., Travis, M., Cen, D. and Chen, B., 1995, Human T, B, natural killer, and dendritic cells arise from a common bone marrow progenitor cell subset. Immunity. 3:459.

Inaba, K., Inaba, M., Deguchi, M., Hagi, K., Yasumizu, R., Ikehara, S. and Muramatsu, S., 1993, Granulocytes, macrophages, and dendritic cells arise from a common major histcompatibility complex class II-negative progenitor in mouse bone marrow. Proc Natl Acad Sci USA. 90:3038.

Kaplan, G., Walsh. G., Guido, L.S., Meyn, P., Burkhardt, R.A., Abalos, R.M., Barker, J., Frindt, P.A., Fajardo, T.T., Celona, R., Cohn, Z.A., 1992, Novel responses of human skin to intradermal recombinant granulocyte / macrophage colony-stimulating factor: Langerhans cell recruitment, keratinocyte growth, and enhanced wound healing. J Exp Med. 175:1717.

Kimber, I. and Cumberbatch, M., 1992, Stimulation of Langerhans cell migration by tumour necrosis factor alpha (TNF alpha). J Invest Dermatol. 99:48S.

Koch, F., Stanzl, U., Jennewein, P., Janke, K., Heufler, C., Kampgen, E., Romani, N. and Schuler, G., 1996, High level IL-12 production by murine denritic cells: upregulation via MHC class II and CD40 molecules and downregulation by IL-4 and IL-10, J Exp Med. 184:741.

Macatonia, S.E., Hosken, N.A., Litton, M., Vieira, P., Hsieh, C.S., Culpepper, J.A., Wysocka, M., Trinchieri, G., Murphy, K.M. and O'Garra, A., 1995, Dendritic cells produce IL-12 and direct the development of Th1 cells from naive CD4+ T cells. J Immunol. 154:5071.

MacPherson, G.G., Jenkins, C.D., Stein, M.J. and Edwards, C., 1995, Endotoxin-mediated dendritic cell release from the intestine. Characterization of released dendritic cells and TNF dependence. J Immunol. 154:1317.

Matsuno, K., Ezaki, T., Kudo, S. and Uehara, Y., 1996, A life stage of particle-laden rat dendritic cells in vivo: their terminal division, active phagocytosis and translocation from the liver to hepatic lymph. J Exp Med. 183:1865.

McWilliam, A.S., Nelson, D., Thomas, J.A., Holt, P.G., 1994, Rapid dendritic cell recruitment is a hallmark of the acute inflammatory response at mucosal surfaces. J Exp Med. 179:1331.

Roake, J.A., Rao, A.S., Morris, P.J., Larsen, C.P., Hankins, D.F., Austyn, J.M., 1995, Systemic lipopoly-saccharide recruits dendritic cell progenitors to nonlymphoid tissues. Transplantation. 59:1319.

Roake, J.A., Rao, A.S., Morris, P.J., Larsen, C.P., Hankins, D.F., Austyn, J.M., 1995, Dendritic cell loss from non-lymphoid tissues after systemic administration of lipopolysaccharide, tumour necrosis factor, and interleukin-1. J Exp Med. 181:2237.

Sallusto, F. and Lanzavecchia, A., 1994, Efficient presentation of soluble antigen by cultured human dendritic cells is maintained by granulocyte/macrophage colony stimulating factor plus interleukin 4 and down regulated by tumor necrosis factor alpha. J Exp Med. 179:1109.

Steinman, R.M., 1991, : The dendritic cell system and its role in immunogenicity. Annu. Rev.Immunol. 9:271.

Tazi, A., Bouchonnet, F., Grandsaigne, M., Boumsell, L., Hance, A.J., Soler, P., 1993, Evidence that granulocyte macrophage-colony-stimulating factor regulates the distribution and differentiated state of dendritic cells / Langerhans cells in human lung and lung cancers. J Clin Invest. 91:566.

Young, J.W., Szabolcs, P., Moore, M.A.S., 1995, Identification of dendritic cell colony-forming units among normal CD34+ bone marrow progenitors that are expanded by *c-kit* ligand and yield pure dendritic cell colonies in the presence of granulocyte / macrophage colony-stimulating factor, and tumor necrosis factor alpha. J Exp Med. 182:1111.

CONTROL OF HIV ENTRY AND TRANSCRIPTION, AS A POSSIBLE MECHANISM OF THE ANTIVIRAL EFFECTS OF T LYMPHOCYTES IN HIV INFECTION

J.-L.Virelizier, A. Amara, E. Oberlin, D. Rousset,
M. Rodriguez, and M. Kroll

Unité d'Immunologie Virale, Institut Pasteur, Paris, France

INTRODUCTION

For decades it has generally been assumed that T cell-mediated antiviral immunity acts through lysis of infected cells by specific T lymphocytes recognizing viral epitopes in the context of major histocompatibility antigens class I. Indeed, MHC class I restricted-, CD8 T cells are found in infected animals and do lyse infected cells in vitro in a highly specific manner. The MHC-dependence of this phenomenon was a remarkable discovery by Rolf Zinkernagel and Peter Dogherty (Nature, 1974) ,who were awarded a Nobel prize in 1996 precisely for this important finding. The "CTL assay" remains the best tool of research to asses the fine specificity and MHC restriction of antiviral CD8 T lymphocytes. The in vivo relevance of the CTL assay as a host defence mechanism, however, is not yet fully ascertained in most cases of viral infection or immunization.

An alternative mechanism whereby antiviral T cells, whether class I-(CD8) or class II (CD4)-restricted , may control viral infections in vivo is cytokine secretion. For exemple, it was shown that the protective effect of "CTL" clones transfered to mice expressing as a transgene the hepatitis B (HBV) genome, is not mediated by cytolytic mechanisms, but is due rather to the production by these specific clones of interferon gamma (IFNγ) and tumor necrosis factor (TNFα). Examination of liver in the experimental animals showed very little cell destruction, which contrasted whith an intense decrease in HBV genome transcription (Guidotti et al , 1994). In the case of HIV infection, CD8 T cells capable of inducing specific cytolysis in vitro are also found in infected individuals (Klenerman et al, 1996), but no decisive evidence could yet confirm their role in protection against HIV infection in vivo. Moreover, a series of recent evidence from many laboratories including ours (for review see D'Souza and Harden, Nature Medicine, 1996) indicate that chemokines, secreted by specific CD8 T cells or produced non-specifically, protect lymphocytes against HIV infection in vitro. Although chemokine-

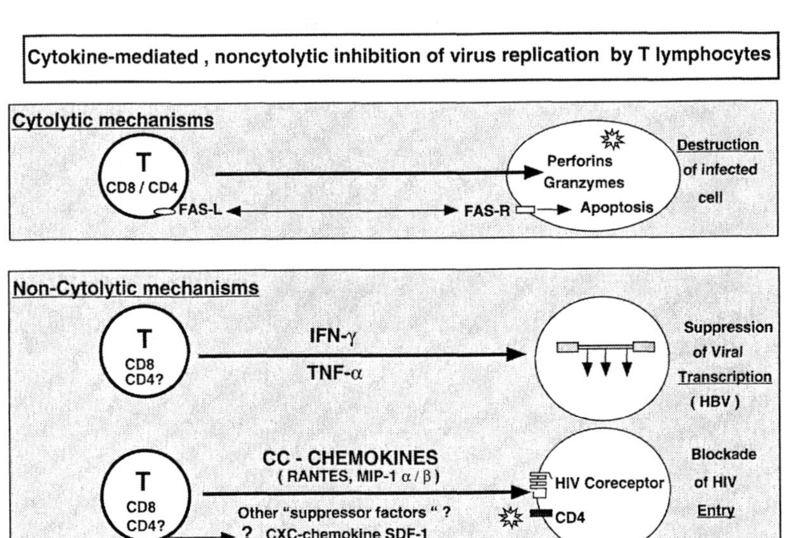

Figure 1. Two alternative mechanisms used by T lymphocytes to protect cells against virus infection. The first is cytolysis of infected cells, through either secretion and introduction into infected cells of toxic mediators (perforins and/or granzymes), or Fas receptor-induced apoptosis induced by ligation of the Fas ligand, expressed on the T cell membrane or secreted . The second is noncytolytic, and mediated by interferon γ and tumor necrosis factor α, both shown to suppress transcription of the hepatitis B genome, or chemokines such as RANTES, MIP-1α_/_β , shown to suppress HIV replication by blocking virus coreceptors .

mediated, anti-HIV effects of specific T lymphocytes remain to be established in vivo, an alternative, noncytolytic mechanism of protection against HIV infection must now be envisaged. Its potential relevance to future vaccines to HIV deserves discussion, in the light of present knowledge on HIV entry and transcription in lymphocytes and macrophages. Figure I is a diagramatic representation of the two main mechanisms, one cytolytic and the other cytokine-mediated, thought to be used by specific T lymphocytes to protect against virus infections.

HIV productively infects cells of two main leukocyte lineages. One is the myelo-monocytic lineage, including tissue macrophages, Langerhans cells and dendritic (but not follicular dendritic) cells. This macrophage tropism is common to most lentiviruses, including visna virus and SIV. The other cell lineage showing active HIV infection is that of T lymphocytes. Analysis of the molecular mechanisms controling HIV tropism and HIV genome transcription in immunocompetent cells is essential for our efforts to understand the pathogenesis of HIV infection and design future antiviral therapies aimed at controlling progression to AIDS, in conjunction whith available chemotherapies. In particular, the new concept that specific T lymphocytes may exert their antiviral effects through secretion of cytokines capable of interfering with either virus entry into cells or genome transcription, rather than cytolytic mechanisms, should be borne in mind when designing future antiviral vaccines.

CONTROL OF HIV ENTRY INTO CELLS

It has been known for long that CD4, but not CD8, lymphocytes are productively infected by HIV. This led to the erroneous notion that the CD4 molecule is the only receptor for the virus. Indeed both CD4 T lymphocytes and macrophages express this transmembrane antigen, and blockade of CD4 by some antibodies or soluble CD4 does block HIV entry. However, carefull studies using techniques such as quantitative PCR or in situ hybridization showed that only a minority of CD4- bearing lymphocytes or macrophages are actually infected in patients. Improvement of the techniques measuring virus load combined with the use of potent antiviral chemotherapies suggested that the limiting factor could not be virus particle production in infected individuals. Such production indeed is permanent and massive, of the order of 1 to 10^9 particles per day (Ho et al, 1995). These in vivo observations , together with in vitro data obtained by fusion of murine and human cells (Dragic et al, 1996), suggested that HIV co-receptor(s) were needed to permit, in addition to attachement to CD4, efficient virus entry. The mystery was solved by the recent identification of a series of receptors, normally used by chemokines, as co-receptors for HIV fusion and entry. Two major chemokine-receptor types are used by HIV as co-receptors. One is mainly represented by the CC chemokine receptor 5 (CCR5) (Dragic et al, 1996), which expression after transfection in CD4+, CCR5-negative cells is sine qua non for HIV entry and infection in vitro. Neither CD4 or CCR5 expression is sufficient, both are necessary. A mutation (deletion of 32 bp) in the CCR5 gene occurs on the 2 alleles in about 1% of caucasian people. People homozygous for this asymptomatic mutation show natural resistance to HIV infection (Samson et al, 1996), demonstrating the in vivo relevance of HIV usage of the CCR5 coreceptor. CCR5-dependent HIV entry is efficiently blocked by addition to PBL cultures of the natural ligands of CCR5, namely the CC-chemokines RANTES, MIP1α and MIP1β, and the antiviral effect of CD8 cells can be blocked by neutralization of the three chemokines (Cocchi et al, 1995). The second type of co-receptor used by HIV is LESTR, also called fusin (Feng et al, 1996), and for which we have proposed the name of CXCR4 (Oberlin et al, 1996). HIV entry through this receptor is blocked by a novel type of CXC-chemokine, namely SDF, the natural ligand of CXCR4 (Oberlin et al, 1996), (Bleul et al, 1996).

The therapeutic potential of such observations is obvious, but remains to be investigated. Interestingly, the use of the two co-receptors described above is not redundant. HIV isolates unable to induce syncitia (NSI strains) and tropic for both macrophages and CD4 T lymphocytes mainly use CCR5 as co-receptor. Such strains apparently predominate for many years of asymptomatic HIV infection. HIV viruses inducing syncytia (SI) and able to infect and fuse cells of lymphoblastoid cell lines, use the CXCR4 co-receptor. The variability of the HIV genome makes it possible that the *env* gene adapts its sequence, and the gp120 envelope antigen its conformation, to the CXCR4 receptor, without necessarily losing its ability to use CCR5 (dual tropism frequently observed in primary isolates from patients during the symptomatic phase of HIV infection). This adaptation to CXCR4 usage appears to provide HIV with a clear biological advantage in terms of number of potential target cells available for active replication. Indeed, while CCR5 expression seems to be very poor in resting CD4 lymphocytes (unpublished results), that of CXCR4 is very intense in all leukocyte types, including CD4 T lymphocytes in their resting state. Preliminary evidence in our laboratory suggest that CD4 T cell activation is associated not only with up-regulation of CCR5 expression, but also with a down-regulation of CXCR4 membrane expression. The remarkable efficiency of SDF-1 to protect lymphocytes against CXCR4-dependent HIV viruses appears to be due to both occupancy and down-regulation of this receptor (to be reported elsewhere). The in vivo emergence of CXCR4-dependent , SI HIV viruses frequently coincides with or precedes progression to AIDS (Keet et al, 1994), an observation consistent with the concept that adaptation of HIV *env* gene to virus entry through CXCR4 is a critical factor in progression from asymptomatic infection to disease. Thus HIV tropism for co-receptors, rather than variability *per se*, appears to be a pivotal factor in the pathogenesis of AIDS. If ever used, future immunotherapies or gene therapies using CC or CXC chemokines as antivirals will probably have to be adapted to the tropism of HIV strains isolated from each patient, in terms of adaptation to one or more of these co-receptors, and the endogenous status of chemokine production.

In addition to secretion of RANTES and MIP 1 α/β,_it was shown that specific T cell can suppress HIV transcription in vitro through other, yet uncharacterized mediators (Paliard et al, 1996). This intriguing phenomenom deserves to be discussed in the light of recent knowledge on the molecular mechanisms regulating transcription of integrated HIV proviruses, as described below.

CONTROL OF HIV GENOME TRANSCRIPTION

Once HIV particles have fused through the cell membrane, other levels of control of virus replication are observed. The *ds* DNA provirus, associated with viral and cellular proteins, must be transported into the nucleus, where the viral integrase will permit integration into cellular DNA. These steps do not appear to be limiting in most cells, except possibly in resting lymphocytes (Zack et al, 1990) .The fate of the integrated provirus will then depend on the cellular environment, in particular the cell lineage infected and the activation status of the cell bearing an integrated copy of the HIV genome (Virelizier,1990; Fauci et al, 1991; Gaynor, 1992).

In CD4 T cells, the viral genome remains latent in resting cells, whereas T cell activation results in HIV genome transcription and virus replication. Using transfection of reporter genes under the control of the regulatory region (the LTR) of HIV, or that of whole HIV provirus with specific mutations, it was shown that the HIV enhancer sequences have an essential role in the decision to transcribe or not the integrated provirus. What triggers the HIV enhancer is the transcription factor NF-κB (Nabel and Verma,1993; Ghosh et al, 1995) a p50/p65 heterodimer normally retained in the cytoplasm by the inhibitor protein IκBα_ (Nabel and Baltimore, 1987; Cullen and Garrett, 1992). Membrane stimulation by either cytokines such as TNF (Poli *et al*, 1994), or antigen recognition through the TCR /CD3 complex (Hazan *et al*, 1990), leads to IκBα degradation through a yet poorly defined kinase phosphorylating the protein at serine residues 32 and 36, followed by IκBα ubiquitination and rapid IκBα degration by the 26S proteasome. IκBα degradation uncovers the nuclear localisation sequences (NLS) of NF-κB, resulting in the immediate translocation of NF-κB into the nucleus (Baeuerle and Henkel, 1994; Israël, 1995). There, the heterodimer binds to and activates the HIV enhancer, thus triggering HIV genome transcription and activating replication.

Resting CD4 T lymphocytes appear to be an ideal niche for HIV genome latency, since no HIV LTR activity is observed in such cells lacking functional nuclear NF-κB. Normal CD4 T lymphocytes thus do not provide HIV with an appropriate environment for transcription and replication (Alcami et al, 1995). The situation entirely changes after phorbol ester stimulation in circulating lymphocytes, or antigen recognition in human CD4, IL2-dependent T cell clones (Hazan et al, 1990). NF-κB is activated, and in association with other transcription factors (Gaynor, 1992; Verdin et al, 1993) will launch HIV transcription, soon to be amplified by the transactivating effects of HIV Tat on LTR activity (Gaynor, 1992; Greene, 1991).

It should be underlined that the activation of NF-κB is itself tightly regulated. As soon as NF-κB is translocated into the nucleus, it triggers the transcription of many NF-κB-dependent genes (Greene, 1992), in particular that of the IκBα gene (Ten et al, 1992). Neosynthesized IκBα proteins migrate to the nucleus, where they bind NF-κB heterodimers, dissociate them from the HIV enhancer DNA sequences, and transport them in a retrograde manner towards the cytoplasm, thus terminating NF-κB function (Arenzana-Seisdedos et al, 1995, and in press, 1997). The balance between NF-κB and IκBα expression in the nucleus thus controls HIV LTR activity. Nuclear IκBα expression also suppresses HIV-Rev function, through competition with common export pathways. This is due to competitive interference between the nuclear export sequence (NES) of IκBα (Bachelerie et al, in preparation,1997) , which is highly similar to that of HIV Rev. Thus induction of IκBα transcription in infected cells by cytokines may control HIV transcription and replication through termination of NF-κB function and/or competition for HIV Rev-mediated transport towards the cytoplasm of viral RNA, the latter being critical for virus replication (Pomerantz et al, 1992; Malim and Cullen, 1993). Whether this type of antiviral effect could be induced by activation of HIV-specific lymphocytes remains to be determined.

The pivotal role of NF-κB in the control of HIV transcription is shown by the inability of HIV proviruses with specific mutations in NF-κB-responsive elements to establish infection in normal T lymphocytes (Alcami et al, 1995). Intervention at the level of NF-κB-dependent HIV transcription might be of therapeutic interest, but is limited by the fact that NF-κB plays important roles in cell physiology, particularly in lymphocyte activation. For example, inhibition of NF-κB activation by antioxidants (Matthews et al, 1992; Hay et al, 1993) indeed blocks TNF or phorbol ester-induced HIV transcription, but also results in suppression of IL2-induced T cell proliferation (Aillet et al, 1994).

The strategy used by HIV to chronically infect macrophages differs from that observed in lymphocytes. In monocytic cell lines, it was shown that HIV replication itself activates NF-κB, a phenomenon which ensures chronic, self-perpetuating HIV transcription and replication (Bachelerie et al, 1991). Indeed interruption (by the use of the specific proteasome inhibitor MG132) of the constitutive activation of NF-κB observed in chronically infected monocytic cells promptly aborts the indefinite, high level HIV transcription observed in cells of the monocytic lineage (Jacqué et al, 1996). This is in keeping with in vivo observations showing that brain macrophages actively replicate HIV in patients and SIV in experimental macaques, and that HIV infection in the brain is associated with increased nuclear immunoreactivity for NF-κB in microglia and macrophages (Rattner et al, 1993).

CONCLUSION

Analysis of the multiple levels of control of HIV replication, and study on the peculiar strategy developped by HIV to escape immune responses and use immunocompetent cells for the benefit of its own latency and replication, shed usefull light on the pathogenesis of HIV infection and AIDS. Understanding better the basic mechanisms of HIV entry into cells and its inhibition by appropriate chemokines, and the molecular events associated with HIV reactivation from latency is likely to provide new molecular targets and strategies for antiviral intervention. In addition, future anti-HIV candidate vaccines may have to use chemokine production by T lymphocyte as a parameter of efficient immunization, and the supernatant of antigen-stimulated lymphocyte cultures from immunized individuals should be tested for their ability to prevent HIV entry and /or transcription in vitro.

REFERENCES

Aillet, F, Gougerot-Pocidalo, M.A., Virelizier, J.L. and Israel, N.,1994, AIDS Res.Hum.Retrovirus, 10:405.

Alcami, J., Lain de Lera, T., Folgueira, L., Pedraza, M.A., Jacqué, J.M., Bachelerie, F., Noriega, A.R., Hay, R.T., Harrich, D., Gaynor, R.B., Virelizier, J-.L. and Arenzana-Seisdedos, F., 1995, Absolute dependence on κB responsive element for initiation and Tat-mediated amplification of HIV transcription in blood CD4 T lymphocytes, EMBO J., 14:1552.

Arenzana-Seisdedos, F., Thompson, J., Rodriguez, M.S., Bachelerie, F., Thomas, D. and Hay, R.T., 1995, Inducible nuclear expression of newly synthesized IkB-alpha negatively regulates DNA-binding and transcriptional activities of NF-kB, Molecular And Cellular Biology, 15:2689.

Bachelerie, F., Alcami, J., Arenzana-Seisdedos, F. and Virelizier, J. L., 1991, HIV enhancer activity perpetuated by NF-kB induction on infection of monocytes, Nature, 350:709.

Baeuerle, P. A., and Henkel, T., 1994, Function and activation of NF-kB in the immune system, Annual Review of Immunology, 12:141.

Baltimore, D., and Beg, A. A., 1995, DNA-binding proteins - a butterfly flutters by, Nature, 373:287.

Cocchi, F., Devico, A. L., Garzinodemo, A., Arya, S. K., Gallo, R. C. and Lusso, P., 1995, Identification of rantes, mip-1-alpha, and mip-1-beta as the major hiv-suppressive factors produced by CD8(+) T cells, Science, 270:1811.

Cullen, B. R., and Garrett, E. D., 1992, A comparison of regulatory features in primate lentiviruses, Aids Research And Human Retroviruses, 8:387.

Dragic,T, Litwin,V., Allaway, G.P., Martin, S.R., Huang, Y, Nagashima, K.A., Cayanan,C., Maddon, P.J., Koup, R.A., Moore, J.P., and Paxton, W. A., 1996, HIV-1 entry into CD4+ cells is mediated by the chemokine receptor CC-CKR-5, Nature, 381:667.

D'Souza,M.P. and Harden, V. A., 1996,Chemokines and HIV second receptors.Confluence of two fields generates optimism in AIDS research, Science, 12:1293.

Fauci, A. S., Schnittman, S. M., Poli, G., Koenig, S. and Pantaleo, G., 1991, Immunopathogenic mechanisms in human-immunodeficiency-virus (HIV) infection, Annals Of Internal Medicine, 114:678.

Feng, Y., Broder, C. C., Kennedy, P. E. and Berger, E. A., 1996, HIV-1 entry cofactor - functional cDNA cloning of a seven-transmembrane, G protein-coupled receptor, Science, 272:872.

Gaynor, R., 1992, Cellular transcription factors involved in the regulation of HIV-1 gene expression, AIDS, 6:347.

Ghosh, G., van Duyne, G., Ghosh, S. and Sigler, P. B., 1995, Structure of NF-kappa B p50 homodimer bound to a kappa B site, Nature, 373:303.

Greene, W. C., 1991, NF-kB and the activation of HIV-1 gene-expression, Journal of Acquired Immune Deficiency Syndromes, 4:312.

Guidotti, L. G., Ando, K, Hobbs, M. V, Ishikawa, T, Runkel, L., Schreiber, R. B., and Chisari, F., 1994, Cytotoxic T lymphocytes inhibit hepatitis B virus gene expression by a noncytolytic mechanism in transgenic mice, Proc.Natl.Acad.Sci.USA, 91:3764.

Hay, R. T., Wakasugi, N., Virelizier, J. L. and Matthews, J., 1993, Regulation of the DNA-binding activity of the transcription factor NF-kB, Journal of Cellular Biochemistry, 10:144.

Hazan, U., Thomas, D., Alcami, J., Bachelerie, F., Israel, N., Yssel, H., Virelizier, J. L. and Arenzana-Seisdedos, F., 1990, Stimulation of a human T-cell clone with anti-CD3 or tumor necrosis factor induces NF-kB translocation but not human immunodeficiency virus 1 enhancer-dependent transcription, Proceedings of The National Academy of Sciences USA, 87:7861.

Ho, D. D., Neuman, A.U., Perelson, A.S., Chen, W., Leonard, J. M. and Markowitz, M., 1995, Rapid turnover of plasma virions and CD4 lymphocytes in HIV-1 infection, Nature, 373:123.

Israel, A., 1995, The rel/NF-kB and I-kB proteins - recent data on structure, function and regulation, M S-Medecine Sciences, 11:1017.

Keet, I. P., Krol, A., Roos, M .T., de Wolf, F., Miedema, F. and Coutinho, R. A., 1994, Predictors of disease progression in HIV-infected homosexual men with CD4+ cells 200.10.6 but free of AIDS-defining clinical disease, AIDS, 11:1577.

Klenerman, P, Phillips, R. and McMichael, A.,1996, Cytotoxic T cell antagonism in HIV, Semin. Virol., 7:31.

Jacque, J. M., Fernandez, B., Arenzana-Seisdedos, F., Thomas, D., Baleux, F., Virelizier, J. L. and Bachelerie, F., 1996, Permanent occupancy of the human immunodeficiency virus type 1 enhancer by NF-kappa B is needed for persistent viral replication in monocytes, Journal of Virology, 70:2930.

Malim, M. H. and Cullen, B. R., 1993, Rev and the fate of pre-mRNA in the nucleus: implications for the regulation of RNA processing in eukaryotes, Molecular & Cellular Biology, 13:6180.

Matthews, J. R., Wakasugi, N., Virelizier, J. L., Yodoi, J. and Hay, R. T., 1992, Thioredoxin regulates the DNA-binding activity of NF-kB by reduction of a disulfide bond involving cysteine 62, Nucleic Acids Research, 20:3821.

Nabel, G., and Baltimore, D., 1987, An inducible transcription factor activates expression of human immuno-deficiency virus in T cells, Nature, 326:711.

Nabel, G. J., and Verma, I. M., 1993, Proposed NF-kB/I-kB family nomenclature, Genes & Development, 7: 2063.

Oberlin, E., Amara, A., Bachelerie, F., Bessia, C., Virelizier, J. L., Arenzana-Seisdedos, F., Schwartz, O., Heard, J. M., Clark-Lewis, I., Legler, D. F., Loetscher, M., Baggiolini, M. and Moser, B., 1996, The CXC chemokine SDF-1 is the ligand for Lestr/Fusin and prevents infection By T-cell-line-adapted HIV-1, Nature, 382:833.

Paliard, X, Lee, A.Y., and Walker, C. M., 1996, RANTES,MIP-1 α and MIP-1β are not involved in the inhibition of HIV-1sf33 replication mediated by CD8+ T cell clones, AIDS, 10:1317.

Poli, G., Kinter, A. L., Vicenzi, E. and Fauci, A. S., 1994, Cytokine regulation of acute and chronic HIV-infection *in vitro* from cell-lines to primary mononuclear-cells, Research In Immunology, 145:578.

Pomerantz, R. J., Seshamma, T. and Trono, D., 1992, Efficient replication of human-immunodeficiency-virus type-1 requires a threshold level of rev - potential implications for latency, Journal Of Virology, 66: 1809.

Rattner, A., Korner, M., Walker, M. D. and Citri, Y., 1993, NF-kB activates the HIV promoter in neurons, EMBO J., 12:4261.

Samson, M., Libert, F., Doranz, B.J., Rucker, J., Liesnard, C., Farber, C. M., Saragosti, S., Lapoumeroulie, C., Cognaux, J., Forceille, C., Muyldermans, G., Verhofstede, C., Burtonboy, G., Georges, M., Imai, T., Rana, S., Yi, Y. J., Smyth, R. J., Collman, R. G., Doms, R. W., Vassart, G. and Parmentier, M., 1996, Resistance to HIV-1 infection in caucasian individuals bearing mutant alleles of the CCR-5 chemokine receptor gene, Nature, 382:722.

Ten, R. M., Paya, C. V., Israel, N., Lebail, O., Mattei, M. G., Virelizier, J. L., Kourilsky, P. and Israel, A., 1992, The characterization of the promoter of the gene encoding the p50 subunit of NF-kB indicates that it participates in its own regulation, EMBO J, 11:195.

Verdin, E., Paras, P. and Van Lint, C., 1993, Chromatin disruption in the promoter of human immunodeficiency virus type 1 during transcriptional activation, EMBO J., 12:3249.

Virelizier, J. L., 1990, Cellular activation and human-immunodeficiency-virus infection, Current Opinion In Immunology, 2:409.

Zack, J. A., Arrigo, S. J., Weitsman, S. R., Go, A. S., Haislip, A. and Chen, I. S. Y., 1990, HIV-1 entry into quiescent primary lymphocytes - molecular analysis reveals a labile, latent viral structure, Cell, 61:213.

DEVELOPMENT OF AN INFLUENZA-ISCOM™ VACCINE

John Cox, Alan Coulter, Rod Macfarlan, Lorraine Beezum,
John Bates, Tuen-Yee Wong and Debbie Drane

CSL Ltd, 45 Poplar Road, Parkville, Victoria, 3052, Australia

INTRODUCTION

Annual immunisation of the elderly with trivalent influenza vaccines is an important public health measure (Mullooly et al, 1994). The efficacy of currently available vaccines ranges from 60 to 80% in young healthy adults, but is usually lower in the elderly (Fedson et al, 1993; Govaert et al. 1994). Vaccine uptake is less than optimal (CDC 1995; Nguyen-Van-Tam and Nicholson, 1993) especially in this target group. Various ways have been investigated to increase vaccine efficacy including the use of adjuvants (Salk et al. 1952; Salk et al. 1953; Davenport et al. 1968; Glück et al. 1994; Martin, 1996), increased antigen dose (Arden et al. 1986; Palache et al. 1993), use of cell-culture rather than egg-grown viral antigen (Cox et al. 1995; Burnet, 1935) and temperature-sensitive (Subbarao et al. 1995) and cold-adapted (Khan et al. 1996) live virus vaccines. Of these approaches, adjuvants have been the only one to show increased protective efficacy, the most outstanding being the water-in-oil formulations of Salk et al. (1951), which clearly established the feasibility of this approach even though the reactivity of these vaccines was considered unacceptable (Beebe et al. 1964). This paper will describe our rationale for the choice of certain adjuvants with the potential to improve the efficacy of a human influenza vaccine, then give an overview of the initial evaluative studies in mice, and the optimisation steps for Immunostimulating Complexes (Iscom™ and Iscomatrix™, Iscotec AB, Sweden), our chosen adjuvant formulations for progress into clinical trial.

ADJUVANT SELECTION

Cox and Coulter (1997) have defined five properties of adjuvants which may exist either alone or in various combinations and which permit a substance or formulation to be described as "adjuvant-active." These properties are:

(i) immunomodulation, the ability of a substance to influence the cytokine network in such a way as to upregulate an immune response. This upregulation may be general (eg. stimulation of IL-1) or selective (stimulation of either Th1 or Th2 cytokines).

Vaccine Design: The Role of Cytokine Networks
Edited by Gregoriadis *et al.*, Plenum Press, New York, 1997

(ii) presentation, the ability to preserve native antigen structure and present it, usually in multimeric configuration, so that production of neutralising antibody is maximised.
(iii) targeting, the ability to deliver antigen with maximum efficiency to antigen-presenting cells (APC) especially dendritic cells (DC) and macrophages.
(iv) cytotoxic T-lymphocyte (CTL) induction, which requires the ability to deliver antigen to the cytosol of APC resulting in class 1 processing and presentation to CD_8^+ T cells.
(v) depot generation, where vaccine is retained near the dose site to give a short term trickle release or a longer term pulsed release.

The most immediate immune response required of an effective influenza vaccine is the ability to neutralise infectious virus at the respiratory mucosal surface and hence prevent infection. For this reason, importance was placed on selection of an adjuvant which would give good presentation. Immunomodulation was also important, provided there was not an overt Th1 bias which could result in inflammatory cellular responses and complement-fixing antibodies which could cause damage of mucosal barriers. Based on this rationale, Iscoms™ (Morein et al. 1984) and oil-in-water (o/w) emulsions (Hunter et al. 1981; Snippe et al. 1981; Kenney et al. 1989), possibly in association with non-ionic block copolymers (Hunter et al. 1981) were identified as prime adjuvant candidates. There are a number of ways in which influenza virus infection may occur even when an effective vaccine has been used. These include exposure at a stage when vaccine-induced antibody titres are declining, exposure to an overwhelming challenge, exposure at the time of some other respiratory infection and exposure to a strain which shows antigenic drift from the vaccine strain. Under these circumstances, cellular immune responses will be important, with an effective CTL response possibly being the best way to limit then clear the infection (Rimmelzwaan and Osterhaus, 1995). This argument formed a further reason to evaluate Iscoms™, an adjuvant with the ability to induce strong CTL responses (Mowat et al. 1991). In addition, γ-inulin (Cooper, 1995) an adjuvant which induces strong cellular responses and algammulin (Cooper and Steele, 1988; Cooper and Steele, 1991;), a combination of γ-inulin and aluminium hydroxide (strong Th2 responses and the potential for a short term depot effect), were also chosen for evaluation.

MATERIALS AND METHODS

Vaccine Formulations

Phosphate buffered saline, pH 7.2 (PBS) was the base buffer used for all formulations.

(i) Monovalent o/w vaccines were made by simultaneous microfluidisation (Ott et al. 1995) of all components. Five passes through a model 110Y microfluidiser (Microfluidics Corp., USA) was used routinely. Formulation variables were type and level of stabiliser (0.2% Tween 80 or a combination of 0.5% Tween 80 and 0.5% Span 85) and use of the non-ionic block copolymer L121 (BASF, USA) at concentrations of 1.0 and 25mg/ml.
(ii) Iscoms™ were prepared by the method of Morein et al. (1989). To a preparation of viral antigen, about one third haemagglutinin (HA), was added concentrated solutions of cholesterol and phospholipid in detergent (MEGA-10, Bachem, Switzerland) and aqueous saponins (Quil-A, Superfos, Denmark or isolated fractions of Quillaia saponin, Iscotec AB, Sweden) to yield final concentrations of cholesterol, 800μg/ml; phospholipid, 800μg/ml; saponin, 4mg/ml; protein, 4mgHA/ml and MEGA-10, 16mg/ml. The reaction mixture was stirred overnight at 24°C then dialysed extensively against PBS, initially at 24°C then at 4°C. Figure 1 shows a typical HPLC profile of Quil-A and the approximate positions of fractions QH-A, QH-B and QH-C. Iscoprep™ 703 which was used in later experiments is a mixture of 7 parts QH-A and 3 parts QH-C. Figure

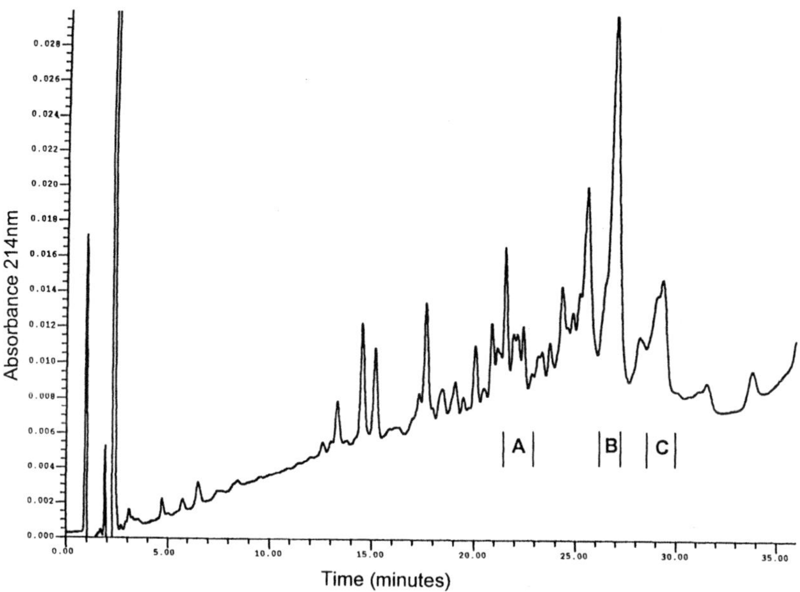

Figure 1. Quil-A (Superfos, Denmark) was subjected to reverse-phase HPLC analysis on a Polymer Labs PLRP-S column. The column was run in 0.10% TFA in an acetonitrile gradient from 20% (0 min) to 48% (35 min).

2 shows the typical cage-like 40nm Iscom™ structures. This formulation, prepared at a higher-than-normal protein concentration, shows spikes of influenza HA radiating from the Iscom™ surface. Iscomatrix™ (Barr & Mitchell, 1996) was formed similarly except that viral antigen was excluded from the process.

(iii) γ-inulin and Algammulin were kindly supplied by Dr Peter Cooper, Australian National University, Canberra, Australia. Formulations were made by simple mixing with viral antigen.

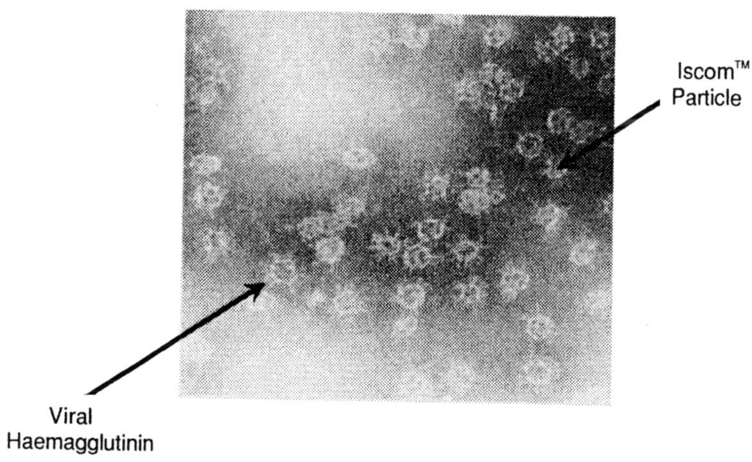

Figure 2. Influenza virus Iscoms, formed at a high HA:saponin ratio were prepared for EM examination as described in the text.

Virus

The mouse adapted H1N1 strain of influenza virus, A/PR/8/34 (Gerhard et al. 1991) was kindly supplied by Dr Margot Anders, University of Melbourne, Australia. B/Panama/45/90 was a 1994 human vaccine strain kindly supplied by Dr Michael Hocart, CSL Limited.

(i) Virus for vaccine preparation was grown in the allantoic cavity of embryonated hens' eggs, inactivated with ß-propiolactone, purified on a sucrose gradient, disrupted with sodium tauro-deoxycholate and ultrafiltered to yield a disrupted, detergent-free viral antigen preparation.
(ii) Virus for enzyme immunoassay was grown in MDCK cell culture, released by freeze-thawing, concentrated by centrifugation in the presence of polyethylene glycol 6000 and stored at -70°C.
(iii) Virus for challenge was grown in embryonated hens' eggs, harvested and stored, aliquoted, at -70°C.
(iv) Virus for haemagglutination inhibition assay was grown in embryonated hens' eggs, clarified and stored frozen at -70°C.
(v) Virus for CTL assay was the same as that used for challenge.

Assay Procedures

Enzyme immunoassay (EIA): Sera were assayed for the presence of antibody to whole A/PR/8/34 virus by indirect EIA. Microtitre plates were coated with virus diluted to 10μg/ml protein in 0.05M carbonate buffer, pH 9.6, washed, blocked, stabilised and stored dry at 4°C. Sera were tested at five-fold dilutions from 1/100 to 1/12500 along with controls and standards on every plate. All samples were diluted in the plate to a final volume of 100μl, and incubated at room temperature for 60 mins. The plates were washed 5 times in PBS/Tween 20, 100μl/well of horse-radish peroxidase conjugated anti-species IgG (γ chain specific) added and incubated at room temperature for 60 mins. The plates were washed again and 100μl/well substrate, a freshly prepared combination of H_2O_2 and 3, 3', 5, 5' tetramethylbenzidine was added. The reaction was stopped by the addition of 50μl/well of 0.5 M H_2SO_4 when the OD 620nm of the well containing the highest concentration of standard reached 0.600. Plates were read at 450nm with Kineticalc Junior (Biotek, USA) installed on a Ceres 900 plate reader (Biotek, USA). Sample potencies were determined from a standard curve, generated on each plate, using 4-parameter fit calculations. The results were expressed in units/ml with 1 U/ml equivalent to an endpoint titre of 10^{-2}. A positive and negative control were tested on each plate for assay validation. The negative control OD at 450 nm needed to be <0.1 and the positive control potency within a predetermined range for any plate used in the assay to be considered valid.

CTL assay: CTL activity was assayed following *in-vitro* restimulation of spleen cells from vaccinated and control mice (Macfarlan *et al.* 1986). Spleen cells were cultured in 2 ml volumes at 2.5 x 10^6 cells/ml together with 'stimulator' cells at 0.5 x 10^6 cells/ml. Stimulator cells were spleen cells from non-vaccinated (BALB/c) mice, that had been infected *in-vitro* with A/PR/8/34. (This mixture of cells is known as 'effector' cells).

Cells were cultured in RPMI 1640 (CSL Ltd.) containing 10% v/v inactivated foetal bovine serum (FBS), 5 x 10^{-5} M 2-mercaptoethanol and 40 μg/ml gentamycin. After 5 days incubation at 37°C in 5% CO_2, cells were recovered, washed, counted and tested for CTL activity.

Effector cells at various concentrations were mixed with 10^4 uninfected or A/PR/8/34 virus-infected ^{51}Cr-labelled P815 cells, together with a 20 fold excess of uninfected unlabelled P815 cells (for cold target inhibition of natural killer-like cytotoxic activity). Assays were in 96 well plates in 0.2ml of RPMI 1640 with 10% FBS. After 4 hours at 37°C in 5% CO_2, the plates were centrifuged and the cell-free supernatant sampled for released ^{51}Cr. The data is expressed as % specific ^{51}Cr release at various effector/target ratios. Results take into account the spontaneous release in medium alone (0%), and the maximum release in 0.1% Triton X100 (100%). Spleen cells from mice that had recovered from challenge after significant weight loss were used as positive controls for the CTL assay.

Haemagglutination inhibition (HAI) activity: Sera were assayed, together with appropriate controls, for HAI antibody using a standard microtitre technique. The test is one used routinely in the Quality Control department, CSL Ltd. Non-specific serum inhibitors were inactivated by heating at 56°C for 30 minutes and treatment with receptor-destroying enzyme (RDE). The HAI titre for each serum was expressed as the last serum dilution that gave complete inhibition of haemagglutination.

Challenge procedure: Full details of the challenge procedure is described elsewhere (Wong *et al.* submitted). Briefly, mice were exposed over a period of 10 minutes to an aerosol of infectious virus (A/PR/8/34) derived from a virus suspension containing $10^{7.3}$ tissue culture infectious dose ($TCID_{50}$) per ml. They were weighed prior to challenge and also, where relevant, 5 days after challenge. Mice were kept for 14 days after challenge, the survivors tallied and euthanased.

Haemolytic assay: The haemolytic activity of Quillaia saponin fractions either in solution or as Iscomatrix™ was determined using group O human red blood cells (RBC) diluted in PBS as substrate. The concentration of the RBC was adjusted so that when 50% were lysed, an absorbance at 405nm of 0.5 would be obtained. Saponin or Iscomatrix™ samples were serially diluted in 96-well U-bottom plates, RBC were added and the plates incubated at 37°C for 1 hour in a water bath. Plates were centrifuged at 1000g for 5 minutes and the haemolytic titre was determined by measuring the absorbance of the supernatant at 405nm. Results were expressed as the amount of saponin required to induce 50% haemolysis, thus the greater the amount of saponin required, the lower its haemolytic activity.

Measurement of dose-site reactivity: Dose-site reactivity of various vaccine formulations were determined by dosing sheep subcutaneously with a small (0.25ml) and a large (1ml) volume of various adjuvant formulations containing 5μg of virus antigen. Each formulation at both the small and large volumes was tested in triplicate in sheep. The coded dose sites were examined by a qualified veterinarian at 1, 2, 3, 4, 7, and 14 days after injection.

Reactivity was scored according to the following scale: 0 = no observable reaction; 1 = pimple; 2 = raised flat area; 3 = soft lump; 4 = hard lump; 5 = abscess

Cholesterol assay: Cholesterol was measured with the Boehringer Mannheim enzymatic colorimetric assay. The assay was adapted for use in 96-well microtitre plates by scaling down the standard method. Values were read on the CERES 900 plate reader at the recommended wavelength.

Qualitative estimation of lipid in Iscoms™: Diphenylhexatriene (DPH) was used to determine the position of lipid (Haugland, 1996) when Iscom™ formulations were fractionated on a sucrose gradient. Briefly, to 50μl of sample in a microtiter plate was added 50μl of 20μg/ml DPH in PBS, pH 7.2. This is freshly prepared by dilution from 1mg/ml solution in acetone. The mixture was left at room temperature for 2.5 hours. The plate was then read in a Labsystems Fluoroskan II using an excitation wavelength of 355nm and an emission detection wavelength of 460nm. Results were expressed as fluor units.

Table 1. Immunogenicity and efficacy of oil-in-water formulations

HA (μg/dose)	Oil	Emulsifier	L121 (mg/dose)	Median EIA Titre		Challenge Outcome	
				1°	2°	% survivors	% wt change
1	squalene	Tween	0	34	233	67	-16
0.1				11	ND	70	-29
0.01				3	ND	10	-24
1	squalene	Tween/Span	0	82	550	100	-14
0.1				42	ND	90	-17
0.01				8	ND	33	-16
1	squalane	Tween	0	19	79	70	-26
0.1				18	ND	70	-23
0.01				3	ND	11	-26
1	squalane	Tween	0.1	63	348	90	-16
0.1				50	ND	100	-17
0.01				3	ND	20	-23
1	squalane	Tween	2.5	149	403	100	-8
0.1				16	ND	100	-20
0.01				4	ND	60	-28
1		unadjuvanted		2	14	30	-24
0.1		unadjuvanted		0	ND	20	-19

ND= Not Done

BALB/c mice were immunised with formulations prepared as described in the text. Primary titres (15/group) were determined 4 weeks after a single dose. Secondary titres (5/group) were determined 1 week after a second dose (administered at week 4). Mice (10/group) were challenged 5 weeks after their primary dose. Challenge mice did not receive a second dose.

Quantitation of Quillaia components: The Quillaia content of Iscom™ vaccines was determined by reverse-phase HPLC in the Quality Control department of the Pharmaceutical Division, CSL Ltd. Conditions were selected so that other vaccine components and potential contaminants were eluted as discrete peaks.

Basic Experimental Protocol

BALB/c mice were dosed with 0.1ml of a vaccine formulation containing inactivated detergent-disrupted, viral antigen derived from the mouse-adapted H1N1 strain of A/PR/8/34 influenza virus. Group size was generally 15, with 10 mice used for challenge and the remaining 5 used for secondary antibody response and CTL assay: Day 0, weigh and primary dose all mice; Day3, weigh all mice; Day 28, bleed all mice and redose subset of mice (for secondary response); Day 35, weigh and challenge primary dose mice; bleed secondary dose mice; Day 40, weigh challenge mice; Day 49, terminate challenge; remove spleens of secondary dose mice for CTL activity.

Electron Microscopy (EM)

Iscom™ preparations were negatively stained by the agar diffusion filtration method of Hayat and Miller (1990) and grids examined with a Philips EM301 transmitting electron microscope.

Statistical Analysis

Results were analysed by use of the Epistat Statistical Package. Samples were compared by the Wilcoxon rank sum test (for independent samples). Comparisons were considered significantly different for probabilities less than 0.05.

RESULTS

The Immunogenicity and Efficacy of an O/W Emulsion Vaccine is Affected by its Components

Three component variations were investigated in these studies - the nature of the oil (squalene or squalane), the nature and amount of emulsifier (0.2% Tween 80 or 0.5% each of

Table 2. Comparison of γ-inulin, algammulin, Iscom[tm] and o/w formulations

HA (µg/dose)	Adjuvant	Median EIA Titre		Challenge Outcome	
		1°	2°	% survivors	% wt change
1	γ-inulin	3	135	100	-12
0.1	20µg/dose	3	16	90	-11
0.01		1	1	30	-18
1	γ-inulin	5	178	100	-9
0.1	100µg/dose	3	19	90	-9
0.01		1	1	50	-12
1	γ-inulin	9	97	100	-4
0.1	500µg/dose	4	53	70	-11
0.01		1	1	40	-15
1	Algammulin	5	69	80	-12
0.1	20µg/dose	1	16	70	-12
0.01		1	6	40	-18
1	Algammulin	7	79	100	-4
0.1	100µg/dose	1	41	60	-14
0.01		1	1	40	-16
1	Algammulin	5	91	90	-9
0.1	500µg/dose	1	46	70	-11
0.01		1	1	60	-12
1	Iscom[TM]	58	1233	100	-1
0.1	15µg saponin/dose	40	460	100	-6
0.01		6	73	100	-11
1	o/w	76	ND	100	-5
0.1	squalane	75	164	100	-2
0.01	0.1mg L121/dose	22	72	100	-4
1	unadjuvanted	1	11	70	-12

ND = Not Done

BALB/c mice were immunised with formulations prepared as described in the text. Primary titres (15/group) were determined 4 weeks after a single dose. Secondary titres (5/group) were determined 1 week after a second dose (administered at week 4). Mice (10/group) were challenged 5 weeks after their primary dose. Challenge mice did not receive a second dose.

Tween 80 and Span 85) and the amount of the non-ionic block copolymer L121 present (0, 1mg/ml and 25mg/ml). Typical results from a number of experiments are shown in Table 1. The change from squalene to squalane made no significant difference in the efficacy parameters measured ($p=0.5$). The change from Tween to a Tween/Span combination however led to a consistent and significant improvement ($p=0.02$) in immunogenicity, survival and weight change thus supporting the earlier report on this emulsifier combination (Valensi et al. 1994). Similarly, addition of L121 at 1mg/ml led to a significant improvement in efficacy, again as expected from earlier reports (Hunter et al. 1981). The further increase to 25mg/ml (the level chosen for the Syntex adjuvant formulation, SAF-1, Kenney et al. 1989) did not lead to any added benefit in this model..

Comparison of Iscoms™, O/W Emulsions, γ-inulin and Algammulin

The squalane o/w emulsion containing 1mg/ml L121 was compared with Iscoms™, γ-inulin and algammulin each at three levels of HA. The outcomes are summarized in Table 2. Iscoms™ and o/w emulsions behave similarly at all three levels by all measured parameters. γ-inulin and algammulin demonstrated significant adjuvant activity by comparison with unadjuvanted controls ($p=0.03$), but in turn were significantly less active than Iscoms™ ($p<0.0001$) or o/w emulsions ($p=0.0001$). Interestingly, the adjuvant activity of the γ-inulin and algammulin was seemingly unaffected by adjuvant dose in the range of 20 to 500μg/dose.

CTL Induction

The preferred formulations of the four adjuvants from Section 2 above at 1μg HA/dose were tested for their ability to induce CTL. The results (Figure 3) show that Iscoms™ consistently gave the best CTL responses, although they were clearly not as good as those seen in experimentally infected mice.

Dose Site Reactivity

Dose site reactivity was evaluated by subcutaneous injection of selected vaccines into sheep and examination of the dose site both visually and by touch for 2 weeks. Iscoms™ and o/w emulsions based on squalane and without L121 showed minimal reactivity and less than that of the unadjuvanted vaccine. Substitution of squalane with squalene led to a substantial increase in dose-site reactivity. Addition of L121 to squalane or squalene-based o/w emulsion vaccines led to a dose-dependent increase in dose site reactivity. The results are shown in Figure 4.

Selection of Defined Saponin Fractions and Phospholipid for Iscom™ Formulation

Iscoms™ and Iscomatrix ™ have traditionally been prepared using Quil-A (Dalsgaard, 1981) or saponin preparations of similar purity. Although this material had been defined as homogenous, based on analytical procedures available at that time, more sophisticated HPLC analysis revealed considerable complexity (Figure 1). Fractions from this mixture were studied for biological activity and from these, 3 fractions (QH-A, B and C) were selected for further study (Rönnberg *et al.* 1995). These three fractions, along with a mixture of 7 parts QH-A and 3 parts QH-C (subsequently named Iscoprep™ 703) were used to form Iscomatrix™. The haemolytic activity of saponin solutions and of Iscomatrix™ prepared from each is recorded in Figure 5. This figure shows the amount of saponin required to induce 50% haemolysis in a suspension of group O RBC. Thus the greater the amount of saponin required to induce haemolysis, the less the haemolytic activity of that saponin preparation. It can be seen that QH-A has the lowest haemolytic activity, QH-B is highly haemolytic and QH-C is intermediate. Iscoprep™ 703 has the activity which is expected of the blend. When used to form Iscomatrix™,

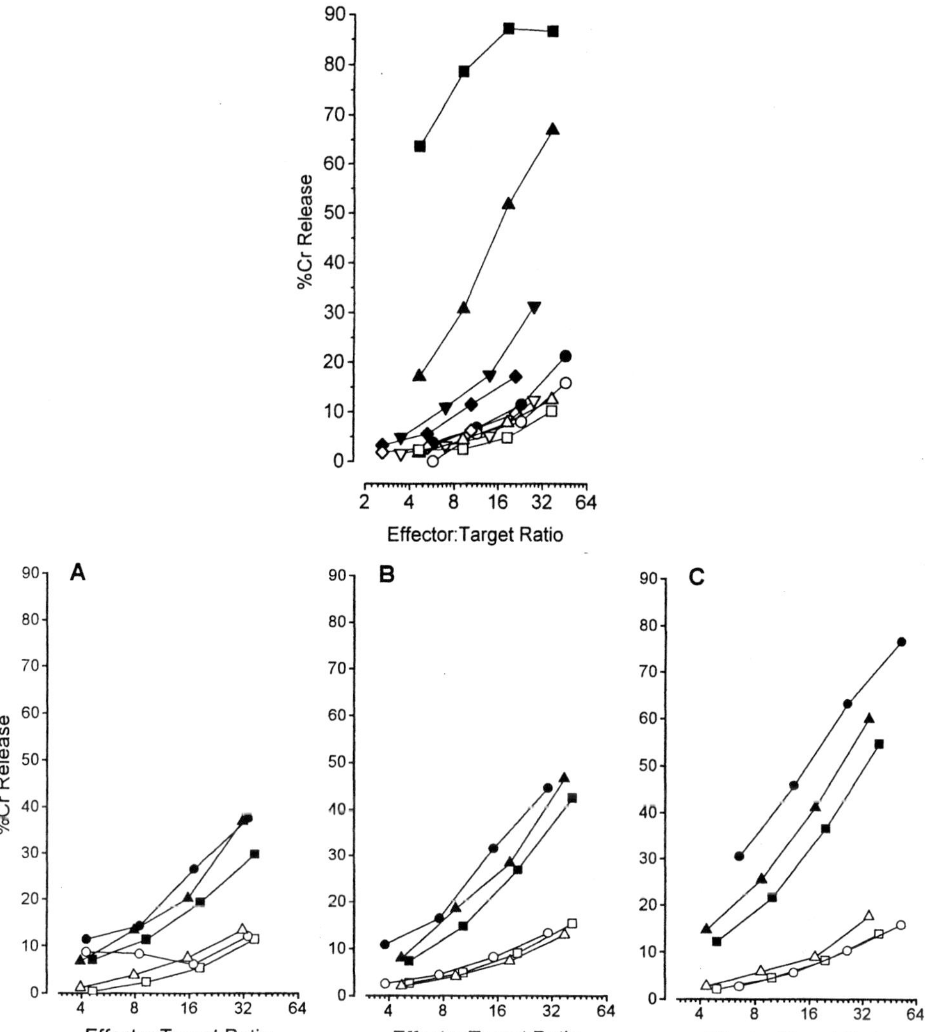

Figure 3. CTL Responses induced by Iscoms and oil-in-water adjuvanted vaccines (upper level): BALB/c mice were vaccinated twice subcutaneously, four weeks apart, with 1μg of HA formulated with various adjuvants. Three weeks after the final immunization, spleen cells pooled from three mice were restimulated *in vitro* with A/PR/8/34 virus, and after 5 days of culture, CTL were assayed against A/PR/8/34-infected (solid symbols) or uninfected (open symbols) P815 cells. CTL responses following no immunization (●); or immunization with 6μg ISCOPREP™ 703 as viral antigen-ISCOMs containing 1μg HA (▲); oil-in-water emulsion with squalane, 100μg L121, and 1μg HA (▼); 1μg HA in PBS (◆); or following recovery from infection with A/PR/8/34 virus (■).

CTL Responses induced by Iscoms, algammulin, and γ-inulin (lower level): BALB/c mice were vaccinated twice subcutaneously, four weeks apart, with 1μg of HA formulated with various adjuvants. Three weeks after the final immunization, spleen cells were restimulated *in vitro* with A/PR/8/34 virus, and after 5 days culture, CTL were assayed against A/PR/8/34-infected (solid symbols) or uninfected (open symbols) P815 cells. Panel A shows CTL responses of individual mice following immunization with 100μg of γ-inulin and 1μg of HA; Part B with 100μg of algammulin and 1μg of HA; Panel C, with 15μg Quil A as viral antigen-ISCOMS containing 1μg HA.

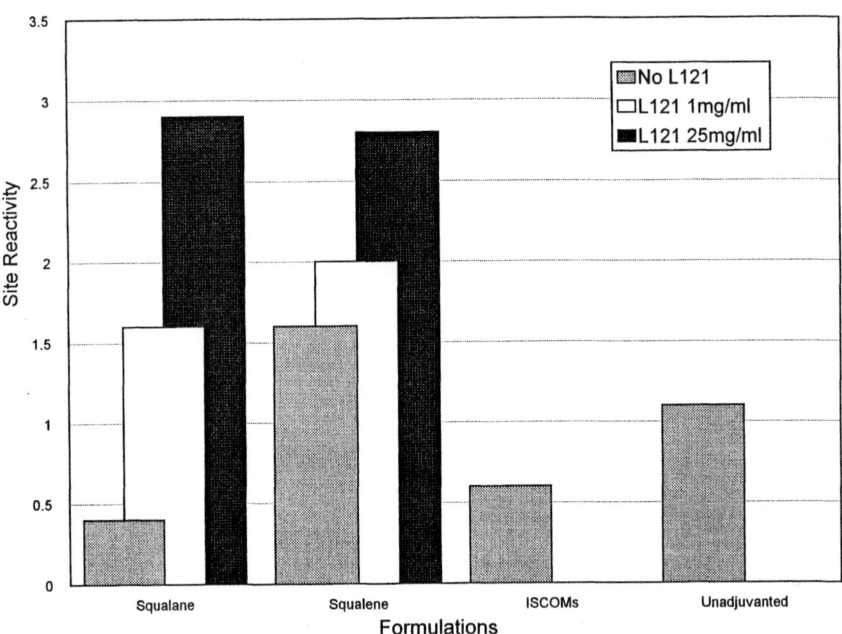

Figure 4. Each formulation was injected subcutaneously into sheep at six sites and the average score for six observations at each site over 14 days was calculated.

Reactivity Scale

0 = no reaction	1 = pimple
2 = raised flat area	3 = soft lump
4 = hard lump	5 = abscess

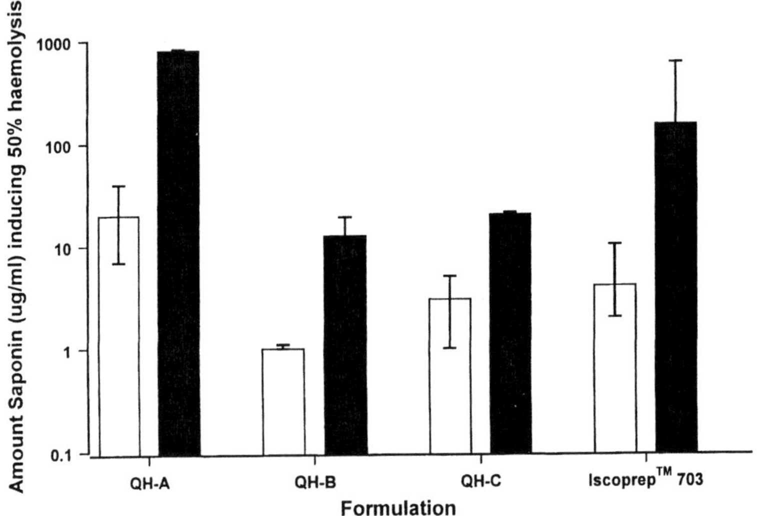

Figure 5. Relative haemolytic activities expressed as amount of saponin required to induce 50% haemolysis for Iscoprep™703 fractions as solutions (□) and as Iscomatrix™ (■).

Table 3. Immunogenicity and efficacy of influenza Iscoms™ formed from quil-a and various saponin fractions

HA (μg/dose)	Formulation	Median EIA titre		Challenge Outcome	
		1°	2°	% survivors	% wt change
1	QH-A Iscoms™	19	305	90	-7
0.1		10	57	70	-14
1	QH-B Iscoms™	52	690	100	-3
0.1		22	245	90	-8
1	QH-C Iscoms™	11	122	100	-4
0.1		17	53	100	-9
1	Iscoprep™ 703 Iscoms™	64	484	100	0
0.1		40	697	100	-4
0.1	Quil-A Iscoms™	32	226	90	-8
0.1	o/w, squalane,0.1mg/dose L121	91	322	100	-7
1	unadjuvanted	2	4	90	-13
0.1		2	3	50	-16

BALB/c mice were immunised with formulations prepared as described in the text. Primary titres (15/group) were determined 4 weeks after a single dose. Secondary titres (5/group) were determined 1 week after a second dose (administered at week 4). Mice (10/group) were challenged 5 weeks after their primary dose. Challenge mice did not receive a second dose.

essentially the same ordering was observed except that the Iscoprep™ 703 Iscomatrix™ was substantially less haemolytic than would have been expected.

Immunogenicity and efficacy studies on Iscoms™ made from these four saponins are summarized in Table 3 and compared with Quil-A Iscoms™, o/w emulsions and unadjuvanted vaccine. It can be seen that QH-A Iscoms™ performed marginally less well by efficacy markers compared with the other adjuvanted formulations. Iscoprep™ 703 Iscoms™ performed at least

Table 4. Immunogenicity and efficacy of Iscoprep™ 703 influenza Iscoms™ formed with different phospholipids

HA (μg/dose)	Formulation	Median EIA titre		Challenge Outcome	
		1°	2°	% survivors	% wt change
1	Egg PC Iscoms™	33	912	100	-3
0.1		13	764	80	-12
1	Soya PC Iscoms™	34	775	90	-14
0.1		13	159	100	-9
1	Hydrogenated Soya PC Iscoms™	22	871	100	0
0.1		18	413	100	-9
1	DPPC Iscoms™	19	805	90	-3
0.1		32	347	100	-6
0.1	o/w, squalane, 0.1mg/dose L121	47	352	100	-1
0.1	Quil-A Iscoms™	28	602	100	-6
1	Unadjuvanted	4	52	60	-8

BALB/c mice were immunised with formulations prepared as described in the text. Primary titres (15/group) were determined 4 weeks after a single dose. Secondary titres (5/group) were determined 1 week after a second dose (administered at week 4). Mice (10/group) were challenged 5 weeks after their primary dose. Challenge mice did not receive a second dose.

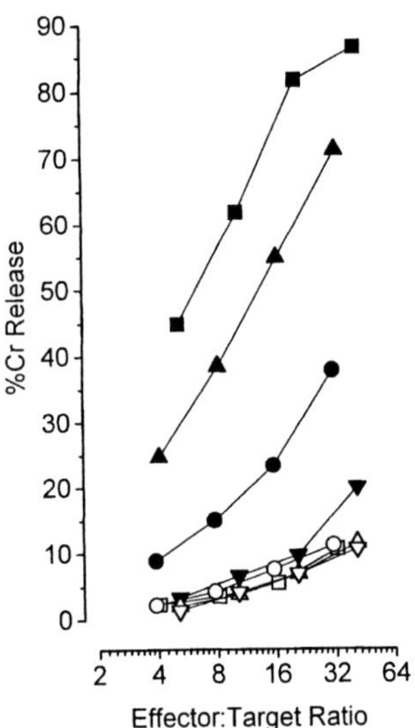

Figure 6. CTL Responses induced by Iscoms and Iscomatrix vaccines. BALB/c mice were vaccinated twice subcutaneously, four weeks apart, with 1μg of HA formulated with various adjuvants. Three weeks after the final immunization, spleen cells pooled from three mice were restimulated *in vitro* with A/PR/8/34 virus, and after 5 days of culture, CTL were assayed against A/PR/8/34 infected (solid symbols) or uninfected (open symbols) P815 cells. CTL responses following no immunization (▼); or immunization with 6μg ISCOPREP™ 703 as viral antigen - ISCOMs containing 1μg HA (▲); 6μg ISCOPREP™ 703 as ISCOMATRIX mixed with viral antigen containing 1μg HA (●) or following recovery from infection with A/PR/8/34 virus (■).

Table 5. Immunogenicity and efficacy of influenza vaccines formulated Iscomatrix™ as Iscoms™ or with

HA (μg/dose)	Formulation	Median EIA Titre		Challenge Outcome	
		1°	2°	% survivors	% Wt Change
0.1	Iscom™	21	733	100	4
0.01		8	160	100	-1
0.1	Iscomatrix™	22	575	100	-1
0.01		3	157	70	-14
0.1	Unadjuvanted	2	20	90	-14
0.01		1	4	30	-18

BALB/c mice were immunised with formulations prepared as described in the text. Primary titres (15/group) were determined 4 weeks after a single dose. Secondary titres (5/group) were determined 1 week after a second dose (administered at week 4). Mice (10/group) were challenged 5 weeks after their primary dose. Challenge mice did not receive a second dose.

as well by all markers, and this led to the selection of Iscoprep™ 703 as the preferred saponin mixture to progress to clinical trial.

Four different phosphatidyl choline (PC) lipid preparations were used to form Iscoprep™ 703 Influenza Iscoms™ ie. egg PC, soya PC, hydrogenated soya PC and dipalmitoyl phosphatidyl choline (DPPC). The results, summarised in Table 4 showed comparable immunogenicity and efficacy for all four phospholipid formulations, suggesting the nature of the lipid was not important for the range of lipids selected for this study. The fully hydrogenated and purified DPPC was chosen because of its comparative stability and ready characterisation.

Comparison of Iscom™ and Iscomatrix™ Vaccines

Influenza Iscom™ vaccines (where the influenza antigens are incorporated into the Iscom™ structure during formation) and Iscomatrix™ vaccines (where the Iscomatrix™ is preformed and influenza antigens are subsequently added) were compared for immunogenicity, efficacy and CTL induction in the mouse model and for immunogenicity in sheep. Mouse and sheep results are shown in Tables 5 and 6 respectively; the CTL data is in Figure 6. The sheep data shows that influenza Iscoms™ give both a higher response and a longer duration of response compared with Iscomatrix™. Both adjuvanted vaccines were vastly more immunogenic than the unadjuvanted control. Group size in this experiment was 8. At low antigen levels, similar results were observed in mice although the Iscom™ vaccine was not superior at higher antigen dose. CTL responses of mice to Iscom™ vaccines were about 2 to 3 times that of Iscomatrix™ vaccines as evidenced by ^{51}Cr release at various dilutions. Although the assay variability is too great to claim significance for this conclusion, the difference was consistently observed.

Re-Examination of the Reactant Ratios for Iscomatrix™ Formation

Having changed two of the three basic components of Iscomatrix™ ie. the saponin from Quil-A to Iscoprep™ 703 and the phospholipid from egg PC to DPPC, it was important to re-examine the reactant ratios to ensure they were still optimal. In the experiment summarized in Table 7, various ratios of lipid:cholesterol:saponin in the Iscomatrix™ reaction mixture were investigated, the readout was haemolytic activity, opalescence, appearance by electron microscopy and percentage of free saponin by HPLC. It can be seen that haemolytic activity is directly related to saponin:cholesterol ratio but inversely related to saponin:lipid ratio at constant cholesterol. The former is the more important marker and supports the observation of the high affinity of saponins for cholesterol (Bangham and Horne, 1962). As the saponin:cholesterol ratio increases, the percentage of free saponin and the haemolytic activity of the resultant Iscomatrix™

Table 6. Comparison in sheep of the immunogenicity of influenza vaccines formulated as Iscoms™ or with Iscomatrix™

HA µg/dose	Formulation	Median EIA (HAI) titres at week:			
		4	5	13	42
10	Iscom™	25 (1280)	1650 (7680)	77 (480)	55 (240)
10	Iscomatrix™	11 (480)	440 (1920)	21 (240)	<2 (100)
10	Unadjuvanted	<2 (30)	6 (60)	<2 (<20)	<2 (<20)

Sheep (8/group) received two doses at week 0 and 4, containing 10µg B/Panama HA and, where appropriate 60µg Iscoprep™ 703 as Iscoms™ or Iscomatrix™.

Table 7. Characteristics of Iscomatrix™ formed with different reactant ratios of lipid, cholesterol and saponin

Preparation	Saponin	Lipid	Lipid:Chol:Saponin	Haemolysis (μg/mL)	Opalescence*	EM**	Free Saponin (%)
1	Iscoprep™ 703	DPPC	1.00:1:2.5	>800	3+	P	2
2	"	"	.50:1:2.5	"	3+	P	2
3	"	"	.25:1:2.5	"	3+	P	1
4	"	"	1.00:1:3.3	600	1+	E	3
5	"	"	.67:1:3.3	>800	2+	E	2
6	"	"	.33:1:3.3	"	3+	E	1
7	"	"	1.00:1:5.0	40	1+	A	8
8	"	"	.50:1:5.0	300	1+	A	5
9	"	"	.25:1:5.0	800	3+	P	4
10	"	"	1.00:1:10.0	10	1+	G	17
11	"	"	.50:1:10.0	20	0	A	16
12	Quil-A	"	1.00:1:5.0	40	0	G	ND
13	Iscoprep™ 703	Egg PC	1.00:1:5.0	200	0	G	ND
14	Quil-A	"	1.00:1:5.0	20	0	G	ND

* Increasing opalescence, 0 → 3+
** E = Excellent A = Adequate
G = Good P = Poor
ND = Not determined

Iscomatrix™ was made as detailed in the text using the stated saponins and lipids at a range of reactant ratios. The resultant preparations were analysed for haemolytic activity, opalescence, appearance by EM and presence of free saponin.

is also found to increase. This free saponin may exist as undialysable micelles or alternatively it may be loosely associated with the Iscomatrix™ structure. This "undialysable" saponin is removed by ultrafiltration on a 30kD membrane (W. Woods, CSL Ltd, personal communication). Opalescence was inversely correlated with amount of lipid in the reaction mix and may in fact suggest that Iscomatrix™ formed in a shortage of lipid has an increased tendency for aggregation possibly as a result of a reduced surface negative charge. Certainly Iscomatrix™ of typical appearance and showing minimal haemolysis or free saponin was formed when the ratio of cholesterol:saponin was 1:3.3 over a wide range of lipid. This is supported by the sucrose gradient examination of preparation 5 (Figure 7) where a sharp symmetrical peak is obtained with overlapping readings for cholesterol assay and saponin assay (by DPH estimation).

CONCLUSIONS

The studies described here were undertaken to select, from an initially extensive list (Cox and Coulter, 1992), a preferred adjuvant for development of a human influenza vaccine. The rationale for selection of adjuvants evaluated here was based on attempts to understand the basis of adjuvant activity (Cox and Coulter, 1997) and to select on this basis, adjuvants which might be suitable for humans and would induce responses appropriate to the predicted requirements of a good influenza vaccine. The principal method chosen for the evaluation was the lethal mouse model of A/PR/8/34 strain of influenza virus in BALB/c mice. This model permitted measurement of efficacy in terms of immunogenicity, CTL responses, survival and weight loss at day 5 post challenge as markers of resistance to challenge. Reactogenicity and limited immunogenicity studies were also performed in sheep. Comparison of o/w emulsions and

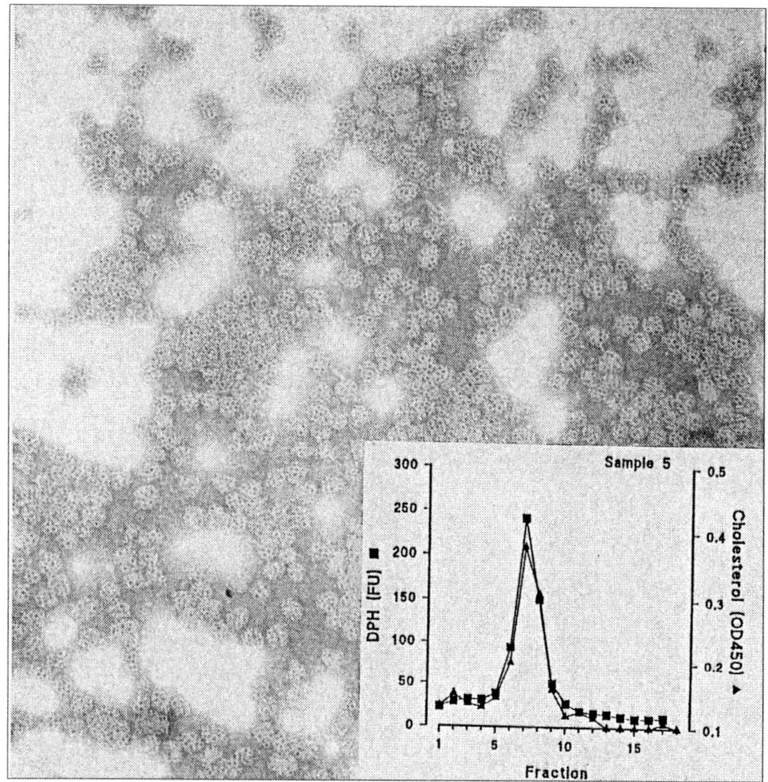

Figure 7. Iscomatrix™ formed at a phospholipid:cholesterol:saponin reactant ratio of 1:1:3.3 was subjected to sucrose-gradient (10 to 60%) centrifugation. Fractions were analysed for cholesterol and saponin (by DPH measurement) and the peak fraction examined by EM.

Iscoms™ showed that the selected o/w emulsion formulations using either squalane and L121 at a minimum level of 1mg/ml or squalene and a Tween/Span emulsifier were as efficacious as Iscoms™. There were however two factors in favour of Iscoms™, their substantially lower dose-site reactivity in sheep and their ability to induce consistently good CTL responses in mice. γ-inulin and algammulin formulations were more efficacious than unadjuvanted vaccines but substantially less so than the Iscom™ and o/w formulations. They also induced lesser CTL responses. For these reasons Iscoms™ were selected for further development.

The selection of Iscoprep™ 703 components resulted from examination of a range of chromatographic fractions from Quil-A. These fractions were chosen for their important biological properties, in particular the ability to form Iscoms™, general adjuvant activity and relative lack of haemolytic activity. From these studies, a mixture of 7 parts QH-A and 3 parts QH-C (Iscoprep™ 703) was selected for its high adjuvant activity, ease of Iscom™ formation and surprisingly low haemolytic activity. Selection of DPPC as the preferred lipid resulted from its positive attributes of being fully hydrogenated and hence stable and defined, and from its similarity to egg PC in all aspects of Iscom™ formation and evaluation. A re-examination of the reaction mixture used to form Iscomatrix™ using these new components then identified small but important changes required to prepare consistent, high-quality product. The need for modified reaction mixtures when using Iscoprep™ 703 has also been observed by others (K. Lövgren-Bengtsson and B. Sundquist, Iscotec AB, personal communication).

Finally, immunogenicity, resistance to challenge and CTL studies in mice and immunogenicity studies in sheep using a human vaccine strain (B/Panama) at predicted human dosing levels (60μg saponin as Iscoprep™ 703 and 10μg viral HA/dose) supported the decision to proceed with this basic formulation through to clinical trial.

Acknowledgements

The authors thank Ian Gust for his constructive scrutiny of this manuscript and Catherine Cole for its excellent preparation. The technical assistance of Rodney Harris, Greg Turner, Dianna Hocking and Sarina Camuglia is also gratefully acknowledged. In addition, we thank Ross Hamilton, who performed all the electron microscopy relating to this work.

REFERENCES

Arden, N.H., Patriarca, P.A., Lui, K.-J., Harmon, M.W., Brandon, F. and Kendal, A.P., 1986, safety an immunogenicity of a 45-ug supplemental dose of inactivated split-virus influenza B vaccine in the elderly. J.Infect. Dis. 153:805.

Bangham, A.D. and Horne, R.W., 1962, Action of saponin on biological cell membranes. Nature 196:952.

Barr, I.G. and Mitchell, G.F., 1996, ISCOMS (immunostimulating complexes) The first decade. Immunol.Cell. Biol,.74:8.

Beebe, G.W., Simon, A.H. and Vivona, S., 1964, Follow-up study on army personnel who received adjuvant influenza virus vaccine 1951-1953. Am.J.Med.Sci. 247:385.

Burnet, F.M., 1935, Propagation of the virus of epidemic influenza on the developing egg. Med. J. Aust. 2:687.

Centers for Disease Control, 1995, Influenza and pneumococcal vaccination coverage levels among persons aged >65 years - United States, 1973-1993. MMWR 44:506.

Cooper, P.D., 1995, Vaccine adjuvants based on gamma inulin. In: "Vaccines: New Generation Immunological Adjuvants". G. Gregoriadis, B. McCormack and A.C. Allison (eds.). Plenum Press, New York, p. 35.

Cooper, P.D. and Steele, E.J., 1988, The adjuvanticity of gamma inulin. Immunol.Cell Biol. 66:345.

Cooper, P.D. and Steele, E.J., 1991, Algammulin, a new vaccine adjuvant comprising gamma inulin particles containing alum: Preparation and in vitro properties. Vaccine 9:351

Coulter, A., Cox, J., Drane, D., Bates, J. and Macfarlan, R. Studies on adjuvanted influenza vaccines: Comparison of immune stimulating complexes (Iscoms) and oil-in-water vaccines. Submitted.

Cox, J.C. and Coulter, A.R., 1992, Advances in adjuvant technology and application. In: "Animal Parasite Control Utilizing Biotechnology". W.K.Yong (ed.), CRC Press, Boca Raton, p. 49.

Cox, J.C. and Coulter, A.R., 1997, Adjuvants - a classification and review of their modes of action. Vaccine, 15:248.

Cox, N., Hannoun, C., Hay, A., Kaverin, N.V., Kilbourne, E.D., Webster, R., Levandowski, R.A., Schild, G., Wood, J., Ghendon, Y., Grachev, V., Griffiths, E. and Martinez, L.J., 1995, Cell culture as a substrate for the production of influenza vaccines: Memorandum from a WHO meeting. 73:431.

Dalsgaard, K., 1981, The application of the Saponin adjuvant Quil A in foot-and-mouth disease vaccines. In: Report and Proceedings from the Symposium on Vaccine Adjuvants held in London on the 30th March, 1981. p. 11.

Davenport, F.M., Hennessy, A.V. and Askin, F.B., 1968, Lack of adjuvant effect of AlPO4 on purified influenza virus hemagglutinins in man. J. Immunol. 100:1139.

Fedson, D.S., Wajda, A., Nicol, J.P., Hammond, G.W., Kaiser, D.L. and Roos, L.L., 1993, Clinical effectiveness of influenza vaccination in Manitoba. JAMA 270:1956.

Gerhard, W., Haberman, A.M., Scherle, P.A., Taylor, A.H., Palladino, G. and Caton, A.J, 1991, Identification of eight determinants in the hemagglutinin molecule of influenza virus A/PR/8/34 (H1N1) which are recognized by class II-restricted T cells from BALB/c mice. J. Virol. 65:364.

Glück, R., Mischler, R., Finkel, B., Que, J.U., Scarpa, B. and Cryz, S.J., Jr., 1994, Immuno-genicity of new virosome influenza vaccine in elderly people. Lancet 344:160.

Govaert, T.M.E., Thijs, C.T.M.C.N., Masurel, N., Sprenger, M.J.W., Dinant, G.J. and Knottnerus, J.A., 1994, The efficacy of influenza vaccination in elderly individuals. A randomized double-blind placebo-controlled trial. JAMA 272:1661.

Haugland, R. P., 1996, Non-polar and Amphiphilic Membrane Probes. In: "Handbook of Fluorescent Probes and Research Chemicals". M. Spence,T.Z. (ed.), Sixth edition, Molecular Probes Inc., Eugene, Oregan, p. 309.

Hayat, M. A. and Miller, S. E., 1990, Negative Staining. McGraw-Hill, New York.

Hunter, R., Strickland, F. and Kezdy, F., 1981, The adjuvant activity of nonionic block polymer surfactants. I. The role of hydrophile-lipophile balance. J. Immunol. 127:1244.

Kenney, J.S., Hughes, B.W., Masada, M.P. and Allison, A.C., 1989, Influence of adjuvants on the quantity, affinity,isotype and epitope specificity of murine antibodies. J. Immunol. Methods 121:157.

Khan, A.S., Polezhaev, F., Vasiljeva, R., Drinevsky, V., Buffington, J., Gary, H., Sominina, A., Keitel, W., Regnery, H., Lonskaya, N.L., Doroshenko, E., Gavrilov, A., Ivakhov, I., Arden, N., Schonberger, L.B., Couch, R., Kendal, A. and Cox, N., 1996, Comparison of US inactivated split-virus and Russian live attenuated, cold-adapted trivalent influenza vaccines in Russian schoolchildren. J. Infect. Dis. 173:453.

Macfarlan, R.I., Dietzschold, B. and Koprowski, H., 1986, Stimulation of cytotoxic T-lymphocyte responses by rabies virus glycoprotein and identification of an immunodominant domain. Mol. Immunol. 23:733.

Martin, T.J., 1996, Enhanced immunogenicity of Chiron Biocine adjuvanted influenza vaccine in the elderly. In: "Options for the Control of Influenza". L.E. Brown, A.W. Hampson and R.G. Webster (eds.), Elsevier Science B.V. Amsterdam, p. 647.

Morein, B., Sundquist, B., Hoglund, S., Dalsgaard, K. and Osterhaus, A., 1984, Iscom, a novel structure for antigenic presentation of membrane proteins from enveloped viruses. Nature 308:457.

Morein, B., Lövgren, K. and Hoglund, S., 1989, Immunostimulating complex (ISCOM). In: "Vaccines: Recent Trends and Progress". G.Gregoriadis, A.C. Allison and G. Poste (Eds.), Plenum Press, New York, p. 153.

Mowat, A.M., Donachie, A.M., Reid, G. and Jarrett, O., 1991, Immune-stimulating complexes containing Quil A and protein antigen prime class I MHC-restricted T lymphocytes in vivo and are immunogenic by the oral route. Immunology 72:317.

Mullooly, J.P., Bennett, M.D., Hornbrook, M.C., Barker, W.H., Williams, W.W., Patriarca, P.A. and Rhodes, P.H., 1994, Influenza vaccination programs for elderly persons: cost-effectiveness in a health maintenance organization. Ann. Intern. Med. 121:947.

Nguyen-Van-Tam, J.S. and Nicholson, K.G., 1993 Influenza immunization; vaccine offer, request and uptake in high-risk patients during the 1991/2 season. Epidemiol. Infect. 111:347.

Ott, G., Barchfeld, G.L., Chernoff, D., Radhakrishnan, R., van Hoogevest, P. and Van Nest, G. 1995, MF59: Design and evaluation of a safe and potent adjuvant for human vaccines. In: "Vaccine Design. The Subunit and Adjuvant Approach". M.F. Powell and M.J. Newman (eds.), Plenum Press, New York, p. 277.

Palache, A.M., Beyer, W.E.P., Sprenger, M.J.W., Masurel, N., de Jonge, S., Vardy, A., Charpentier, B., Noury, J., van Beek, W.C.A., Borst, R.J.A., Ligthart, G.J., Keren, G. and Rubinstein, E., 1993, Antibody response after influenza immunization with various vaccine doses: a double-blind, placebo-controlled, multi-centre, dose-response study in elderly nursing-home residents and young volunteers. Vaccine 11: 3.

Rimmelzwaan, G.F. and Osterhaus, A.D.M.E., 1995, Cytotoxic T lymphocyte memory: Role in cross-protective immunity against influenza? Vaccine 13:703.

Rönnberg, B., Fekadu, M. and Morein, B., 1995, Adjuvant activity of non-toxic Quillaja saponaria Molina components for use in ISCOM matrix. Vaccine 13:1375.

Salk, J.E., Laurent, A.M. and Bailey, M.L., 1951, Direction of research on vaccination against influenza - new studies with immunologic adjuvants. Am. J. Pub. Hlth. 41:669.

Salk, J.E., Bailey, M.L. and Laurent, A.M., 1952, The use of adjuvants in studies on influenza immunization. II. Increased antibody formation in human subjects inoculated with influenza virus vaccine in a water-in-oil emulsion. Am. J. Hyg. 55:439.

Salk, J.E., Contakos, M., Laurent, A.M., Sorensen, M., Rapalski, A.J., Simmons, I.H. and Sandberg, H., 1953, Use of adjuvants in studies on influenza immunization. 3. Degree of persistence of antibody in human subjects two years after vaccination. JAMA 151:1169.

Snippe, H., De Reuver, M.J., Strickland, F., Willers, J.M.N. and Hunter, R.L., 1981, Adjuvant effect of nonionic block polymer surfactants in humoral and cellular immunity. Int.Arch.Allergy Appl.Immunol. 65:390.

Subbarao, E.K., Park, E.J., Lawson, C.M., Chen, A.Y. and Murphy, B.R., 1995, Sequential addition of temperature-sensitive missense mutations into the PB2 gene of influenza A transfectant viruses can effect an increase in temperature sensitivity and attenuation and permits the rational design of a genetically engineered live influenza A virus vaccine. J. Virol. 69:5969.

Valensi, J.-P.M., Carlson, J.R. and Van Nest, G.A., 1994, Systemic cytokine profiles in BALB/c mice immunized with trivalent influenza vaccine containing MF59 oil emulsion and other advanced adjuvants. J. Immunol. 153:4029.

Wong, T.-Y., Turner, G., Cox, J., Pye, D., Bates, J. and Coulter, A. Studies on adjuvanted influenza vaccines: A consistent murine model for evaluating vaccine efficacy. Submitted.

DEVELOPMENT OF PARAINFLUENZA VIRUS AND RESPIRATORY SYNCYTIAL VIRUS SUBUNIT VACCINES

M. Ewasyshyn[1], G. Cates[1], G. Jackson[2], A. Symington[2], N. Scollard[1], R. P. Du[1] and M. Klein[1]

[1]Connaught Centre for Biotechnology Research, [2]Connaught Product Development Centre, Pasteur Mérieux Connaught Canada, 1755 Steeles Ave. W., North York, Ontario, Canada M2R 3T4

INTRODUCTION

Human respiratory syncytial virus (RSV) (McIntosh and Chanock, 1990) and parainfluenza virus (PIV) types 1,2,3 (Chanock and McIntosh, 1990) have been identified as the major viral pathogens responsible for severe respiratory tract infections in infants and young children. In the United States alone, approximately 4,500 infants and young children are expected to die each year as a result of severe respiratory tract infections caused by RSV (Katz, 1985). The global annual infection and mortality figures for RSV are estimated to be 65 million and 160,000, respectively (Robbins and Freeman, 1988). Recent epidemiological data has indicated that RSV also causes significant morbidity and mortality in the elderly (Falsey et al., 1995), the immunocompromised (Englund et al., 1988) as well as in hospitalized adults with lower respiratory tract infections (Dowell et al., 1996). With respect to the parainfluenza viruses, PIV-3 is second only to RSV as the causative agent of bronchiolitis and pneumonia in infants less than 6 months of age. Annually, approximately 1,000 infants may die in the United States from severe respiratory tract infections caused by PIV-3. Furthermore, it is estimated that 600,000 children under the age of 6 develop laryngotracheobronchitis (croup) each year as a result of infection with PIV-1 and 2 (Katz, 1985). It has also been recently reported that the parainfluenza viruses can cause life threatening pneumonia in adult bone marrow transplant recipients (Lewis et al., 1996).

The significant morbidity and mortality figures as well as the substantial health care costs for managing PIV and RSV infections have provided the incentive for aggressively pursuing the development of efficacious PIV-1,2,3 and RSV vaccines. Previous attempts to produce safe and effective vaccines against these viral pathogens were unsuccessful. A formalin-inactivated (FI) trivalent PIV-1,2,3 and RSV vaccine prepared in the 1960's (Chin et al., 1969; Fulginiti et al., 1969) failed to provide adequate protection in clinical trials. In fact, immunization of seronegative infants with the FI-RSV vaccine resulted in the exacerbation of RSV disease in some vaccinees following exposure to wild-type virus. Enhanced disease was not observed

Vaccine Design: The Role of Cytokine Networks
Edited by Gregoriadis *et al.*, Plenum Press, New York, 1997

with the FI-PIV,1,2,3 vaccine; however the vaccine was not efficacious. Over the past several years alternate vaccine strategies have been evaluated for their ability to produce safe and effective PIV and RSV vaccines. Such vaccine strategies have included the production of live attenuated mutants, subunit vaccines produced either from native virus or by recombinant DNA technology, live recombinant viruses and synthetic peptides containing selected B and T-cell epitopes. Although promising results have been obtained with some of these vaccine approaches, this article focuses on recent advances in the development of PIV and RSV subunit vaccines. These subunit vaccines should possess the properties of an ideal RSV/PIV subunit vaccine. They should i) be immunogenic in the presence of maternal antibodies, ii) be capable of reducing the number of hospitalizations resulting from severe respiratory tract infections caused by infection with PIV-1,2,3 and the two major subtypes of RSV (designated A and B), iii) ultimately protect against infection and disease and iv) not cause enhanced disease in vaccinees following exposure to wild-type virus.

An understanding of the fundamental virological and immunological properties of PIV and RSV has provided the scientific basis for pursuing a subunit approach to vaccine development. It is recognized that a protective response is contingent on the induction of neutralizing antibodies against the two major PIV and RSV surface glycoproteins, namely the PIV fusion (F) and hemagglutinin-neuraminidase (HN) (Spriggs, et al., 1987) and the RSV fusion (F) and attachment (G) proteins (Walsh et al., 1987) The PIV (Ewasyshyn and Klein, 1994) and RSV-F proteins (Walsh and Hruska, 1983) are typical type I glycoproteins that are responsible for fusion of the viral envelope with the cell membrane and cell-to-cell spread of the virus. The RSV and PIV F proteins are synthesized as inactive precursors (F0) that are proteolytically cleaved into F1 and F2 moieties that are disulfide-linked. Viral infectivity is dependent on proteolytic cleavage of the F protein. The type II PIV-HN and RSV-G proteins function as the PIV and RSV attachment proteins, respectively. These viral attachment proteins possess unique properties. The PIV-HN protein exhibits both haemagglutination and neuraminidase activities while the RSV G glycoprotein lacks both these activities. The G glycoprotein is heavily glycosylated with O-linked oligosaccharides. The non-glycosylated form of the G protein has a molecular weight of only 33 kDa while the molecular weight of the fully glycosylated protein is 80-90 kDa (McIntosh and Chanock, 1990).

Although the respective HN and F proteins of the PIV types are structurally similar, they are antigenically distinct. Therefore, the HN and F proteins from each type of parainfluenza virus must be included in a trivalent PIV vaccine (Chanock and McIntosh, 1990). In the case of RSV, the F protein is highly conserved between two RSV subtypes A and B (Wertz and Sullender, 1992) and is thus a cross-protective antigen. Anti-F antibodies can cross-neutralize virus from subtypes A and B and protect immunized animals against infections with viruses from both subtypes (Johnson et al., 1987). The F protein has also been identified as a major target for RSV-specific cytotoxic T cells (Pemberton et al., 1987). Although the amino acid sequence of the G protein is conserved within a subtype, significant sequence divergence has been observed between subtypes A and B. Antigenic variation can occur in the G protein within a subtype (Sanz et al., 1994); however, the immunological significance of variations has not been determined. It is well established that the protective immune response elicited by the G glycoprotein is directed primarily at viruses belonging to the same subtype (Johnson et al., 1987). Thus, a universal RSV vaccine should include the G glycoproteins from the two major subtypes.

DEVELOPMENT OF A PIV-1,2,3 SUBUNIT VACCINE

Experimental work at Pasteur Mérieux Connaught Canada has focused on the development of a trivalent PIV-1,2,3 subunit vaccine that contains the HN and F glycoproteins from each parainfluenza virus. The major steps involved in producing such a vaccine from native virus involved: i) preparing validated master and working seed of each virus from PIV clinical isolates in vaccine-quality VERO cells, ii) propagating the virus in VERO cells that were grown on microcarrier beads in 150 L fermentors, iii) purifying the viral glycoproteins from detergent-solubilized viral proteins by affinity or ion-exchange chromatography and iv) evaluating the immunogenicity and protective ability of the purified proteins in suitable animal models.

Our initial studies were directed at producing a PIV-3 subunit vaccine by co-purifying the HN and F proteins from detergent-solubilized viral proteins by lectin-affinity chromatography. This vaccine was highly immunogenic and protective in cotton rats and hamsters. In cotton rats, (Ambrose et al., 1991) the minimum immunogenic dose of the vaccine was 0.1 μg when administered alone and 0.01 μg when adsorbed to aluminum phosphate. Antibody responses in animals immunized twice with 1 μg of HN and F proteins formulated with aluminum phospate were similar to those observed in control animals infected with live PIV-3. Virus titres in both nasal washes and lung lavages were significantly reduced in cotton rats immunized with >0.1 μg of the co-purified HN and F proteins. This vaccine was also highly immunogenic in hamsters (Ewasyshyn et al., 1992). The immunoprotective dose of the co-purified proteins could be reduced to 0.1 μg by the addition of aluminum phosphate, Syntex's MAF-MF formulation or Freund's adjuvant. Deglycosylation of the lectin-purified HN and F proteins with endoglycosidase F did not affect the ability of the alum-adjuvanted proteins to protect hamsters against live virus challenge. These results suggested that the carbohydrate moieties of the HN and F proteins were not necessary for eliciting a protective response in hamsters (Ewasyshyn et al., 1993).

A trivalent prototype PIV-1,2,3 vaccine was recently prepared at Pasteur Mérieux Connaught Canada by purifying the HN and F proteins from detergent-solublized viral proteins of PIV-1,2,3 by ion-exchange chromatography followed by adsorption to aluminum phosphate. In the case of PIV-1, the HN and F proteins were co-purified by ion-exchange chromatography while the PIV-2 HN and F antigens were purified separately and then combined. Sera from mice that were immunized with doses of the alum-adjuvanted trivalent PIV-1,2,3 formulation ranging from 0.3 μg to 10 μg had significant levels of PIV-1,2 and 3 neutralizing antibodies that were similar to those obtained with the corresponding monovalent vaccine. Experimental work is in progress to develop PIV-1 and PIV-2 viruses that can propagate in hamster lungs in order to evaluate the ability of the trivalent PIV-1,2,3 vaccine to protect animals against live virus challenge. A PIV-3 challenge virus is currently available. (Ewasyshyn et al., 1993). The encouraging immunogenicity results provide the basis for the continued development of this prototype PIV-1,2,3 vaccine.

RSV SUBUNIT VACCINES

The most extensively studied RSV subunit vaccines were prepared by Lederle-Praxis. Two vaccine formulations consisting of the RSV-F protein purified from cell lysates of virus-infected VERO cells by either immunoaffinity chromatography (PFP-1) or ion exchange chromatography (PFP-2) have been prepared. The immunoaffinity-purified F protein formulated with alum was highly immunogenic in cotton rats (Murphy et al., 1989) and protected the lower respiratory tract of cotton rats against live virus challenge. In the initial studies, there was no evidence of exacerbated pulmonary pathology in the lungs of immunized cotton rats when animals were challenged 7 days after the final dose. However, there are conflicting reports in the literature regarding the ability of the PFP-1 vaccine to cause enhanced pathology in the lungs of immunized cotton rats when animals are challenged with live virus 3 months after the booster dose. Murphy et al.,. (1990) reported similar histopathological changes in the lungs of animals immunized with either the F-protein or formalin-inactivated (FI) RSV when animals were challenged 3 months post-immunization. In contrast, Hildreth et al. (1993) reported that the F protein formulation did not induce enhanced pulmonary pathology in cotton rats following virus challenge. No definitive reasons were given for these discrepancies; however, additional testing will undoubtly be required before clinical evaluation in seronegative infants is initiated.

Both the PFP-1 and 2 vaccines adjuvanted with alum were safe and immunogenic in seropositive children (Tristram et al., 1993) However, efficacy of the PFP-1 vaccine has not been consistently demonstrated (Belshe et al., 1993). The PFP-2 vaccine has recently been shown to be immunogenic in RSV-seropositive children with cystic fibrosis (Piedra et al.,1996). Although protection against RSV infection was not observed in PFP-2 vaccinees infected with RSV, there was a significant reduction in the clinical manifestations of acute lower respiratory tract infections when compared with the saline control group. Experimental work has also been conducted to improve the quality and quantity of the immune response by formulating the PFP-2 vaccine with alternative adjuvants such as QS-21 (the purified fraction 21 of Quillaja saponaria). Results indicate that formulating the PFP-2 vaccine with QS-21 enhanced both humoral and cell- mediated immune responses and induced a protective response in mice that was similar to that elicited by experimental infection (Hancock et al., 1995).

The Upjohn Co. has produced soluble forms of the RSV F-protein (rF) (Wathen et al., 1989) and a fusion F-G (rF-G) protein (Wathen et al, 1989) in insect cells using the baculovirus expression system. The alum-adjuvanted rF-G chimera proved to be more immunogenic and protective than the rF protein formulated with alum (Brideau et al., 1989). Serum neutralizing antibody titres in animals immunized with the chimera were approximately 5-fold higher than levels induced by the rF protein. The rF protein partially protected immunized animals against live virus challenge whereas <1 ug dose of the rF-G protein completely protected the lower respiratory tract of animals against RSV infection. Conflicting results were obtained regarding the ability of the rF-G protein to cause enhanced pulmonary pathology in immunized cotton rats (Connors et al., 1992; Wathen et al., 1991). Discrepancies were attributed to the vaccine dose, immunization schedule and method used to score histopathology. Unlike FI-RSV, the rF-G protein did not induce augmented pathology in immunized African Green monkeys after live virus challenge (Kakuk et al., 1993). It is anticipated that additional testing will be necessary to confirm the safety of rF-G protein, especially prior to evaluation in seronegative infants.

Elucidation of the mechanism(s) involved in the exacerbation of RSV disease following exposure to wild-type virus will be of primary importance in designing safe RSV vaccines especially for the seronegative population. Experimental evidence suggests that induction of a Th-2 type response may play a role in disease potentiation. Enhanced histopathology observed in mice that were immunized with FI-RSV and challenged with virus could be abrogated by depletion of $CD4^+$ T cells (Connors et al., 1992) or depletion of both interleukin-4 (IL-4) and IL-10 (Connors et al., 1994). BALB/c mice given live virus intranasally or intramusculary elicited a Th-1 type response, whereas FI-RSV induced a Th-2 type of response. Graham et al. (1993) reported a high ratio of IL-4 to IFNγ mRNA in the lungs of animals that were immunized with FI-RSV and challenged with live RSV, thereby indicating a Th-2 type response. In contrast, mice immunized with live RSV either intranasally or intramuscularly had a low IL-4 to IFNγ ratio that is suggestive of a Th-1 type response. Waris et al. (1996) have recently extended the findings of Graham et al. (1993) and reported that cells in bronchoalveolar lavages (analyzed 4 and 8 days after challenge) of mice that were immunized with FI-RSV contained an increased number of total cells, granulocytes, eosinophils and $CD4^+$ cells as compared to the cells observed in the lavages of animals that were immunized with live RSV. There was also a significant increase in the expression of mRNA for the Th-2 cytokines IL-5, IL-13 and a moderate increase in IL-10 expression in the cells of the bronchoalveolar lavages of FI-RSV immunized animals. In contrast, there was a reduction in the expression of the Th-1 type cytokine IL-12. The distinct differences in the pulmonary inflammatory response observed between FI-RSV and live RSV immunized BALB/c mice not only contributes to our understanding of the immunological mechanism of immunopotentiation but also provides a possible model for evaluating the immunopotentiating capability of candidate RSV vaccines. However, one must keep in mind that the clinical significance of these results still remains to be determined. An immunological response to cellular and/or contaminating serum proteins in the vaccine may also contribute to disease potentiation (Vaux-Peretz, 1992; Piedra et al. 1989). Additional research is required to define the precise mechanism(s) involved in immunopotentiation. However, considerable immunological data have been generated over the past few years that should assist in defining the critical parameters involved in controlling the balance between protective immunity and disease potentiation.

DEVELOPMENT OF CHIMERIC PIV-3/RSV PROTEINS

As an alternate approach to PIV-3/RSV vaccine development, we engineered two chimeric RSV/PIV-3 proteins in an attempt to generate single recombinant immunogens capable of simultaneously protecting vaccinees against infection with PIV-3 and RSV. The first chimera consisted of the extracellular domain of the RSV-F protein (amino acids 1-526) linked to the PIV-3 HN protein (amino acids 54-573) (Du et al., 1994). A smaller, predominantly unprocessed, F_{RSV}-HN_{PIV-3} chimera was also produced in *Spodoptera frugiperda* (Sf9) cells using the baculovirus expression system by Homa et al., 1993. The second type of chimera was composed of the external domain of the PIV-3 F protein (amino acids 1-493) linked to the RSV G protein (amino acids 94-299). The chimeric RSV/PIV-3 proteins were produced as soluble, secreted proteins in insect cells using the baculovirus expression system. It was found that the yield of the F_{RSV}-HN_{PIV-3} could be increased approximately 2-fold by using *Trichoplasia ni* (High Five) insect cells in place of the conventional Sf9 cells for expression. The ability of immunoaffinity-purified F_{RSV}-HN_{PIV-3} and F_{PIV-3}-G_{RSV} proteins to induce RSV and PIV-3 neutralizing antibodies and protect immunized cotton rats from challenge with PIV-3 and RSV was evaluated. Both the RSV and PIV-3 moieties of the chimeric proteins were immunogenic in cotton rats. Significant RSV and PIV-3 specific neutralizing antibody titres were detected in the sera of cotton rats that were immunized with either the F_{RSV}-HN_{PIV-3} or F_{PIV-3}-G_{RSV} proteins. The upper and lower respiratory tracts of cotton rats that were immunized with two 1 µg doses of the immunoaffinity-purified F_{RSV}-HN_{PIV-3} or two 9 µg doses of F_{PIV-3}-G_{RSV} proteins were protected against challenge with PIV-3 and RSV. Thus, these chimeras have the potential of being used as dual protective immunogens that are capable of controlling the severe respiratory tract infections caused by PIV-3 and RSV. It will be important to ensure that these chimeras do not cause enhanced pulmonary pathology following live virus challenge.

CONCLUDING REMARKS

Significant progress has been made in the development of subunit vaccines for protection against infection with PIV-1,2,3 and RSV. However, points that should be considered in the rationale design and delivery of future PIV-1,2,3 and RSV subunit vaccines include the dose and route of administration of the vaccine, the importance of inducing a mucosal response, the role of cellular immunity in both recovery from infection and RSV disease potentiation and the immunological mechanism(s) involved in the potentiation of RSV disease. The relevance of the current animal models to humans must also be considered.

REFERENCES

Ambrose, M.W., Wyde, P., Ewasyshyn, M., Bonneau, A.-M., Caplan, B., Meyer, H.L. and Klein, M., 1991, Evaluation of the immunogenicity and protective efficacy of a candidate parainfluenza virus type 3 subunit vaccine in cotton rats, Vaccine, 9:505.

Belshe, R.B., Anderson, E.L. and Walsh, E.E., 1993, Immunogenicity of purified Flycoprotein of respiratory syncytial virus: clinical and immune responses to subsequent natural infection in children, J. Infect. Dis., 168:1024.

Brideau, R.J., Walters, R.R., Stier, M.A. and Wathen, M.W., 1989, Protection of cotton rats against human respiratory virus by vaccination with a novel chimeric FG glycoprotein, J.Gen.Virol., 70:2637.

Chanock, R.M. and McIntosh, K., 1990, Parainfluenza viruses, in: "Virology", B.N. Fields, and D.M. Knipe, eds., Raven Press, New York.

Chin, J., Magoffin, R.L., Shearer, L.A., Schieble, J.H. and Lennette, E.H., 1969, Field valuation of a respiratory syncytial virus vaccine and a trivalent parainfluenza virus vaccine in a pediatric population, Am. J. Epidemiol., 89: 449.

Connors, M., Collins, P.L., Firestone, C.-Y., Sotnikov, A.V., Waitze, A., Davis, A.R., Hung, P.P., Chanock, R.M. and Murphy, B., 1992, Cotton rats previously immunized with a chimeric RSV FG glycoprotein develop enhanced pulmonary pathology when infected with RSV, a phenomenon not encountered following immunization with vaccinia-RSV recombinants or RSV, Vaccine,10:475.

Connors, M., Giese, N.A., Kulkarni, A.B., Firestone, C.Y., Morse, H.C., Sotnikov, A.V. and Murphy, B.R., 1992, Pulmonary histopathology induced by respiratory syncytial virus (RSV) challenge of formalin-inactivated RSV-immunized BALB/c mice is abrogated by depletion of $CD4^+$ cells, J. Virol., 66: 7444.

Connors, M., Giese, A.B., Firestone, C.Y., Morse, H.C. and Murphy, B.R., 1994, Enhanced pulmonary histopathology induced by respiratory syncytial virus (RSV) challenge of formalin-inactivated RSV-immunized BALB/c mice is abrogated by depletion of interleukin-4 (IL-4) and IL-10, J. Virol., 68:5321.

Dowell, S.F., Anderson, L.J., Gary, H.E., Erdman, D.D., Plouffe, J.E., File, T.M., Marston, B.J. and Breiman, R.F., 1996, Respiratory syncytial virus is an important cause of community-acquired lower respiratory infection among hospitalized adults, J. Infect. Dis., 174:456.

Du, R-P., Jackson, E.D., Wyde, P.R., Yan, W.-Y., Wang, Q., Gissoni, L., Sanhueza, S.E., Klein, M.H. and Ewasyshyn, M.E., 1994, A prototype recombinant vaccine against respiratory syncytial virus and parainfluenza virus type 3, Biotechnology, 12:813.

Englund, J.A., Sullivan, C.J., Jordan, M.C., Dehner, L.P., Vercellotti, G.M. and Balfour, H.H., 1988, Respiratory syncytial virus infection in immunocompromised adults, Ann. Intern. Med., 109:203.

Ewasyshyn, M., Caplan, B., Bonneau, A.-M., Scollard, N., Graham, S., Usman, S. and Klein, M., 1992, Comparative analysis of the immunostimulatory properties of different adjuvants on the immunogenicity of a prototype parainfluenza virus type 3 subunit vaccine, Vaccine, 10:412.

Ewasyshyn, M.E., Bonneau, A.-M., Usman, S., Scollard, N. and Klein, M., 1993, Comparative analysis of the immunoprotective abilities of glycosylated and deglycosylated parainfluenza virus type 3 surface glycoproteins. J. Gen. Virol., 74:2781.

Ewasyshyn, M.E. and Klein, M., 1994, "Development of Paramyxoviridae vaccines", in: Modern Vaccinology, E. Kurstak, ed., Plenum Publishing Corporation, New York.

Falsey, A.R., Cunningham, C.K. and Barker, W.H., 1995, Respiratory syncytial virus and influenza A infections in the hospitalized elderly, J. Infect. Dis., 172:389.

Fulginiti, V.A., Eller, J.J., Siever, O.F., Joyner, J.W., Minamitani, M. and Meiklejohn, G., 1969, respiratory virus immunization. A field trial of two inactivated virus vaccines: an aqueous trivalent parainfluenza virus vaccine and an alum-precipitated respiratory syncytial virus vaccine. Am. J. Epidemiol., 89: 435.

Graham, B. S., Henderson, Y.-W., Tang, S., Lu, Neuzil, K.M. and Colley, D.G., 1993, Priming immunization determines T helper cytokine mRNA expression patterns in lungs of mice challenged with respiratory syncytial virus, J. Immunol., 151:2032.

Hancock, G. E., Speelman, D.J., Frenchick, P.J., Mineo-Kuhn, M.M., Baggs, R.B. and Hahn, D., 1995, Formulation of the purified fusion protein of respiratory syncytial virus with the saponin QS-21 induces protective immune responses in BALB/c mice that are similar to those generated by experimental infection, Vaccine, 13:391.

Hildreth, S.W., Baggs, R.R., Brownstein, D.G., Castleman, W.L. and Paradiso, P.R., 1993, Lack of detectable enhanced pulmonary histopathology in cotton rats immunized with purified F glycoprotein of respiratory syncytial virus (RSV) when challenged at 3-6 months after immunization, Vaccine, 11:615.

Homa, F.L., Brideau, R. J., Lehman, D.J., Thomsen, D. R., Olmsted, R.A. and Wathen, M.W., 1993, Development of a novel subunit vaccine that protects cotton rats against both human respiratory syncytial virus and human parainfluenza virus type 3. J. Gen. Virol., 74:1995.

Johnson, P.R., Olmsted, R.a., Prince, G.A., Murphy, B.R., Alling, D.W., Walsh, E.E. and Collins, P.L., 1987, Antigenic relatedness between glycoproteins of human respiratory syncytial virus subgroups A and B: evaluation of the contributions of the F and G glycoproteins to immunity, J. Virol., 61:3163.

Kakuk, T. J., Soike K., Brideau, R. J., Zaya, R. M., Cole, S.L., Zhang, J.-Y., Roberts, E.D., Wells, P.A. and Wathen, M.W., 1993, A human respiratory syncytial virus (RSV) primate model of enhanced pulmonary pathology induced with a formalin-inactivated RSV vaccine but not a recombinant FG subunit vaccine. J. Infect. Dis., 167:553.

Katz, S.L. 1985, Prospects for immunizing against parainfluenza and respiratory synyctial viruses, in: "New Vaccine Development Establishing Priorities", National Academic Press, Washington.

Lewis, V.A., Champlin, R., Englund, J., Couch, R., Goodrich, J.M., Rolston, K., Przepiorka, D., Mirza, N.Q., Yousuf, H.A., Luna, M., Bodey, G.P. and Whimbey, E.,1996,Respiratory diseases due to parainfluenza virus in adult bone marrow transplant recipients, Clinical Infect. Dis., 23:1033.

McIntosh, K. and Chanock, R.M., 1990, Respiratory syncytial virus, in: "Virology", B. N. Fields, and D.M. Knipe, eds., Raven Press, New York.

Murphy, B.R., Sotnikov, A., Paradiso, P.R., Hildreth, S.W., Jenson, A.B., Baggs, R.B., Lawrence, L., Zubak, J.J. Chanock, R.M., Beeler, J.A. and Prince, G.A., 1989, Immunization of cotton rats with the fusion (F) and large (G) glycoproteins of respiratory syncytial virus (RSV) protects against RSV challenge without potentiating RSV disease, Vaccine, 7:533.

Murphy, B.R., Sotnikov, A., Lawrence, L., Banks, S. and Prince, G., 1990, Enhanced histopathology is observed in cotton rats immunized with formalin-inactivated respiratory syncytial virus (RSV) or purified F glycoprotein and challenged with RSV 3-6 months after immunization, Vaccine ,8:497

Pemberton, R.M., Cannon, M.J., Openshaw, L.A., Ball, G.W., Wertz, G.W. and Askonas, A., 1987. Cytotoxic T cell specificity for respiratory syncytial virus proteins: fusion protein is an important target antigen, J. Gen. Virol., 68:2177

Piedra, P.A., Camussi, F. and Ogra, P.L., 1989. Immune response to experimentally induced infections with respiratory syncytial virus: possible role in the development of pulmonary disease, J.Gen.Virol., 70:325.

Piedra, P.A., Grace, S., Jewell, Al., Spinelli, S., Bunting, D., Hogerman, D.A., Malinoski, F. and Hiatt, P.W., 1996, Purified fusion protein vaccine protects against lower respiratory tract illness during respiratory syncytial virus season in children with cystic fibrosis, Pediatr. Infect. Dis.J., 15:23.

Robbins, A. and Freeman, P., 1988, Obstacles for developing vaccines for the third world. Sci.Am., 259:126.

Sanz, M. C., Kew, O.M. and Anderson, L.J., 1994, Genetic heterogeneity of the attachment glycoprotein G among group A respiratory syncytial viruses, Virus Research, 33:203.

Spriggs, M.K., Murphy, B.R., Prince, G.A., Olmsted, R.A. and Collins, P.L., 1987, Expression of the F and HN glycoproteins of human parainfluenza virus type 3 by recombinant vaccinia viruses: contributions of the individual proteins to host immunity, J. Virol., 61:3416.

Tristam, D.A., Welliver, R.C., Mohar, C.K., Hogerman, D.A., Hildreth, S.W. and Paradiso, P., 1993, Immunogenicity and safety of respiratory synyctial virus subunit vaccine in seropositive children 18-36 months old, J. Infect. Dis., 167:191.

Vaux-Peretz, F., Chapsal, J.-M. and Meignier, B., 1992, Comparison of the ability of formalin-inactivated respiratory syncytial virus, immunopurified F,G, and N proteins and cell lysates to enhance pulmonary changes in BALB/c mice, Vaccine, 10:113.

Walsh, E.E. and Hruska, J., 1983. Monoclonal antibodies to respiratory syncytial virus proteins:identification of the fusion protein, J. Virol., 47:171.

Walsh, E.E., Hall, C.B., Briselli, M., Brandriss, M.W. and Schlesinger, J.J., 1987, Immunization with glyco-protein subunits of respiratory syncytial virus to protect cotton rats against viral infection, J. Infect. Dis.,155:1198.

Waris, M.E., Tsou, D., Erdman, D.D., Zaki, S. and Anderson, L.J., 1996, Respiratory syncytial virus infection in BALB/c mice previously immunized with formalin-inactivated virus induced enhanced pulmonary inflammatory response with a predominant Th2-like cytokine pattern, J. Virol., 70:2852.

Wathen, M.W., Brideau, R.J. and Thomsen, D.R., 1989a, Immunization of cotton rats with the human respiratory syncytial virus F glycoprotein produced using a baculovirus vector, J. Infect. Dis., 159: 255.

Wathen, M.W., Brideau, R.J. and Thomsen, D.R., 1989b, Characterization of a novel human respiratory syncytial virus chimeric FG glycoprotein expressed using a baculovirus vector, J. Gen. Virol., 70: 2625.

Wathen, M.W., Kakuk, T.J., Brideau, R. J., Hausknecht, E.D., Cole, S.L. and Zaya, R.M., 1991, Vaccination of cotton rats with a chimeric FG glycoprotein of human respiratory syncytial virus induces minimal pulmonary pathology on challenge, J. Infect. Dis., 163:477.

Wertz, G.W. and Sullender, W.M., 1992, Approaches to immunization against respiratory syncytial virus, Biotechnology, 20:151.

MUCOSAL VACCINES: PERSPECTIVES ON THE DEVELOPMENT OF ANTI-H.PYLORI VACCINES

Paolo Ghiara

Chiron Vaccines, Immunobiological Research Institute Siena,
Dept of Immunology, Siena, Italy

INTRODUCTION

Chronic infection of the gastric mucosa by the Gram negative organism Helicobacter pylori causes chronic active gastritis, peptic ulcer and increases the risk of gastric cancer (Parsonnet et al., 1991; Parsonnet et al., 1994; Blaser and Parsonnet, 1994). The risk of infection is high in childhood and is directly correlated to hygienic conditions and overcrowded homes (Webb et al., 1994). Once established, a successful colonization may be lifelong. Due to significant improvement in hygienic conditions the risk of exposure to infection is now decreasing in the developed contries, where the prevalence of infection approximately increases 1% per year of age and is about 40-50% in the over 50 year old population. However as high as 80% of the young population can be infected in developing countries before the adolescence, and nearly all elderly individuals are infected (Megraud, 1994).

Current antibiotic therapies are quite successful (Tytgat, 1994) but still have many drawbacks consisting of quite high costs, poor patient compliance and, more importantly, selection of resistant strains (Malfertheiner, 1993: Rautelin et al., 1994).

The development of a vaccine to prevent or to eradicate the infection is therefore very attractive. Ideally a vaccine against an infection in the stomach would be a mucosal vaccine, probably an oral vaccine. An exciting challenge involving several laboratories has thus started that exploits the present knowledge on mucosal immunity and vaccination technology to develop a vaccine formulation suitable for tests in humans.

Necessary steps to develop a H.pylori vaccine are: a) the understanding of the pathogenesis of infection, b) the development of good animal models of infection and disease and c) identification of good antigen formulation and delivery.

THE PATHOGENESIS OF H.PYLORI INFECTION

Although the infection is very common, only about 10-20% of the infected develop a symptomatic severe disease. Duodenal ulcer patients rarely develop gastric adenocarcinoma although both diseases are associated with the infection (Hansson et al., 1996). The age of acquisition seems to be relevant to the disease outcome, with cancer being more frequent in individuals who had contracted the infection in early childhood (Blaser et al., 1995).

While some role for the host's genetic background is feasible, but not yet defined, it is now clearly established that a subset of bacteria with enhanced virulence, called Type I, are more frequently isolated from patients with peptic ulcer (Telford et al., 1994).

Type I strains differ from the other Helicobacter pylori bacteria (Type II) because they are able to express a toxin which induces epithelial cell vacuolization and also because they can induce the release of the cytokine IL8, which is chemotactic for neutrophils, from gastric epithelial cells. The toxic activity has been associated to the product of the vacA gene, encoding a 140kDa precursor protein that is actively secreted by the bacteria and cleaved to a mature form of about 95kDa. This 95kDa toxin is further split into two subunits of 58 and 37kDa respectively, which remain associated. This toxin has been shown to play an important role in the pathogenesis of ulcer (Telford et al., 1994). Type II strains also bear the vacA gene but cannot express it or can express an antigenic but not biologically active molecule (Xiang et al., 1995).

The capacity to express toxic activity in Type I strains is associated with the presence of the cagA gene (cytotoxin associated gene A). However the genes encoding for CagA and VacA are not functionally linked (Xiang et al., 1995). Studies by Covacci and coworkers (Covacci et al., 1993) have shown that the cagA gene encodes for a highly immunogenic protein that can be exploited as a serological marker antigen to identify patients who are infected by the more virulent strains (Xiang et al., 1993). More recent results obtained examining the genomic regions flanking the cagA gene (Censini et al, in press), show that this gene is a part of a 40kb pathogenicity island (PAI) containing several other genes, including those involved in the induction of IL8 synthesis, that are responsible for the observed enhanced virulence. Similar mechanism of enhanced pathogenicity have been described for other microorganisms like salmonella (Shea et al., 1996).

A prominent histopathological hallmark of the gastric biopsies of chronically infected patients is a marked infiltration of the lamina propria by inflammatory cells. In chronic active gastritis polymorphomuclear leukocytes are the prominent infiltrating cells. This may be an asymptomatic condition but it is thought to precede the occurrence of peptic ulcer The selective ability to induce IL8 synthesis by gastric epithelial cells (Crabtree et al., 1995) confers to this subset of bacteria the capacity to elicit a more evident inflammation in the gastric mucosa.

The chronic infection is thus characterized by a continuous mucosal injury that also causes antigen sampling and processing by the leucocytes present in the mucosal lamina propria. As a result an intense immune response can be easily observed in infected people (Crabtree et al., 1991a). However activation of the immune system upon H.pylori colonization of the gastric mucosa is apparently inefficient in eliminating the infection. Although an evident antibody response is elicited, both systemically and locally, there is no clear relationship between cellular and humoral responses in infected people (Sharma et al., 1994). H.pylori-specific CD4+ T cell clones may be isolated from both seronegative and seropositive patients (Di Tommaso et al., 1995). Recent observations show that Th1 CD4+ T cell clones (producing IFNγ and IL2) can be more frequently isolated from infected patients with peptic ulcer. Interestingly, most of the clones are specific for the antigen encoded by the cagA gene (D'Elios et al, in press). The proinflammatory effects exerted by the cytokine pattern produced by this T cell subset may play a role in the exacerbation of the disease observed in chronically infected patients. The cellular infiltration that occurs in chronic infection is sustained by the expression of soluble mediators, such as TNFα, IL6 and IL8 (Crabtree et al.,1991b: Crabtree et al., 1993). It can therefore be hypothesized that the only outcome of the immune response during H.pylori infection is to sustain the disease rather that efficiently fight off the infection.

A VACCINE AGAINST H.PYLORI?

Thus there seems to be major drawbacks for the success of active immunotherapy against H.pylori. However a number of observations should also induce us to be more optimistic. First of all the evident cellular immune response that can be frequently detected in individuals that are apparently not infected and seronegative suggests the possibility of the occurrence of a transient infection that has been spontaneously resolved but that has elicited immunological memory in the host. Spontaneous resolution of infection has been also reported in some study describing voluntary or accidental ingestions of H.pylori (Marshall 1988).

Epidemiological studies in developed countries report that about 50% of the over 50 year olds are not infected, suggesting that although being exposed to the same high risk of infection in their childhood, they could acquire resistance to chronic infection. It is tempting to speculate that they might have developed the 'right' immunity against H.pylori.

The recent evidence of a prominent Th1-type of cellular immunity that can be detected in infected patients (D'Elios et. Al, in press), also prompt us to speculate that possibly the induction of a Th2-type of response could be the 'right' immunity to fight off the infection.

To define the protective immunity against H.pylori infection, and thus identify effective vaccination strategies, it is important to develop good animal models of infection that are relevant to the human disease.

DEVELOPMENT OF THE MOUSE MODEL OF PERSISTENT H.PYLORI INFECTION

H.felis infection of mice has been the most extensively used and characterized model so far. Chen and coworkers reported for the first time that vaccination against helicobacter was feasible, immunizing the mice orally with bacterial lysates plus CT as mucosal adjuvant (Chen et al., 1992). Urease, an antigen that is necessary for colonization of all H.pylori strains, has been recently shown to induce good protection in this model (Lee et al., 1995). This model has however poor relevance to the human disease because a) it uses a bacterium that is not a human pathogen, b) H.felis is not able to express the pathogenic determinants (i.e. VacA and CagA) that have been demonstrated as important in human pathology, and , c) chronic infection does not induce ulcerations in the host. This model, although having been the first conveniently available model of infection with a Helicobacter, is not ideal for giving insight into the pathogenesis of human infection and for the development of human vaccines.

Previous attempts to establish persistent infection in normal mice had only poor success. Persistent infection could be obtained only using nude or germ-free mice, whose peculiar immune systems limits their use in developing relevant vaccination systems. Normal mice could bear only a transient infection (2-4 weeks) even using fresh isolates (Karita et al., 1991; Cellini et al., 1994).

We have been able to obtain infections detectable for at least 12 weeks by using very fresh clinical isolates cultured in microaerophylic conditions for no more that three weeks after isolation from patients' biopsies. Bacteria isolated from infected mice two weeks after the primary inoculum were then orally inoculated to other mice. Several cycles of isolation-reinoculation were then performed with an apparent increase in colonization efficiency. This suggests that 'good colonizers' could be selected and maintained by passaging the bacteria in vivo. Using these 'mouse adapted' H.pylori strains we can now observe infections that persist for a long time (≥ 12 months) with no signs of decrease.

Infections were performed with phenotypically characterized H.pylori strains. Cytotoxic (Type I) strains were able to establish gastric colonization of mouse gastric mucosa more quickly than non cytotoxic (Type II) strains. A moderate gastritis was observed in all infected

Table 1. Protection induced by intragastric immunizations in mice

Immunization with	Infected/total	% protected mice
		Challenge with Type I bacteria
saline	14/14	0
LT	13/14	7.1
urease + LT	2/13	84.6
VacA + LT	3/14	78.6
Lysate + LT	1/20	95
		Challenge with Type II bacteria
saline	8/8	0
LT	6/8	25
urease + LT	1/8	87.5
VacA + LT	7/7	0
Lysate + LT	0/10	100

Mice received three weekly intragastric immunizations of saline alone or saline containing 10ug of LT alone or together with 100ug of the indicated antigens. 1 week after the last immunization mice were challenged with 10^9 CFU of bacteria as indicated and the colonization was assessed two weeks later (Marchetti et al., 1995)

mice after 4-8 weeks, but in mice infected with Type I strains the gastric pathology was much more evident and consisted of both cell infiltration in the lamina propria and superficial erosions of epithelium (Marchetti et al., 1995).

The availability of this greatly improved mouse model of H.pylori infection and disease allows us to study the pathogenesis and to assess for the first time the feasibility of a vaccine in animal models that is highly relevant to human disease.

We have reported successful protection of mice from infection by H.pylori following intragastric immunization with H.pylori antigens together with the heat-labile enterotoxin of E.coli (LT) as mucosal adjuvant (Marchetti et al., 1995). Table 1 summarizes the results obtained. While immunization with urease or total bacterial lysates was able to protect mice from infection by both Type I and Type II strains, the VacA induced a Type I specific protection. This indicated that the observed protection was due to antigen specific immune mechanisms.

FEASIBILITY OF VACCINATION IN HUMANS: DEVELOPMENT OF A SAFE VACCINE

The mouse model of persistent infection has been further exploited to address two major issues: a) the identification of a non toxic mucosal adjuvant, and b) the identification of other H.pylori antigens as vaccine candidates.

The highly toxic activity of LT is a major drawback to its use as adjuvant in humans. The adjuvant activity of this molecule, as one of its homologous cholera toxin (CT), has been linked to its strong ADP-ribosylating activity (Lycke et al., 1992). In spite of these published data, the group of M.Pizza and R. Rappuoli at Chiron Biocine was able to obtain by site-directed

Table 2. Comparison between the adjuvant effect of LT and non toxic mutant LTK63

Immunization with	Infected/total	% protected mice
saline	20/20	0
LT	13/18	27.7
LTK63	13/16	18.7
VacA	12/16	25
VacA + LT	3/12	75
VacA + LTK63	4/19	78.9
Lysate	7/10	30
Lysate + LT	1/10	90
Lysate + LTK63	1/10	90

see legend to table 1

mutagenesis a number of non-toxic and non-enzymatically active mutants of LT that retained good adjuvant activity to antigens co-delivered at mucosal sites (Pizza et al., 1994; Douce et al., 1995). The initial observation has been subsequently extended to many antigens including ovalbumin, KLH, tetanus toxin C fragment, the hemagglutinin of influenza virus, and HIV gp120 (Di Tommaso et al., 1996 and unpublished observations).

These non-toxic molecules have been therefore used as adjuvants in oral immunizations of mice. One of them, LTK63, was selected for its high stability to proteases. Table 2 shows representative experiments in which the toxin VacA, or a total bacterial lysate, together with LTK63 induced indistinguishable levels of protection from infection.

The adjuvant LTK63 was then used to assess the potential of other H.pylori antigens as vaccine candidate. Table 3 shows that the antigen CagA and the antigen TOX100, a recombinant non toxic form of VacA expressed in E.coli, corresponding to the mature unprocessed 95kDa VacA, were able to induce good protection (Marchetii et al, 1997).

Table 3. CagA and recombinant non toxic VacA as protective antigens

Immunization with	Infected / Total	% protection
saline	10/10	0
CagA	6/10	40
CagA + LTK63	2/10	80
TOX100	6/10	40
TOX100 + LTK63	2/10	80

see legend to table 1

Table 4. Therapeutic vaccination

Therapeutic immunization with	Infected / Total	% eradication
saline	10/10	0
LTK63	8/10	20
TOX100 + LTK63	1/10	90

Mice infected for 6 weeks by a H.pylori Type I strain received three weekly intragastric immunizations. Eradication of infection was assessed 1 week after the last treatment (Ghiara et al, 1997, submitted).

ERADICATION OF INFECTION IN MICE BY THERAPEUTIC IMMUNIZATION

Mucosal vaccination strategies can be exploited also for eradication of otherwise chronic infections. The first evidence of the feasibility of this therapeutic approach in the helicobacter field was obtained by Doidge and coworkers, who showed that an established infection by H.felis in the mouse could be eradicated by therapeutic vaccination using whole cell sonicates and CT (Doidge et al., 1994). This result was then reproduced in the same animal model using recombinant urease as antigen (Corthesy-Theulaz et al.,1995).

More recent results in our laboratory using the new model of H.pylori infection in the mouse showed that a completely non toxic vaccine formulation consisting of LTK63 and the recombinant non toxic VacA (TOX100) could efficiently eradicate the infection (Table 4). Moreover the immunised mice were resistant to subsequent re-infection with live bacteria indicating that therapeutic immunization not only eradicates the infection but also can induce protective memory (Ghiara et al, 1997, submitted).

CONCLUSIONS

The mouse model of persistent H.pylori infection has established the concept of the feasibility of vaccination against H.pylori, an idea that was previously only inferred by using the H.felis model. This new model is a poweful tool to dissect the pathogenesis and to identify other protective antigens.

The next challenge will be to identify a vaccine formulation to be tested in human efficacy trials and to identify the target population of a candidate H.pylori vaccine as well as to test the efficacy and the safety of therapeutic immunization. Thus the next decade will witness the transfer of experience accumulated on laboratory animals to clinical trials that will assess the feasibility of human vaccination against this important human pathogen.

REFERENCES

Blaser, M.J. and Parsonnet, J., 1994. Parasitism by the "slow" bacterium Helicobacter pylori leads to altered gastric homeostasis and neoplasia. J Clin Invest. 94:4.

Blaser, M.J., Chyou, P.H., and Nomura, A., 1995. Age at establishment of Helicobacter pylori infection and gastric carcinoma, gastric ulcer, and duodenal ulcer risk. Cancer Res. 55:562.

Cellini, L., Allocati, N., Angelucci, D., Iezzi, T., Dicampli, E., Marzio, L., and Dainelli, B., 1994. Coccoid Helicobacter pylori not culturable in vitro reverts in mice. Microbiol. Immunol. 38:843.

Censini, S., Lange, N. Xiang, Z., Crabtree, J.E., Ghiara, P., Borodovsky, M., Rappuoli, R, and Covacci A. cag, a pathogenicity island of Helicobacter pylori, encodes Type I-specific and disease associated virulence factors. Proc.Natl.Acad.Sci.USA. in press.

Chen, M., Lee, A., and Hazell, S., 1992. Immunisation against gastric helicobacter infection in a mouse/ Helicobacter felis model [letter]. Lancet. 339:1120.

Corthesy-Theulaz, I., Porta, N., Glauser, M., Saraga, E., Vaney, A.C., Haas, R., Kraehenbuhl, J.P., Blum, A.L., and Michetti, P., 1995. Oral immunization with Helicobacter pylori urease B subunit as a treatment against helicobacter infection in mice. Gastroenterol. 109:115.

Covacci, A., Censini, S., Bugnoli, M., Petracca, R., Burroni, D., Macchia, G., Massone, A., Papini, E., Xiang, Z., Figura, N., and Rappuoli, R., 1993. Molecular characterization of the 128-kDa immunodominant antigen of Helicobacter pylori associated with cytotoxicity and duodenal ulcer. Proc.Natl.Acad.Sci USA. 90:5791.

Crabtree, J.E., Shallcross, T.M., Wyatt, J.I., Taylor, J.D., Heatley, R.V., Rathbone, B.J., and Losowsky, M.S., 1991a. Mucosal humoral immune response to Helicobacter pylori in patients with duodenitis. Dig. Dis .Sci. 36:1266.

Crabtree, J.E., Shallcross, T.M., Heatley, R.V., and Wyatt, J.I., 1991b. Mucosal tumour necrosis factor alpha and interleukin-6 in patients with Helicobacter pylori associated gastritis. Gut. 32:1473.

Crabtree, J.E., Peichl, P., Wyatt, J.I., Stachl, U., and Lindley, I.J., 1993. Gastric interleukin-8 and IgA IL-8 autoantibodies in Helicobacter pylori infection. Scand.J.Immunol. 37:65.

Crabtree, J.E., Covacci, A., Farmery, S.M., Xiang, Z., Tompkins, D.S., Perry, S., Lindley, I.J.D., and Rappuoli, R., 1995. Helicobacter pylori induced interleukin-8 expression in gastric epithelial cells is associated with CagA positive phenotype. J. Clin. Pathol. 48:41.

D'Elios, M., Manghetti, M., De Carli, M., Costa, F., Baldari, C.T., Burroni, D., Telford, J.L., Romagnani, S., and Del Prete G., 1997. Th1 effector cells specific for Helicobacter pylori in the gastric antrum of patients with peptic ulcer. J.Immunol. 158:962.

Di Tommaso, A., Xiang, Z., Bugnoli, M., Pileri, P., Figura, N., Bayeli, P.F., Rappuoli, R., Abrignani, S., and De Magistris, M.T., 1995. Helicobacter pylori-specific CD4+ T-cell clones from peripheral blodd and gastric biopsies. Infect.Immun. 63:1102.

Di Tommaso, A., Saletti, G., Pizza, M., Rappuoli, R., Dougan, G., Abrignani, S., Douce, G., and De Magistris, M.T., 1996. Induction of antigen-specific antibodies in vaginal secretions by using a nontoxic mutant of heat-labile enterotoxin as a mucosal adjuvant. Infect.Immun. 64:974.

Doidge, C., Gust, I., Lee, A., Buck, F., Hazell, S., and Manne, U., 1994. Therapeutic immunisation against helicobacter infection. Lancet. 343:914.

Douce, G., Trucotte, C., Cropley, I., Roberts, M., Pizza, M., Domenighini, M., Rappuoli, R., and Dougan, G., 1995. Mutants of Escherichia coli heat-labile toxin lacking ADP-ribosyltrasferase activity act as nontoxic, mucosal adjuvants. Proc.Nat.Acad.Sci. USA. 92:1644.

Hansson, L.E., Nyren, O., Hsing, A.W., Bergstrom, R., Josefsson, S., Chow, W.H., Fraumeni, J.F., and Adami, H.O., 1996. The risk of stomach cancer in patients with gastric or duodenal ulcer disease. N.Engl.J.Med. 335:242.

Karita, M., Kouchiyama, T., Okita, K., and Nakazawa, T., 1991. New small animal model for human gastric Helicobacter pylori infection: success in both nude and euthymic mice. Am.J.Gastroenterol. 86:1596.

Lee, C.K., Weltzin, R., Thomas, W.D., Kleanthous, H., Ermak, T.H., Soman, G., Hill, J.E., Ackerman, S.K., and Monath, T.P., 1995. Oral immunization with recombinant Helicobacter pylori urease induces secretory IgA antibodies and protects mice from challenge with Helicobacter felis. J.Infect.Dis. 172:161.

Lycke, N., Tsuji, T., and Holmgren, J. 1992., The adjuvant effect of Vibrio cholerae and Escherichia coli heat-labile enterotoxins is linked to their ADP-ribosyltyransferase activity. Eur.J.Immunol. 22:2277.

Malfertheiner, P. 1993., Compliance, adverse events and antibiotic resistance in Helicobacter pylori treatment. Scand.J.Gastroenterol.Suppl. 196:34.

Marchetti, M., Arico, B., Burroni, D., Figura, N., Rappuoli, R., and Ghiara, P., 1995. Development of a mouse model of Helicobacter pylori infection that mimics human disease. Science. 267:1655.

Marchetti, M., Rossi, M., Giannelli, V., Giuliani, M.M., Pizza, M., Censini, S., Covacci, A., Massari, P., Pagliaccia, C., Manetti, R., Telford, J.L., Douce, G., Dougan, G., Rappuoli, R. and Ghiara, P., 1997. Protection against Helicobacter pylori in mice by intragastric vaccination with H.pylori antigens is achieved using a non toxic mutant of E.coli heat labile enteroxin (LT) as adjuvant. Vaccine, in press

Marshall, B.J., 1988. The Campylobacter pylori story. Scand.J Gastroenterol Suppl. 146:58.

Megraud, F., Epidemiology of Helicobacter pylori infection: where are we in 1995?. 1994. Eur J. Gastroenterol Hepatol. 7:292.

Parsonnet, J., Friedman, G.D., Vandersteen, D.P., Chang, Y., Vogelman, J.H., Orentreich, N., and Sibley,

R.K., 1991. Helicobacter pylori infection and the risk of gastric carcinoma. N.Engl.J.Med. 325:1127.

Parsonnet, J., Hansen, S., Rodriguez, L., Gelb, A.B., Warnke, R.A., Jellum, E., Orentreich, N., Vogelman, H.J., and Friedman, G.D., 1994. Helicobacter pylori infection and gastric lymphoma. New Engl J Med. 330:1267.

Pizza, M., Fontana, M.R., Giuliani, M.M., Domenighini, M., Magagnoli, C., Gianelli, V., Nucci, D., Hol, W., Manetti, R., and Rappuoli, R., 1994. A genetically detoxified derivative of heat-labile Escherichia coli enterotoxin induces neutralizing antibodies against the A subunit. J.Exp.Med. 80:2147.

Rautelin, H., Tee, W., Seppala, K., and Kosunen, T.U., 1994. Ribotyping patterns and emergence of metronidazole resistance in paired clinical samples of Helicobacter pylori. J.Clin.Microbiol. 32:1079.

Sharma, S.A., Miller, G.G., Perez-Perez, G.I., Gupta, R.S., and Blaser, M.J., 1994. Humoral and cellular immune recognition of Helicobacter pylori proteins are not concordant. Clin Exp Immunol. 97:126.

Shea, J.E., Hensel, M., Gleeson, C., and Holden, D.W., 1996. Identification of a virulence locus encoding a second type III secretion system in Salmonella typhimurium. Proc.Natl.Acad.Sci.USA. 95:2593.

Telford, J.L., Covacci, A., Ghiara, P., Montecucco, C., and Rappuoli, R., 1994. Unravelling the pathogenic role of Helicobacter pylori in peptic ulcer: potential for new therapies and vaccines. Trends Biotechnol. 12:420.

Tytgat, G.N.J., 1994. Review Article - Treatments that impact favourably upon the eradication of Helicobacter pylori and ulcer recurrence. Aliment.Pharmacol.Therapeut. 8:359.

Webb, P.M., Knight, T., Greaves, S., Wilson, A., Newell, D.G., Elder, J., and Forman, D., 1994. Relation Between Infection with Helicobacter Pylori and living conditions in childhood - evidence for person to person transmission in early life. Br Med J. 308: 750.

Xiang, Z., Bugnoli, M., Ponzetto, A., Morgando, A., Figura, N., Covacci, A., Petracca, R., Pennatini, C., Censini, S., Armellini, D., and Rappuoli, R., 1993. Detection in an enzyme immunoassay of an immune response to a recombinant fragment of the 128 kilodalton protein (CagA) of Helicobacter pylori. Eur.J Clin Microbiol Infect Dis. 12: 739.

Xiang, Z.Y., Censini, S., Bayeli, P.F., Telford, J.L., Figura, N., Rappuoli, R., and Covacci, A., 1995. Analysis of expression of CagA and VacA virulence factors in 43 strains of Helicobacter pylori reveals that clinical isolates can be divided into two major types and that CagA is not necessary for expression of the vacuolating cytotoxin. Infect.Immun. 63:94.

A SINGLE TREATMENT WITH ADJUVANT STIMULATES TH1-LIKE CYTOKINES AND DOWNREGULATES TH2-MEDIATED PRIMARY AND SECONDARY ALLERGIC RESPONSES

Dorothy E. Scott and Basil Golding

Laboratory of Plasma Derivatives, Division of Hematology,
Office of Blood, Center of Biologics Evaluation and Research,
United States Food and Drug Administration, Bldg 29, Rm 232,
8800 Rockville Pike, Bethesda MD 20892 USA

INTRODUCTION

CD4+ T cells play a central role in most effective immune responses to antigens and pathogens. Since the phenotype of CD4+ T cells induced defines the nature of the subsequent immune response, designing vaccines which favor the appropriate T cell subset is of critical importance. Two subsets of mature Th cells, Th1 and Th2, have been distinguished based upon the pattern of cytokines they produce (Mosmann and Coffman, 1989; Brown et al., 1989). Antigen-presenting cells (APC), which first contact and process antigens, present them to naive "Th0" cells in the context of certain cytokines and costimulatory signals. The microenvironment encountered by naive Th0 cells in conjuction with antigens influences their development towards a Th1 or Th2 direction. In particular, IL-12, IFN-γ and IFN-α favor Th1 cell development, whereas IL-4 promotes differentiation into Th2 cells (Swain, 1993; Hsieh et al., 1993a; Seder et al., 1993; Brinkmann et al., 1993; Wenner et al., 1996). Differentiated, antigen-specific Th1 cells produce IFN-γ, IL-2 and TNF-β (Abbas et al., 1996). Th1 cells promote DTH and complement-fixing, IgG2a antibody production in mice, while the Th2 subset promotes the formation of IgG1 and allergy-mediating IgE antibodies in mice (Finkelman et al., 1990; Snapper and Paul, 1987; Finkelman et al., 1988b; Finkelman et al., 1988a; Finkelman et al., 1986). Evidence for Th1 and Th2-like populations exists in human diseases such as leprosy, leishmaniasis, HIV (progression), atopy, and asthma (Secrist et al., 1993; Parronchi et al., 1991; Clerici and Shearer, 1993; Yamamura et al., 1991; Heinzel et al., 1991). Th1 and Th2 subsets produce factors which enhance their own development and downregulate each other's activity (Maggi et al., 1992; Powrie and Coffman, 1993; Schmitt et al., 1994; Swain et al., 1991; Tanaka et al., 1993). Therefore, pathologic Th2-mediated conditions could theoretically be prevented by vaccines which promote potent Th1 responses.

To test this concept, an in vivo experimental system was used in which a Th2 response normally develops. Mice injected with ovalbumin adsorbed to alum (O/A) develop IL-4-dependent, Th2-mediated responses to ovalbumin which results in formation of anti-ova IgE antibodies (Yang and Hayglass, 1993; Vaz et al., 1971). These anti-ova IgE antibodies are capable of triggering passive cutaneous anaphylaxis in rats (Hayglass and Strejan, 1983). Thus the O/A system is a model for human allergic pathology.

Th1 responses can be induced by a number of adjuvants, most of which are derived from intacellular bacteria, although recombinant IL-12 is also being used for this purpose. Substances with Th1-inducing activity, as evidenced by their ability to promote Th1-like responses and/or IgG2a antibodies, are often components of bacterial cell walls. These include CFA, BCG, monophosphoryl lipid A (MPL), live attenuated listeria, and heat-killed Brucella Abortus (BA) (Grun and Maurer, 1989; Aldovini and Young, 1991; Van de Wijgert et al., 1991; Hsieh et al., 1993a; Svetic' et al., 1993; Finkelman et al., 1988a; Golding et al., 1991; Zaitseva et al., 1995). BA and LPS derived from BA (BA-LPS) are non-toxic in doses which promote high levels of IgG2a secretion (Goldstein et al., 1992). BA induction of IgG2a is largely IFN-γ dependent (Finkelman et al., 1988a); furthermore we and others have shown that BA given with protein/peptide antigen or alloantigen causes formation of Ag-specific Th1 and CTL populations (Street et al., 1990; Lapham et al., 1996).

In this report, we determined whether Th1-promoting BA, given simultaneously with O/A could alter the usual allergic response to O/A. We demonstrate that BA in vivo induces Th1-promoting cytokines IL-12 and IFN-γ within 24 hours of injection, and that BA can indeed abrogate the allergic response even when mice are rechallenged with allergen alone. Furthermore, the requirements for IL-12 and IFN-γ for IgG2a promotion and IgE suppression are examined.

MATERIALS AND METHODS

Animals

Female BALB/c and IFN-γ knockout mice (Dalton et al., 1993) on a BALB/c background were purchased from Jackson Laboratories (Bar Harbor, ME). Mice were used at 8-10 weeks of age. All animals were used in accordance with NIH guidelines for animal use and care.

Immunizations

Mice were immunized i.p. with 2 μg of ovalbumin in 0.5 ml $Al(OH)_3$. Heat-killed BA (Department of Agriculture, Ames IA) was injected i.p. at 10^8 organisms/mouse. BA conjugated to ovalbumin (BA-ova) was synthesized by Dr. John Inman (Golding et al., 1995). The amount of BA in the BA-ova preparation used was 10^8 organisms/mouse conjugated to 2-4 μg/ova/mouse. Anti-IL-12 was a kind gift from Genetics Institute; mice received 200 μg i.p. 24 hours prior to immunizations. As a control for anti-IL-12, mice were given polyclonal sheep IgG (Rockland, Gilbertsville PA).

Detection of antigen-specific immunoglobulins in serum

ELISA assays for IgG1 and IgG2a were performed as previously described (Hayglass and Stefura, 1991). Briefly, 96-well Immulon 4 plates (Dynatech, Chantilly, VA) were coated with 0.2 mg/ml chicken ovalbumin fraction V (Sigma, St. Louis, MO) in carbonate buffer, pH 9.6. Plates were blocked with 1% BSA in PBS. Serum samples were plated in serial 2-fold dilutions. After overnight incubation at 4°C, plates were washed and anti-mouse heavy-chain γ2a or γ1 conjugated to alkaline phosphatase (Southern Biotechnology, Birmingham AL) was added at 1/500 dilution. Plates were developed with diethanolamine buffer and phosphatase-substrate tablets (Kierkegaard and Perry, Gaithersburg, MD). Results were read as positive if the optical density (O.D.) exceeded the mean + 2 SD of the O.D. of control serum from untreated mice for each plate. The method for determination of ova-specific IgE was kindly provided by D. Gajewzcyk (personal communication). Immulon 4 plates were coated with 100 μl of 2 μg/ml rabbit anti-ovalbumin antisera in carbonate buffer, pH 9.6, and incubated overnight at 4°C. After washing X 4 with PBS/.05% tween, plates were blocked with 1% BSA in PBS for 3 hours at 37°. After washing, ovalbumin at 10 μg/ml was added and plates were incubated for 1 hour at 37°C or overnight at 4°C. Serum samples were then added in 2-fold serial dilutions. After incubation at 37°C for 3 hours, plates were washed and alkaline phosphatase conjugated anti-mouse IgE (Pharmingen, San Diego, CA) was added at 1/1500 dilution. Plates were developed after 3 hours at 37°C with a phosphatase substrate as described above. Results of this assay correlated with results obtained with passive cutaneous anaphylaxis in Lewis rats.

Enumeration of cytokine-producing cells

The frequencies of IL-4 and IFN-γ-secreting cells (SC) were determined by Elispot assays that were modified from previously described assays (Taguchi et al., 1990). Immulon 2 plates (Dynatech, Chantilly, VA) were coated overnight at 4°C with 100 μl of the anti-IL-4 antibody RVD4 (Pharmingen, San Diego, CA) or anti-IFNγ antibody (Biosource International, Camarillo, CA) at 10 μg/ml in PBS. After washing, wells were blocked for 1 hour at 37°C with 200 μl/well of RPMI+10% FCS.

Single cell suspensions were prepared from spleens of mice injected with soluble ovalbumin (10 μg i.p.) 3 days prior to Elispot. Enriched CD4+ populations were obtained using αCD4-conjugated Dynabeads (Dynal, Oslo, Norway) according to the manufacturer's instructions. Cells were plated for Elispot at 0.5-1 X 10^6/200μl, and serially diluted (2X dilutions). Plates were incubated for 4 hours at 37°C. The wells were then washed three times with PBS followed by three washes with PBS/0.05% tween. Biotinylated anti-IL-4, or anti-IFN-γ (Pharmingen, San Diego, CA) were added at 10 μg/ml in 100 μl of PBS/0.05% tween + 5% FCS. Plates were incubated overnight at 4°C. The next day plates were washed as before, and streptavidin-alkaline phosphatase (Pharmingen, San Diego, CA) at 1/1500 was added at 100 μl/well. After a 3 hour incubation at 37°C, spots were developed with 200 μl/well

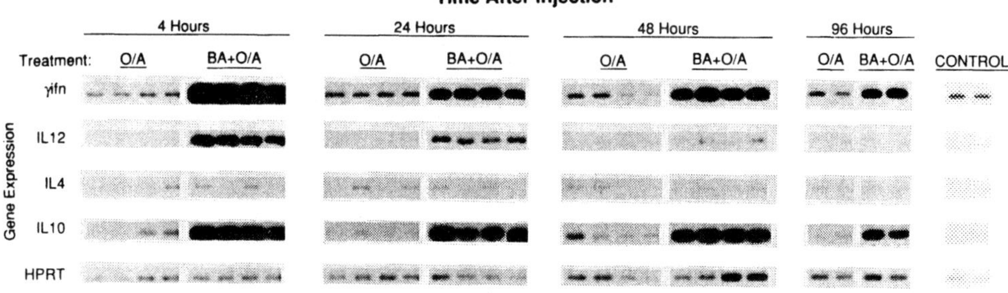

Figure 1. BA+O/A, but not O/A alone, induces Th1-promoting cytokine gene expression. BALB/c mice were injected with O/A, BA + O/A, or HBSS (control mice). Spleens were removed at the indicated time points and RNA was extracted for RT-PCR. Primers specific for IFN-γ, IL-4, IL-10, IL-12 p40, and HPRT were used to amplify the cDNA. The amplified DNA was applied to agarose gels and detected with specific ^{32}P-labeled probes.

of the substrate, 5-bromo-4-chloro-indolyl phosphate (Sigma, St. Louis, MO) at 1 mg/ml, dissolved in 0.1 M 2-amino-2-methyl-1-propanol buffer (Sigma, St. Louis, MO) + 0.6% Seaplaque agarose (FMC Bioproducts, Rockland, ME). Agarose and buffer were boiled, then cooled to 50°C before adding substrate, which was dissolved gradually in a 50°C water bath. Plates were left covered and stationary overnight. On the following day, spots were enumerated in each well using a dissecting microscope. As a positive control, cells were stimulated with PMA+ionomycin.

RT-PCR

The coupled RT-PCR was performed as previously described (Svetic' et al., 1991; Gause and Adamovicz, 1994). Briefly, spleens were removed from mice at the indicated time points after injection and homogenized immediately in RNAzol (Tel-Test, Friendswood, TX). RNA samples (3.0 μl of 1.2 μg/μl sample, diluted in water) were reverse transcribed with Superscript RT (Bethesda Research Laboratories, Bethesda, MD), and cytokine-specific primers were used to amplify selected cytokine messages (19). IL-12 p40 primer sequences were obtained from W. Gause: sense- ACCAGCTTCTTCATCAGG, anti-sense- CTTTGCATTGGACTTCGG, and probe- AGTACCCTGACTCCTGGA. For each gene product, the optimum number of cycles (that which achieves detectable product which is well below plateau concentrations) was determined experimentally. To verify that equal amounts of RNA were added in each RT-PCR

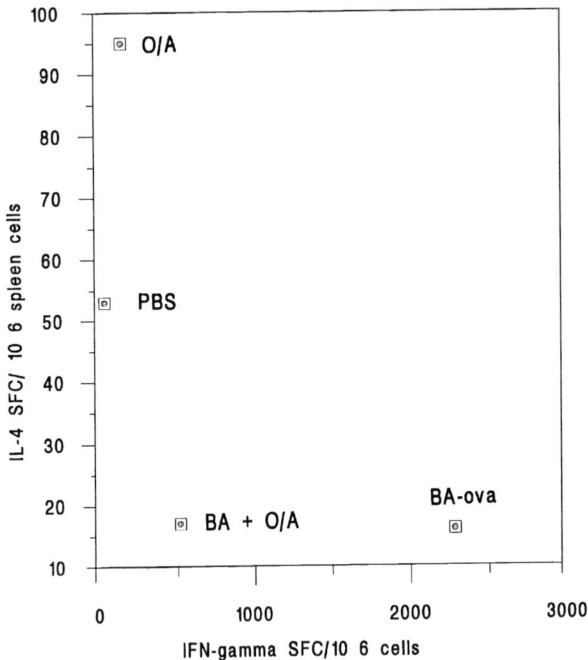

Figure 2. BA given with ovalbumin induces a Th1-like environment in CD4-enriched spleen cells at 1 week. Mice were treated as indicated, and frequencies of splenic IL-4 and IFN-γ-secreting cells were determined by elispot 1 week after immunization without further stimulation. Spleens from 2-3 mice/treatment were pooled and assayed in triplicate. Standard errors were less than 10% of total spots counted for each cytokine.

reaction, primers for a "housekeeping gene," hypoxanthine phosphoribosyl transferase (HPRT), were used in each experiment. Amplified PCR product was detected by Southern blot analysis using ^{32}P-labeled oligonucleotide probes and developed on X-ray film at -60°C.

RESULTS

BA induces Th1 but not Th2-promoting cytokine mRNA early after injection

The cytokine environment present during initial stimulation of naive T cells is important in determining their ultimate phenotype. BA is known to induce IFN-γ mRNA within hours of injection (Svetic' et al., 1993), however IFN-γ alone is not a strong inducer of Th1 responses. To further characterize the cytokine milieu after BA, cytokine mRNA expression was assessed in spleens of mice receiving BA + O/A or O/A (Fig. 1). BA + O/A treated mice expressed high levels of IL-12 p40 mRNA, as well as IFN-γ, whereas O/A treated mice had only constitutive expression of these cytokines. Interestingly, as reported previously, BA also induced IL-10 mRNA, which has been associated with Th2 cells (Svetic' et al., 1993). In other systems, IL-10 secretion can be triggered by IL-12 (Morris et al., 1994). BA + O/A did not result in early expression of IL-4 message. Thus BA + O/A produced an environment favoring development of Th1-like cells. Similar results were seen when BA conjugated to ovalbumin was injected (data not shown).

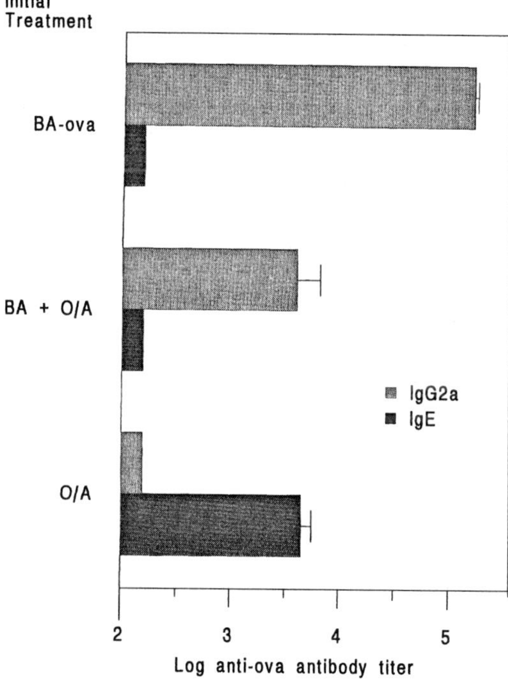

Figure 3. BA given with O/A or as BA-ova inhibits subsequent IgE responses after O/A challenge. Mice were initially treated at indicated, with BA+O/A, BA-ova, or O/A. One month later, all mice were challenged with O/A alone and serum anti-ova responses were assessed 10 days later. PBS-treated mice had no detectable anti-ova antibody levels.

BA induces IFN-γ and suppresses IL-4 secreting T cells

To confirm that CD4+ Th1-like cells developed as a consequence of BA injection, mice received O/A, BA+O/A, or BA-ova i.p. One week post-injection, CD4-enriched spleen cells were assayed by Elispot to determine the frequency of IFN-γ and IL-4 secreting cells in the absence of in vitro stimulation (Fig. 2). Mice which received only PBS had low constitutive numbers of IL-4 secreting cells. Mice which received O/A had an increase in IL-4 secreting cells but not in IFN-γ secreting cells and thus were a Th2-predominant population. In contrast, mice receiving BA+O/A or BA-ova had greatly increased frequencies of IFN-γ secreting cells. BA-ova treated mice had greater numbers of Th1-like cells than BA+O/A treated mice, possibly reflecting the ability of O/A to partially counteract the Th1 promoting effect of BA. Both BA-ova and BA + O/A resulted in a decrease of IL-4 secreting cells, even below constitutive levels. Thus BA has both an IL-4 lowering as well as IFN-gamma-enhancing activity suggesting potential utility in downregulation of Th2-mediated responses.

BA downregulates antigen-specific Th2-mediated IgE responses, even after rechallenge with allergen alone

We next tested the ability of BA to downregulate the IgE response to O/A. Mice were injected initially with O/A alone, BA-ova, or BA+O/A. One month later, all mice were challenged with O/A only. Anti-ova IgE and IgG2a antibodies were assessed ten days after the second injection (Fig. 3). IgE responses were abrogated in mice which received either BA-ova or BA+O/A initially, compared to mice receiving O/A alone. Th1-dependent IgG2a antibodies were elevated in BA-treated mice but not mice which received only allergen. BA-ova treated mice had higher IgG2a responses than BA+O/A treated mice, which correlates with the

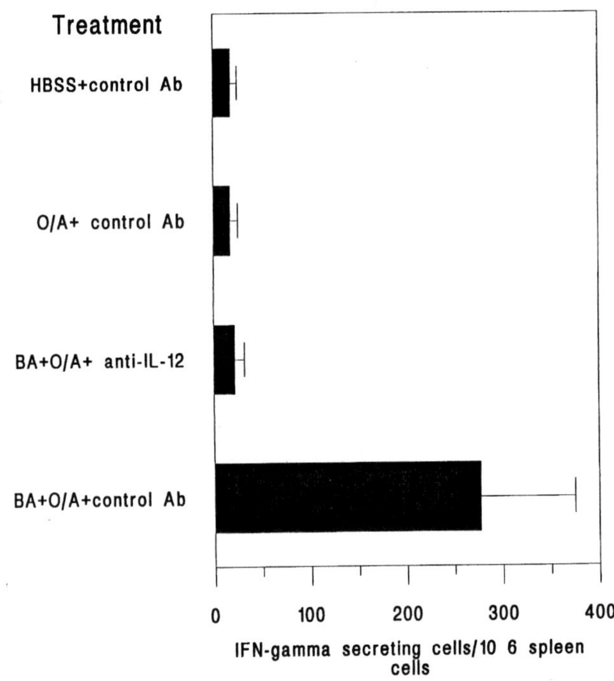

Figure 4. Anti-IL-12 blocks BA-induced splenic IFN-γ secretion. Mice were injected as indicated. Spleens from 2-4 mice/group were removed at 48 hours and assayed in triplicate.

observation that BA-ova also induced more IFN-gamma secreting CD4+cells (Fig. 2). Therefore BA, given with O/A or as a conjugate to soluble ovalbumin, prevented allergic antibody formation after allergen challenge, and instead promoted antigen-specific IgG2a antibodies.

The role of IL-12 in BA-induced Th1 responses and suppression of IgE

IL-12 is a necessary factor in many in vitro and in vivo systems for optimal Th1 development. In addition, IL-12 in vivo can downregulate primary polyclonal IgE responses by an IFN-γ independent mechanism (Morris et al., 1994). To elucidate the role of BA-induced IL-12, mice were treated with O/A, O/A + BA, or O/A + BA + anti-IL-12. To determine the effectiveness of anti-IL-12, the frequency of IFN-γ secreting cells was determined 48 hours after injection (Fig. 4). As expected, mice given BA+O/A had a high frequency of IFN-γ secreting cells whereas O/A treated mice had no increase over constitutive levels. Mice given anti-IL-12 had complete suppression of IFN-γ secretion, indicating that IL-12 is required for BA-induced IFN-γ secretion early after injection. Similar results were obtained at 24 hours (data not shown).

To further examine effects of blocking BA-induced IL-12, spleen cytokine mRNA levels for IL-12, IL-10, and IFN-γ were determined by RT-PCR at early time points (Fig. 5). IFN-γ mRNA levels were reduced by anti-IL-12, at 4 and 24h, although not to baseline levels. Interestingly, maximal IL-10 gene expression was also dependent upon IL-12. IL-12 expression was slightly increased by anti-IL-12, possibly reflecting reduced negative feedback due to less IL-10 production in the presence of anti-IL-12 (Fig. 5C).

The suppression of IFN-γ mRNA and secretion suggested that BA-induced IL-12 is important for Th1 development. To determine whether IL-12 and IFN-γ are required for IgG2a generation and IgE suppression, mice were injected as previously described in the presence or absence of anti-IL-12, and primary antibody responses were determined 14 days later. One month later, all except PBS-treated mice received O/A alone (Fig. 6). IL-12 was needed for optimal secondary IgG2a responses (Fig. 6A), since anti-IL-12 blocked this response. However, IgE suppression occurred in the presence or absence of anti-IL-12 (Fig. 6B), suggesting that BA mediates IgE suppression via an IL-12 and IFN-γ independent pathway. These results imply that IL-12 is required for the induction of memory Th1-like cells which can then drive a secondary IgG2a response. In contrast, BA-mediated downregulation of allergen-induced IgE responses does not appear to be IL-12 or IFN-γ dependent.

Because some IFN-γ message was still apparent even with anti-IL-12 treatment, the possibility that small amounts of IFN-γ (not detectable by Elispot or present at a later time) were contributing to IgE suppression could not be ruled out. To address this question, IFN-γ knockout mice and control BALB/c mice were injected with O/A, BA + O/A or PBS (Fig. 7). O/A-induced IgE was suppressed by BA below detectable levels in the primary response in both wild type and IFN-γ KO mice, thus indicating that IFN-γ is not required for IgE suppression in this system.

DISCUSSION

Our studies use an in vivo model system to show that a strong Th1-promoting substance, BA, can overcome a Th2, allergy-inducing stimulus. The strategy of employing bacterial components as adjuvants which downregulate Th2 responses exploits a well orchestrated, highly evolved defense system which is normally used against intracellular bacteria. BA differs from exogenous administration of recombinant IL-12 in that many more cytokines are induced, and cytokine production occurs in situ. Furthermore, BA induces endogenous IL-10, which can

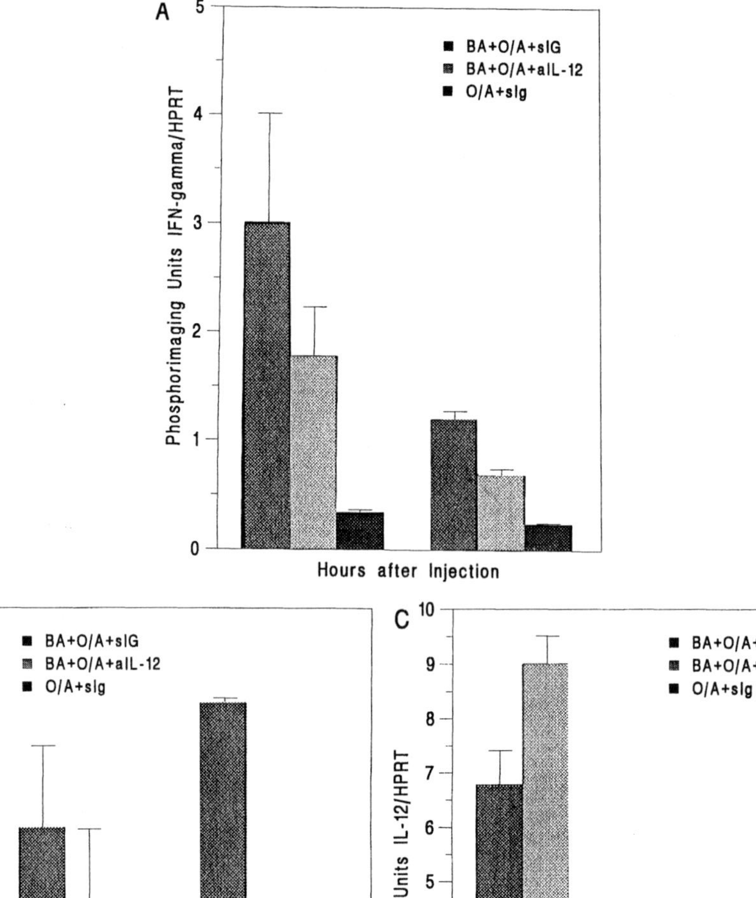

Figure 5. IL-12 is required for optimal IL-10 and IFN-γ gene expression, but does not decrease IL-12 expression. Mice were immunized with BA+O/A+control antibody (sIg), BA+O/A+αIL-12, or O/A+sIg. Splenic cytokine mRNA was assessed 4 and 24 hours post-immunization by RT-PCR in 4 mice/treatment group. Results are expressed as phosphorimaging units (an index of band intensity) of cytokine message divided by phosphorimaging units of the housekeeping gene, HPRT, for that sample. 5A) IFN-γ, 5B) IL-10, 5C) IL-12.

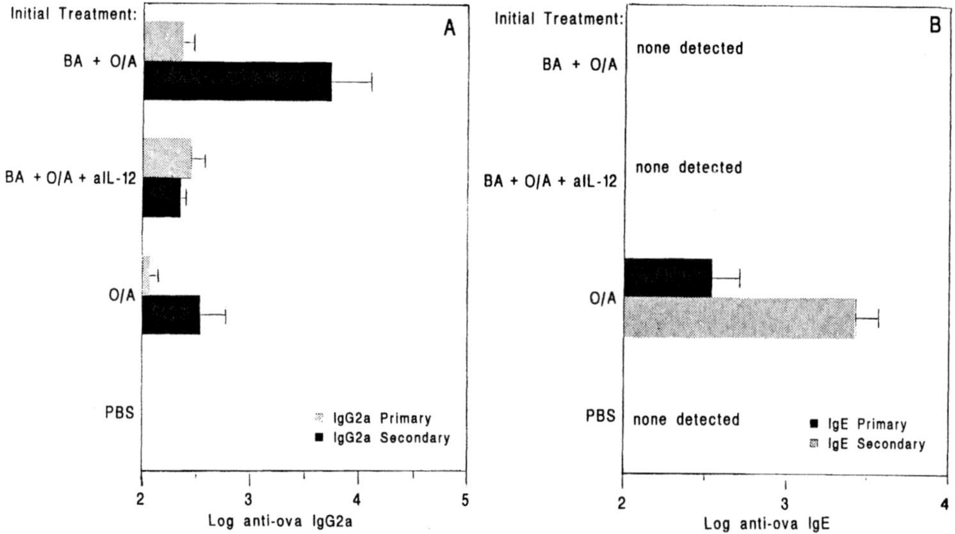

Figure 6. IL-12 is required for optimal Th1-dependent IgG2a secretion, but not IgE suppression. Mice were injected as indicated in the figures (primary immunization). All except PBS-treated mice were challenged 1 month later with O/A alone (secondary immunization). Anti-IL-12 antibody abrogated optimal secondary IgG2a responses (6A), but did not prevent IgE suppression after O/A challenge (6B).

control the level of inflammatory cytokines and thus limits damage to the host (Svetic' et al., 1993; de Waal-Malefyt et al., 1991; Fiorentino et al., 1991). IL-10 has been shown to have important protective effects in models of endotoxic shock (Berg et al., 1995). In support of this idea, we have observed that BA given to IL-10 deficient mice results in lethality at doses which are well-tolerated in normal mice.

Our results appear to contrast with in vitro studies in which murine T cells stimulated

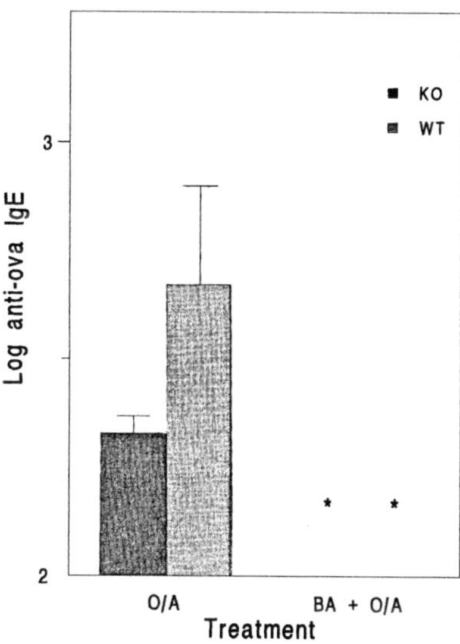

Figure 7. BA suppresses primary IgE responses in WT and IFN-γ KO mice. To rule out the possibility that small amount of BA-induced IFN-γ suppressed IgE responses, WT and KO mice were injected with O/A alone or BA+O/A. KO mice had lower IgE responses than WT mice but BA inhibited IgE in both groups.

with antigen in mixed Th1/Th2-promoting conditions (IL-4 + IL-12) develop into Th2-predominant populations (Hsieh et al., 1993b). However, the relative amounts of IL-4 and IL-12 in vivo may not be reflective of in vitro conditions; also several BA-induced factors may act together to decrease IL-4 in vivo. Other differences between these systems which may influence Th1/Th2 development include the types of APC, their level of function, and costimulatory molecule expression. Altogether, this observation emphasizes that vaccine outcomes in vivo may not be predictable based entirely upon in vitro observations using recombinant cytokines.

Studies using IL-12 or polymerized ovalbumin to promote Th1 responses to proteins have not resulted in longlasting downregulation of IgE in BALB/c mice after allergen challenge (Gieni and Hayglass, 1991; Gieni et al., 1993). In contrast, we have observed that even after two subsequent injections of O/A alone, mice originally receiving BA + O/A are incapable of mounting significant IgE responses. Here we examined the role of BA-induced cytokines in Th1 development and IgE suppression. IL-12, as in many other systems, appears to be necessary for optimal Th1-like responses. However, experiments with anti-IL-12 and IFN-γ KO mice, suggest that long-lasting suppression of Th2-mediated IgE responses does not depend upon either of these factors. Other cytokines which can downregulate IgE include IFN-α, TGF-β, and a recently described ubiquitin-like protein (Finkelman et al., 1990; Nakamura et al., 1996; Meade et al., 1992; Ezernieks et al., 1996; Pene et al., 1988). It is likely that BA injection leads to production of factors which are not induced by either recombinant IL-12 or polymerized ovalbumin, thus explaining the superior ability of BA to suppress IgE.

Heat-killed BA contains constituents such as LPS, other cell wall components, and bacterial DNA, all of which can induce IL-12 and IFN-γ. Purified LPS-BA as well as BA can induce IFN-γ from human T cells, although they are more effective when IL-2 is limiting in culture (Blay et al., 1992). We have recently used PCR methods to confirm that the BA preparations used in these experiments contain bacterial DNA sequences. It may be that optimal Th1-like responses to BA depend upon the presence of several constituents. Current studies are focusing upon the relative contribution of BA components to IL-12 and IL-10 induction. Further understanding of which cells are stimulated, and by which components of BA, could lead to improved design of Th1-promoting vaccines.

In conclusion, we have shown that heat-killed BA used as an adjuvant favors development of Th1-like responses and abrogates deleterious Th2-like responses. The feasibility of this approach has been addressed with toxicity studies. Previous studies in this laboratory with purified LPS-BA have shown that LPS-BA is less toxic than LPS from E. coli.The doses used in the studies herein described were non-toxic in mice. We have recently observed similar lack of toxicity in rhesus macaques receiving BA-peptide conjugates in doses which stimulate anti-peptide IgG responses. Another advantage of using bacterial adjuvants, if toxicity is acceptable, includes low cost, compared with recombinant cytokines. Furthermore, bacterial adjuvants are likely to contain several immune stimulating components which may act together to optimize Th1-like responses (Snapper and Mond, 1996). We have also shown that BA given after IgE responses are established can still act to suppress IgE responses (D. Scott, J. Inman, M. Gober, and B. Golding, 1997). Undesirable Th2-like responses in humans include asthma, anaphylaxis, lepromatous leprosy, and possibly progression of HIV. It is hoped that exploration to determine how BA downregulates Th2-mediated responses will contribute to the development of vaccines which can prevent or treat such conditions.

REFERENCES

Abbas, A.K., Murphy, K.M. and Sher, A. (1996). Functional diversity of helper T lymphocytes. Nature, 383:787.

Aldovini, A. and Young, R.A., 1991. Humoral and cell-mediated responses to live recombinant BCG-HIV vaccines. Nature, 351:479.
Berg, D.J., Kuhn, R., Rajewsky, K., Muller, W., Menon, S., Davidson, N., Grunig, G. and Rennick, D., 1995. Interleukin-10 is a central regulator of the responses to LPS in murine models of endotoxic shock and the Schwartzman reaction but not endotoxin tolerance. J.Clin.Invest., 96:2339.
Blay, R., Hernandez, D., Betts, M., Clerici, M., Lucey, D., Hendrix, C., Hoffman, T. and Golding, B., 1992. Brucella abortus stimulates human T cells from uninfected and infected individuals to secrete IFNg. AIDS Research and Human Retroviruses, 8:479.
Brinkmann, V., Geiger, T., Alkan, S. and Heusser, C.H., 1993. Interferon alpha increases the frequency of interferon-gamma producing human CD4+ T cells. J.Exp.Med., 178:1655.
Brown, K.D., Zurawski, S.M., Mosmann, T.R. and Zurawski, G., 1989. A family of small inducible proteins secreted by leukocytes are members of a new superfamily that includes leukocyte and fibroblast-derived inflammatory agents, growth factors, and indicators of various activation processes. J.Immunol., 142: 679.
Clerici, M. and Shearer, G.M., 1993. A Th1 to Th2 switch is a critical step in the etiology of HIV infection. Immunol.Today, 14:107.
Dalton, D., Pitts-Meek, S., Keshav, S., Figari, I.S., Bradley, A. and Stewart, T.A., 1993. Multiple defects of immune cell function in mice with disrupted interferon-gamma genes. Science, 259:1739.
de Waal-Malefyt, R., Abrams, J., Bennett, B., Figdor, C.G. and de Vries, J., 1991. Interleukin 10 (IL-10) inhibits cytokine synthesis by human monocytes: an autoregulatory role of IL-10 produced by monocytes. J. Exp. Med., 174,:1209.
Ezernieks, J., Schnarr, B., Metz, K. and Duschl, A., 1996. The human IgE germline promoter is regulated by interleukin-4, interleukin-13, interferon-alpha and interferon-gamma via an interferon-gamma activated site and its flanking regions. Eur.J.Biochem., 240:667.
Finkelman, F.D., Katona, I.M., Urban, J.F., Jr., Snapper, C.M., Ohara, J. and Paul, W.E., 1986. Suppression of in vivo polyclonal IgE responses by monoclonal antibody to the lymphokine BSF-1. Proc.Natl.Acad.Sci. USA, 83:9675
Finkelman, F.D., Katona, I.M., Mosmann, T.R. and Coffman, R.L,.1988a. IFN-gamma regulates the isotypes of Ig secreted during in vivo humoral immune responses. Journal of Immunology, 140:1022.
Finkelman, F.D., Katona, I.M., Urban, J.F., Jr., Holmes, J., Ohara, J., Tung, A.S., Sample, J.V. and Paul, W.E., 1988b. IL-4 is required to generate and sustain in vivo IgE responses. Journal of Immunology, 141: 2335.
Finkelman, F.D., Holmes, J., Katona, I.M., Urban, J.F., Jr., Beckman, M.P., Schooley, K.A., Coffman, R.L., Mosmann, T.R. and Paul, W.E., 1990. Lymphokine control of in vivo immunoglobulin isotype selection. Annu.Rev.Immunol., 8:303
Fiorentino, D.F., Zlotnik, A., Mosmann, T.R., Howard, M. and O'Garra, A., 1991. IL-10 inhibits cytokine production by activated macrophages. J.Immunol., 147:3815.
Gause, W.C. and Adamovicz, J., 1994. in: "PCR Methods and Applications" (Cold Spring Harbor, NY: Cold Spring Harbor Laboratory).
Gieni, R.S., Yang, X. and Hayglass, K.T., 1993. Allergen-specific modulation of cytokine synthesis patterns and IgE responses in vivo with chemically modified allergen. Journal of Immunology, 150:302.
Gieni, R.S. and Hayglass, K.T., 1991. Regulation of murine IgE responses: induction of long-lived inhibition of allergen-specific responses is genetically restricted. Cellular Immunology, 138:64.
Golding, B., Golding, H., Preston, S., Hernandez, D., Beining, P.R., Manischewitz, J., Harvath, L., Blackburn, R., Lizzio, E. and Hoffman, T., 1991. Production of a novel antigen by conjugation of HIV-1 to Brucella abortus: studies of immunogenicity, isotype analysis, T-cell dependency, and syncytia inhibition. AIDS Research and Human Retroviruses, 7:435.
Golding, B., Inman, J., Highet, P., Blackburn, R., Manischewitz, J., Blyveis, N., Angus, R.D. and Golding, H., 1995 Brucella abortus conjugated with a gp120 or V3 loop peptide derived from human immunodeficiency virus (HIV) type 1 induces neutralizing anti-HIV antibodies, and the V3-B. abortus conjugate is effective even after CD4+ T-cell depletion. Journal of Virology , 69:3299.
Goldstein, J., Hoffman, T., Frasch, C., Lizzio, E.F., Beining, P.R., Hochstein, D., Lee, Y.L., Angus, R.D. and Golding, B., 1992. Lipopolysaccharide (LPS) from Brucella abortus is less toxic that that from Escherichia coli, suggesting the possible use of B. abortus or LPS from B abortus as a carrier in vaccines. Infection and Immunity, 60:1385.
Grun, J.L. and Maurer, P.H., 1989. Different T helper cell subsets elicited in mice utilizing two different adjuvant vehicles: the role of endogenous interleukin 1 in proliferative responses. Cellular Immunology, 121:134.
Hayglass, K.T. and Stefura, B.P., 1991. Anti-interferon gamma treatment blocks the ability of glutaraldehye-polymerized allergens to inhibit specific IgE responses. J. Exp. Med., 173:279.
Hayglass, K.T. and Strejan, G.H., 1983. Suppression of the IgE antibody response by glutaraldehyde-modified

ovalbumin: dissociation between loss of antigenic reactivitiy and ability to induce suppression. Int.Arch.All.Appl.Immunol., 74:332

Heinzel, F.P., Sadick, M.D., Holaday, B.J., Coffman, R.L. and Locksley, R.M., 1991. Reciprocal expression of interferon gamma or IL4 during the resolution or regression of leishmaniasis. J. Exp. Med., 169:59.

Hsieh, C.-S., Macatonia, S.E., Tripp, C.S., Wolf, S.F., O'Garra, A. and Murphy, K.M., 1993a. Development of Th1 CD4+ T cells through IL-12 produced by listeria-induced macrophages. Science, 260:547.

Hsieh, C.-S., Macatonia, S.E., Tripp, C.S., Wolf, S.F., O'Garra, A. and Murphy, K.M., 1993b. Development of Th1 CD4+ T cells through IL-12 produced by Listeria I-induced macrophages. Science, 260:547

Lapham, C., Golding, B., Inman, J., Blackburn, R., Manishewitz, J., Highet, P. and Golding, H., 1996. Brucella abortus conjugated with a peptide derived from the V3 loop of human immunodeficiency Virus (HIV) Type 1 induces HIV-specific cytotoxic T-cell responses in normal and in CD4+ cell-depleted BALB/c mice. Journal of Virology, 70:3084.

Maggi, E., Parronchi, P., Manetti, R., Simonelli, C., Piccinni, M.-P., Rugiu, F.S., De Carli, M., Ricci, M. and Romagnani, S., 1992. Reciprocal regulatory effects of IFN-gamma and IL-4 on the in vitro develpment of human Th1 and Th2 clones. J. Immunol., 148:2142

Meade, R., Askenase, P.W., Geba, G.P., Neddermann, K., Jacoby, R.O. and Pasternak, R.D., 1992. Transforming growth factor-beta inhibits murine immediate and delayed type hypersensitivity. J. Immunol., 149:521.

Morris, S.C., Madden, K.B., Adamovicz, J.J., Gause, W.C., Hubbard, B.R., Gately, M.K. and Finkelman, F.D. 1994. Effects of IL-12 on in vivo cytokine gene expression and Ig isotype selection. Journal of Immunology, 152:1047.

Mosmann, T.R. and Coffman, R.L., 1989. Th1 and Th2 cells: different patterns of lymphokine secretion lead to different functional properties. Annu.Rev.Immunol., 7:145.

Nakamura, M., Nagata, T., Xavier, R.M. and Tanigawa, Y., 1996. Ubiquitin-like polypeptide inhibits the IgE response of lipopolysaccharide-activated B cells. Int.Immunol., 8:1659.

Parronchi, P., Macchia, D., Piccinni, M.-P., Biswas, P., Simonelli, C., Maggi, E., Ricci, M., Ansari, A.A. and Romagnani, S., 1991. Allergen- and bacterial antigen-specific T-cell clones established from atopic donors show a different profile of cytokine production.. Proc.Natl.Acad.Sci. USA, 88:4538.

Pene, J., Rousset, F., Briere, F., Chretien, I., Bonnefoy, J.Y., Spits, H., Yokota, T., Arai, K., Banchereau, J. and de Vries, J., 1988. IgE production by normal human lymphocytes is induced by interleukin 4 and suppressed by interferons gamma and alpha and prostaglandin E2. Proc.Natl.Acad.Sci.USA, 85:6880.

Powrie, F. and Coffman, R., 1993. IL-4 and IL-10 inhibit DTH and IFN-gamma production. Eur.J.Immunol. 23:2223.

Schmitt, E., Hoehn, P., Huels, C., Goedert, S., Palm, N., Rude, E. and Germann, T., 1994. T helper 1 development of naive CD4+ T cells requires the coordinate action of interleukin-12 and interferon-gamma and is inhibited by transforming growth factor-beta. Eur. J.Immunol., 24:793.

Scott, D.E., Agranovich, I., Inman, J., Gober, M. and Golding, B., 1997. Inhibition of primary and recall allergen-specific T helper cell type 2-mediated responses by a T helper cell type I stimulus. J.Immunol., 159, in press

Secrist, H., Chelen, C.J., Wen, Y., Marshall, J.D. and Umetsu, D.T., 1993. Allergen immunotherapy decreases interleukin 4 production in CD4+ T cells from allergic individuals. J.Exp.Med., 178:2123.

Seder, R.A., Gazinelli, R., Sher, A. and Paul, W.E., 1993. Natural killer cell stimulatory factor (interleukin 12 [IL-12]) induces T helper type 1 (Th1)-specific immune responses and inhibits the development of IL-4-producing cells. Proc.Natl.Acad.Sci.USA, 90:10188.

Snapper, C.M. and Mond, J.J., 1996. A model for induction of T cell-independent humoral immunity in response to polysaccharide antigens. J.Immunol., 157:2229.

Snapper, C.M. and Paul, W.E., 1987. Interferon-gamma and B cell stimulatory factor-1 reciprocally regulate Ig isotype production. Science, 236:944.

Street, N.E., Schumacher, J.H., Fong, T., Bass, H., Fiorentino, D.F., Leverah, J.A. and Mosmann, T.R., 1990. Heterogeneity of mouse helper T cells. Evidence from bulk cultures and limiting dilution cloning for precursors of Th1 and Th2 cells. J.Immunol., 144:1629.

Svetic', A., Finkelman, F.D., Dieffenbach, C.W., Scott, D.E., Steinberg, A.D. and Gause, W.C., 1991. Cytokinegene expression following in vivo primary immunization with goat anti-mouse IgD. Journal of Immunology, 147:2391.

Svetic', A.S., Jian, Y.C., Finkelman, F.D. and Gause, W.C., 1993. Brucella abortus induces a novel cytokine gene expression pattern characterized by elevated IL-10 and IFN-gamma in $CD4^+$ T cells. Int.Immunol,. 5:877.

Swain, S.L., Bradley, L.M., Croft, M., Tonkonogy, S., Atkins, G., Weinberg, A.D., Duncan, D.D., Hedrick, S.M., Dutton, R.W. and Huston, G., 1991. Helper T cell subsets: pheonotype, function, and the role of lymphokines in regulating their development. Immunol.Rev., 123:115

Swain, S.L., 1993. IL-4 dictates T-cell differentiation. Research Immunology,, 144:567.

Taguchi, T., McGhee, J.R., Coffman, R.L., Beagley, K.W., Eldridge, J.H., Takatsu, K. and Kiyono, H., 1990. Detection of individual mouse splenic T cells producing IFN-gamma and IL-5 using the enzyme-linked immunospot (ELISPOT) assay. J.Immunol.Meth., 128:65.

Tanaka, T., Hu-Li, J., Seder, R.A., Fazekas de St.Groth, B. and Paul, W.E., 1993. Interleukin-4 suppresses interleukin-2 and interferon-gamma production by naive T cells stimulated by accessory cell-dependent receptor engagement. Proc.Natl.Acad.Sci.USA, 90:5914

Van de Wijgert, J.H., Verheul, F.M., Snippe, H., Check, I.J. and Hunter, R.I., 1991. Immunogenicity of S. pneumoniae type 14 capsular polysaccharide : influence of carriers and adjuvants on isotype distribution. Infection and Immunity, 59:2750.

Vaz, E.M., Vaz, N.M. and Levine, B.B., 1971. Persistent formation of reagins in mice injected with low doses of ovalbumin. Immunology, 21:11.

Wenner, C.A., Guler, M.L., Macatonia, S.E., O'Garra, A. and Murphy, K.M., 1996. Roles of IFN-gamma and IFN-alpha in IL-12-induced T helper 1 development. J.Immunol., 156:1442.

Yamamura, M., Uyemura, K., Deans, R.J., Weinburg, K., Rea, T.H., Bloom, B.R. and Modlin, R.L., 1991. Defining protective responses to pathogens: cytokine profiles in leprosy lesions. Science, 254:277.

Yang, X. and Hayglass, K.T., 1993. Allergen-dependent induction of interleukin-4 synthesis in vivo. Immunology, 78:74.

Zaitseva, M.B., Golding, H., Betts, M., Yamauchi, A., Bloom, E.T., Butler, L.E., Stevan, L. and Golding, B. 1995. Human peripheral blood CD4+ and CD8+ T cells express Th1-like cytokine mRNA and proteins following in vitro stimulation with heat-inactivated Brucella abortus. Infection and Immunity, 63:2720.

INDUCTION OF IL-12 SECRETION AND ENHANCED SURFACE EXPRESSION OF B7.1/B7.2 AND ICAM-1 IN HUMAN MONOCYTES ACTIVATED BY THE VACCINE CARRIER *BRUCELLA ABORTUS*: CORRELATION WITH IN VIVO GENERATION OF CELLULAR IMMUNE RESPONSES

H. Golding[1], M. B. Zaitseva[1], C. K. Lapham[1] and B. Golding[2]

[1]Laboratory of Retrovirus Research, Division of Viral Products, and [2]Laboratory of Plasma Derivatives, Division of Hematology, Center for Biologics Evaluation and Research, US Food and Drug Administration, 8800 Rockville Pike, Bethesda, MD 20892 USA

INTRODUCTION

It is well established that two cytokines, IFN-γ and IL-4, play an important role in the differentiation of Th0/Tc0 cells into effector types Th1/Tc1 or Th2/Tc2 cells during the initial phase of the immune response (O'Garra and Murphy, 1994). In addition to these lymphokines, it has been demonstrated that another cytokine, IL-12, is a pivotal positive factor in the differentiation of the Th1/Tc1 cell subset (Manetti et al, 1993). IL-12 is a heterodimeric protein consisting of p40 and p35 subunits (Kobayashi et al, 1989; Stern et al, 1990) that binds to its receptor of approximately 110 kDa (Chizzonite et al, 1992). The biologic activities of IL-12 include stimulatory effects on human NK cells and cytotoxic T cells (Bloom and Horvath, 1994; Chouaib et al, 1994; Kobayashi et al, 1989; Wolf et al, 1991), and induction of proliferation of activated, but not resting, $CD4^+$ and $CD8^+$ T cells (Bertagnolli et al, 1992; Gately at al, 1991; Perussia et al, 1992). IL-12 potentiates production of IFN-γ by Th1 and Th0 clones (Manetti et al, 1994), and also by NK and $CD8^+$ cells (Croft et al, 1994; D'Andrea et al, 1992). Studies in the murine system demonstrated an important role for IL-12 in the development of immune protection against infectious agents such as Candida (Romani et al, 1992), Leishmania major (Afonso et al, 1994), Listeria in SCID mice (Tripp et al, 1994) and Schistosomiasis (Wynn et al, 1995). IL-12 was also shown to play an important role in IFN-γ-dependent protection against malaria (Sedegah et al, 1994) and tuberculosis (Zhang et al, 1994) in humans. The ability of IL-12 to induce protective immunity against many infections suggests that this cytokine should be a key component of vaccines designed to elicit strong cell-mediated immunity.

In an attempt to identify a vaccine carrier which is capable of promoting Th1-type cytokines from murine and human T cells, we and others (Finkelman et al, 1988; Golding et al, 1995; Svetic et al, 1993, Zaitseva et al, 1996) have been studying the effects of the gram negative bacterium, Brucella abortus (BA), on immune responses in murine and in human systems. The ability of heat inactivated B. abortus to induce IgG2a subclass of antibody in mice, and the observation that inactivated human immunodeficiency virus type 1 (HIV-1) conjugated to B. abortus induced anti-HIV-1-neutralizing antibodies of mainly the IgG2a subclass suggested that B. abortus can stimulate cells to produce IFN-γ which is necessary for IgG2a switching (Snapper et al, 1988). The latter hypothesis was corroborated by our study which demonstrated that B. abortus and LPS derived from B. abortus can elicit IFN-γ mRNA and protein in human peripheral blood $CD4^+$ and $CD8^+$ cells but not in NK cells (Zaitseva et al, 1995). Since IL-12 is an important regulator in the initiation of Th1-like differentiation, it was of interest to determine if B. abortus or LPS from B. abortus could also induce IL-12 production by human monocytes. In the present study, we tested the effect of B. abortus and its LPS on human elutriated monocytes in vitro. We demonstrated that B. abortus induced IL-12 p40 mRNA and protein secretion by human monocytes. The secreted IL-12 possessed biological activities as was determined by its ability to upregulate IFN-γ mRNA expression in autologous purified T cells and to increase NK-mediated killing activity. In addition, we found that heat-inactivated B. abortus induces upregulation of the costimulatory molecules B7.1/B7.2 and the adhesion molecule ICAM-1 on human monocytes. Thus, the ability of B. abortus to induce IL-12 production and to elevate costimulatory molecules on antigen presenting cells strengthens its potential use as a vaccine carrier when Th1/Tc1 cell activation is desirable (Fig. 1). These predictions were coroborated in a murine model system . An 18 amino acid peptide, based on the V3 loop of HIV-1 MN gp120 that contains both B and CTL (but not Th) epitopes, was chemically conjugated to inactivated BA (BA-MN 18mer). The BA-MN 18mer induced a potent CTL response and long term memory in both normal and $CD4^+$ T cell-depleted BALB/c mice.

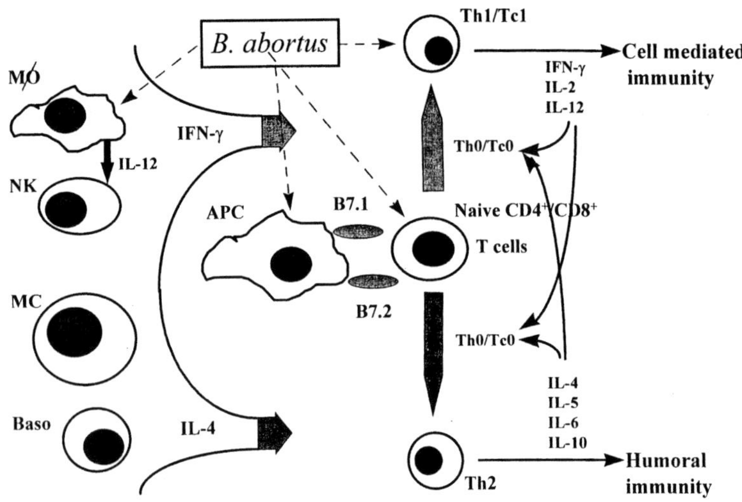

Figure 1. A model of T cell subset differentiation, indicating cell-subpopulations responsive to Brucella abortus.

MATERIALS AND METHODS

Antigens, cytokines, antibodies

Heat-inactivated B. abortus was obtained from the U.S. Department of Agriculture, Ames, Iowa. LPS-BA was purified by butanol extraction as described previously (Goldstein et al, 1992). It contains $\leq$2% protein and $\leq$1% nucleic acids. LPS from E. coli was purchased from List Biological Laboratories, Inc., Campbell, CA. Staphylococcus aureus Cowan I strain (SAC) was obtained from Pansorbin, Calbiochem-Behring Co., La Jolla, CA. Recombinant human IL-12 (rIL-12) was obtained from R & D Systems, Inc., Minneapolis, MN. The following antibodies were used: anti-human IL-12 neutralizing antibody (R & D Systems). FITC-labelled antibodies against CD86 (anti-B7-2), and CD80 (anti-B7-1) were purchased from Pharmingen, San Diego, CA, and monoclonal antibody to CD54 (anti-ICAM) was obtained from AMAC Inc.

Cell purification

Human blood monocytes from normal volunteers were isolated by elutriator as previously described (Lazdins et al, 1990), using a combination of lymphocytopheresis and countercurrent centrifugation elutriation.. The fraction of pure monocytes was collected and contained less than $\leq$1% of T and B cells was collected as verified by flow cytometry. To obtain autologous T cells the fraction of lymphocytes preceding the fraction of pure monocytes was passed through a nylon wool column and subjected to centrifugation on a percoll gradient to remove all B cells and activated T cells. NK cells were purified as previously described (Yamauchi and Bloom 1993) and yielded $\geq$ 90% pure NK cells.

In vitro stimulation of elutriated human monocytes

To induce cytokine production, elutriated monocytes were resuspended at 2×10^6 cells/ml in RPMI 1640 medium supplemented with L-glutamine and 10% fetal bovine serum (FBS, Sigma, St. Louis, MO) and stimulated with: heat-inactivated B. abortus (10^8 organisms/ml), LPS-BA or LPS-E. coli (3 μg/ml, or as indicated), or by Staphylococcus aureus Cowan I strain (SAC, 0.0075% wt/vol). Monocyte cultures were maintained at 37°C in a 5% CO_2 atmosphere. Cells and supernatants were harvested at different time points and assayed for IL-12 p40 mRNA expression, IL-12 protein secretion, and for surface B7.1/B7.2 and ICAM-1 expression. The cell-free culture supernatant fluid from monocytes stimulated with B. abortus (Mo-BA) for 12 hours was collected and concentrated 2.5 - 3 fold using Centricon 30 (Amicon, Inc., Beverly, MA).

Cell culture in transwell plate

Elutriated human monocytes (2×10^6) were placed in the upper chamber of a transwell in a 24-well plate (Corning Costar Corp., Cambridge, MA), and stimulated with (or without) heat-inactivated B. abortus (10^8 organisms) in 1 ml of complete medium. Autologous T cells (2×10^6) were cultured in the lower chamber of the transwells overnight. A 0.1 μm pore size filter separated the upper chamber from the lower chamber and prevented transfer of the killed bacteria to the lower chamber. T cells from the lower chambers were harvested and analyzed for IFN-γ, IL-4 and IL-5 mRNA expression by polymerase chain reaction (PCR) as described before (Zaitseva et al, 1995).

Quantitation of IL-12 p40 in monocyte supernatant

IL-12 p40 secreted by stimulated monocytes was quantified by a double sandwich ELISA using rat anti-human p40 IL-12 Mab, 2-4A1, and peroxidase-conjugated anti-human p40 IL-12 mAb, 4D6 (Hoffmann-La Roche Inc., Nutley, NJ) according to the manufactures's protocol. Recombinant human IL-12 (Hoffmann-La Roche) was used to generate a standard curve ranging from 12.5 pg/ml to 800 pg/ml.

Flow cytometric analysis

Elutriated human monocytes were stimulated by heat-inactivated B. abortus, LPS-BA or LPS-E. coli, washed and stained with FITC-conjugated antibodies to CD86 (anti-B7.2), CD80 (anti-B7.1), and CD54 (anti-ICAM-1) for 1 hour at 4^0C. Flow cytometry was performed on a FACScan (Becton Dickinson & Co.) using Lysis II software.

NK cytotoxic assay

To test the ability of supernatant from B. abortus-stimulated monocytes to enhance NK-cell mediated cytotoxicity, $2x10^6$ NK cells were incubated in 1 ml of media or in the same volume of concentrated supernatant fluid from 18 hour cultures of untreated monocytes, or monocytes stimulated with B. abortus. NK cells were then washed, and tested for their ability to kill ^{51}Cr-labelled K562 target cells (10^4/well) at different effector to target ratios in a total volume of 200 μl as described (Rook et al, 1985).

Synthetic peptides used in the study

Table 1 contains the sequences of the peptides synthesized for the study. The top line depicts the V3 (MN) sequence of the 18mer peptide containing the minimal D^d - restricted CTL epitope The 18mer peptide synthesized, was made up of the 10 amino acid minimal CTL determinant (Shirai et al, 1994) flanked by "linker" residues on both sides that contained 3 other residues from the MN gp120 V3 sequence. Changes were made in the other amino acids to improve solubility, to facilitate synthesis of the peptide, and to allow linkage of the peptide to Brucella abortus. A control 9 amino acid peptide containing the H-2K^d-restricted minimal CTL determinant of influenza nucleoprotein (NP) was synthesized as a specificity control (Table 1 line 2).

In vivo priming of BALB/c mice

Six to eight-week-old BALB/c female mice received two to three intraperitoneal immunizations two weeks apart with 10^7-10^9 Brucella abortus organisms in 100 μl of PBS.

Table 1. Peptide Sequences Used in the Study[a]

MN 18mer	**C-G-R-A-A-I-G-P-G-R-A-F-Y-T-T-K-N-G**
NP peptide	**T-Y-Q-R-T-R-A-L-V**

[a]The MN peptide binds to H-2D^d and the NP peptide binds to H-2K^d. The double underlines indicate anchor residues.

Mice received either unconjugated BA, BA covalently conjugated to MN 18mer peptide (27.6 μg per 10^8 organisms), or BA mixed with 27.6 μg MN 18mer peptide. A separate positive control group was injected with live recombinant vaccinia (10^7 pfu/mouse) expressing the entire MN gp160 envelope (MN Vac, a generous gift from Bernard Moss and Pat Earl, NIAID, NIH). Mice were also immunized with a recombinant vaccinia virus encoding influenza nucleoprotein (NP Vac, generously provided by Jack Bennink and Jonathan Yewdell, NIAID, NIH) to verify that CTL responses generated by MN Vac were directed against the MN protein and not the vaccinia virus itself.

In vitro CTL expansion cultures and cytotoxicity assays

At least 2 weeks after the second immunization, splenocyte suspensions were prepared from mice, and approximately 6 x 10^7 cells were co-cultured with 3 x 10^7 autologous, MN 18mer-pulsed splenocytes for 6 days at 37°C. The cells were grown in Iscove's modified Dulbecco's modified Eagle's medium (IMDM) supplemented with 10% fetal bovine serum, 10% rat Con A supernatant (Rat T stim, Collaborative Research), and 10 μg/ml of gentamycin. At the end of cultures, cells were pelleted and suspended in IMDM supplemented with 10% fetal bovine serum. P815 (H-2D^d) targets were prepared in one of several ways. To infect targets with vaccinia recombinants encoding the gp160 from the MN strain of HIV-1 or influenza nucleoprotein, P815 cells were washed twice with 0.1% BSA in Hanks' balanced salt solution, suspended at a concentration of 10^7 cells /ml, and added to an equal volume of vaccinia virus suspended at a concentration of 1 x 10^8 PFUs/ml. After one hour, 5 volumes RPMI containing 10% fetal bovine serum were added, and the cells were incubated for four more hours. To sensitize with or without peptide, P815 cells were suspended in 0.4 ml of medium containing 0.2 M MN-18mer or 0.4 ml medium alone for 1-2 hr. Peptide-pulsed or vaccinia-infected cells were pelleted and suspended in 100-200 μCi of $Na^{51}CrO_4$ in PBS and incubated for 1 hour at 37°C. Cells were pelleted, washed and suspended at a concentration of 1 x 10^5 cells/ml in IMDM supplemented with 10% fetal bovine serum. Targets were added in 100 μl to the wells of round-bottom, 96-well polystyrene microtiter plates containing CTL effectors in 100 μl IMDM at 4 different E/T ratios. Targets were also added to 100 μl of medium alone for determination of spontaneous release or 100 μl of 15% w/v BRIJ 35 solution for the determination of maximum release. Following a 4-hour incubation, supernatants were

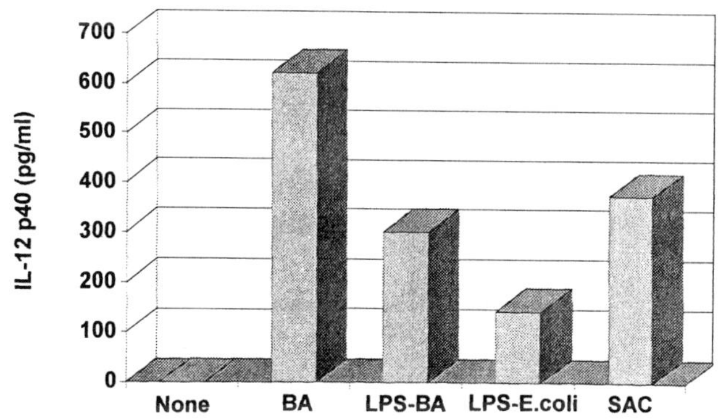

Figure 2. Secretion of IL-12 p40 protein by human elutriated monocytes in response to different stimuli. Monocytes were cultured in medium alone or were stimulated with B. abortus (10^8 organisms/ml), LPS-BA or LPS-E. coli (3 μg/ml), or by SAC (0.0075% wt/vol) for 24 hours. Cell-free supernatants were collected and the amount of free IL-12 p40 chain secreted (pg/ml) was determined by ELISA.

harvested using the Skatron system, and the amount of ^{51}Cr released was determined by gamma counting. The % specific release was defined as [experimental CPM-spontaneous CPM]/[total CPM-spontaneous CPM] x 100.

Anti-L3T4 treatment

Rat anti-mouse L3T4 (CD4) monoclonal antibody (GK1.5) was partially purified from ascites by ammonium sulfate precipitation and dialysed against PBS, as previously described (Golding et al, 1991; Golding et al, 1995)). The batch used in this study killed >70% mouse thymocytes at a 10^{-4} dilution in the presence of rabbit complement (Low-Tox-M, Cedarlane, Ontario, Canada), and contained 2.2 mg/ml rat IgG2b by radial immunodiffusion assay (ICN, Costa Mesa, CA). In order to deplete mice of $CD4^+$ cells they were injected with 0.5 ml of GK1.5 (rat anti-mouse CD4) i.p. daily for three sequential days prior to the first immunization, and then once a week for the remainder of the experiment. Flow cytometry showed that these mice had <1% $CD4^+$ splenic cells. A parallel group of mice, similarly treated, were shown to be incapable of generating T cell help for TNP-KLH or HIV-1 peptide-KLH antibody responses (Golding et al, 1995), confirming the absence of $CD4^+$ T helper function in the anti-L3T4 treated mice.

RESULTS

IL-12 p40 induction in human monocytes stimulated with different doses of LPS from *B. abortus*, LPS from E. coli, and B. abortus

The ability of both B. abortus and LPS from B. abortus to stimulate IL-12 p40 mRNA transcription in human monocytes was measured by RT-PCR (data not shown) and protein ELISA. The supernatant fluids of monocytes incubated with various stimuli for 12 hours were analyzed for the presence of IL-12 p40 chain by double-sandwich ELISA (Fig. 2). Monocytes stimulated with B. abortus produced 600 pg/ml of the free IL-12 p40 chain, whereas LPS from B. abortus, LPS from E. coli and SAC also induced p40 secretion at a lower level (300 pg/ml, 130 pg/ml and 370 pg/ml respectively). Similar results were seen in three separate experiments. There was no detectable p40 chain in the supernatant fluid of untreated monocytes.

BA-treated monocytes secrete a biologically active IL-12 as assayed by its ability to induce IFN-γ mRNA expression in resting T cells

The data, shown above, that B. abortus could induce IL-12 p40 protein secretion suggested, but did not prove, that functional IL-12 heterodimers were secreted. In order to determine if B. abortus can stimulate monocytes to produce biologically active IL-12, we took advantage of a transwell system where two different cell populations are separated by a membrane which do not allow particles with sizes larger than 0.1 μm to pass. In a control experiment, anti-IL-12 antibody abrogated IFN-γ mRNA expression in T cells stimulated directly by 1.0 or 0.01 ng/ml of recombinant IL-12 (Fig. 3A, lane 1,2 and 3,4 respectively). As shown in Fig. 3B, monocytes stimulated with B. abortus in the upper chamber of a transwell induced an increase in the IFN-γ mRNA expression and a decrease in IL-4 mRNA expression in T cells located in the bottom chamber (compare lanes 5 and 6). Anti-IL-12 antibody abrogated and reversed the effects of B. abortus, resulting in a decrease in IFN-γ mRNA and an increase in IL-4 mRNA expression by the T cells (lane 7). These results indicate that B. abortus induced secretion of biologically active IL-12 from human monocytes. In a separate set of experiments it was found that B. abortus-mediated release of IL-12 from human monocytes

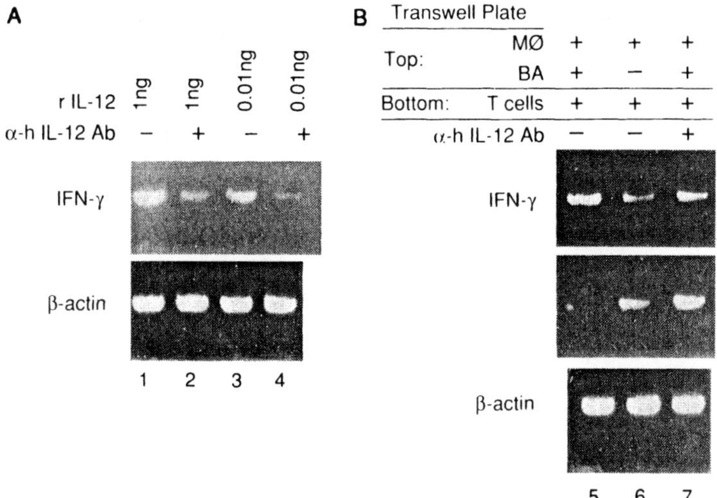

Figure 3. Anti-IL-12 antibody inhibits induction of IFN-γ mRNA expression in T cells by a soluble factor generated from B. abortus-treated monocytes separated by a transwell membrane. (A) Purified human T cells were incubated with the indicated doses of rIL-12 (lanes 1-4 and in the presence (lanes 2,4) or absence (lanes 1,3) of anti-IL-12 antibody (10 μg/ml) in 1 ml of medium. IFN-γ and β-actin RT-PCR were performed using total RNA extracted from T cells. (B) T cells were incubated in the bottom chambers of the transwell plate and autologous monocytes stimulated by B. abortus (10^8 organisms/ml) (lanes 1,3), or unstimulated (lane 2), were placed in the top chamber of each transwell. Cell cultures were maintained in medium alone (lanes 1,2) or with anti-IL-12 antibody (10 μg/ml, lane 3). Total RNA was extracted from T cells after 18 hours, and RT-PCR was performed using primer pairs specific for IFN-γ, IL-4, and β-actin.

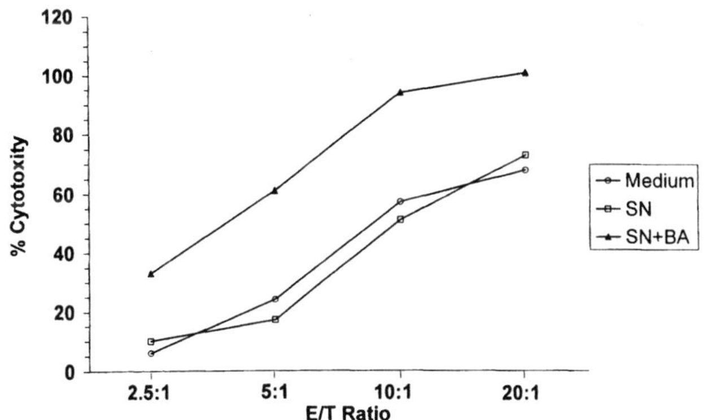

Figure 4. Enhancement of NK-mediated killing of K562 targets by IL-12 containing supernatant from B. abortus-stimulated monocytes. Purified human NK cells were cultured in medium alone (circles) or in the presence of concentrated supernatants from untreated monocytes (quadrants) or monocytes stimulated with B. abortus (triangles) for 24 hours. NK cells were then washed and tested in a 4-h cytotoxic assay against ^{51}Cr-labelled K562 target cells at the indicated E:T ratio.

could act in concert with signaling via TcR to favor expression of IFN-γ and to downregulate IL-5 mRNA in T cells. As a consequence, a Th1-like rather than Th2-like response would be induced (Zaitseva et al. 1996).

Supernatants from BA-stimulated monocytes enhance NK-mediated cytotoxicity

Previous studies demonstrated that recombinant IL-12 has a very strong potentiating effect on the lytic activity of NK cells (Bloom and Horvath, 1994). It was therefore possible to test the supernatants from BA-activated monocytes for the presence of IL-12, using NK killing activity as a biological assay. As shown in Fig. 4 , 2.5-fold concentrated supernatant fluid from monocytes stimulated with B. abortus enhanced NK-mediated cytotoxicity against ^{51}Cr-labled K562 target cells in comparison with similarly concentrated supernatant fluid from unstimulated monocytes or media. This provides additional evidence that B. abortus stimulated human monocytes to release functional IL-12. Similar results were obtained by D'Andrea et al. (1992) using supernatant from SAC-activated human mononuclear cells to enhance the cytotoxic activity of NK cells in vitro.

Expression of costimulatory and adhesion molecules on monocytes stimulated with B. abortus

In addition to the induction of IL-12 release from monocytes, it seemed possible that B. abortus influences expression of monocyte surface molecules involved in interaction with T cells. To study the effect of B. abortus on the expression of costimulatory molecules, we assessed the expression of B7.1/B7.2 by monocytes stimulated with B. abortus, LPS from B. abortus, and LPS from E. coli at different time points (Fig. 5). B7.1 was not detected on monocytes cultured in medium alone for 12 or 36 hours. At the same time points, they did express low levels of B7.2. After stimulation with B. abortus for 12 or 36 hours the

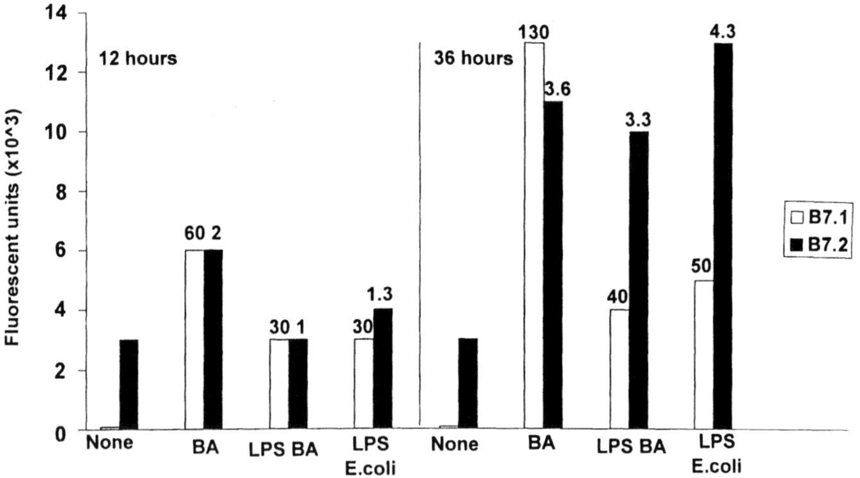

Figure 5. Effect of B. abortus on the expression of B7.1 and B7.2 by human monocytes. Monocytes were cultured in medium alone or stimulated with B. abortus, LPS-BA or LPS-E. coli for 12 or 36 hours, washed, and stained with FITC-conjugated anti-B7.1 (hatched bars) or anti-B7.2 (open bars) mAb, followed by flow cytometry. The numbers above the bars represent the fluorescence fold increase of B7.1/B7.2 expression compared to control monocytes cultured in medium alone.

expression of B7.2 was increased by approximately 2 to 4-fold respectively, whereas the expression of B7.1 was enhanced 60-fold at 12 hours and 130-fold at 36 hours, and was present at similar or higher levels compared with B7.2 at the later time points (Fig. 5). LPS from B. abortus and LPS from E. coli, both induced an increase in B7.1 expression after 12 and 36 hours of culture. An increase in B7.2 molecule expression mediated by LPS-BA and LPS-E. coli was only observed after 36 hours of culture.

In addition to its effect on costimulatory molecules, B. abortus was tested for its ability to stimulate ICAM-1 expression on human monocytes. ICAM-1 is one of the adhesion molecules expressed on monocytes that bind to LFA-1 on T cells, and facilitate monocyte/T cell interactions. Flow cytometric analysis was performed on monocytes stimulated with B. abortus, LPS from B. abortus, and LPS from E. coli and stained with anti-ICAM-1 antibodies. As demonstrated in Fig.6, all these stimuli induced 10, 15 and 18-fold increases in the expression of ICAM-1 molecule by monocytes after 12 and 36 hours. Other surface molecules, such as HLA class II, were not increased following these stimuli (data not shown). The observed increases in ICAM-1 and B7.1/B7.2 expression on B. abortus-treated monocytes are likely to augment the efficiency with which antigen presenting cells can activate naive CD4 and CD8 cells. It may be of particular importance in the activation of $CD8^+$ precursor cytotoxic cells.

CTL induction by BA-MN 18mer conjugate

As Brucella abortus (BA) was shown to stimulate IL-12 production and a Th1 cytokine response from human and murine T cell, we determined whether conjugation of an HIV peptide to BA would induce MHC class I-restricted CTL activity. Mice were immunized with BA alone or with BA conjugated to an 18 amino acid peptide (Table 1) that contained the

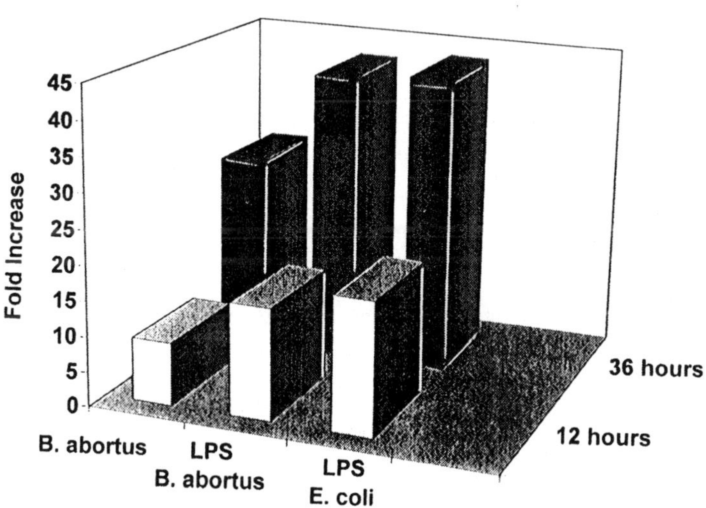

Figure 6. Upregulation of ICAM-1 expression on human monocytes treated with B. abortus, LPS-BA or LPS-E. coli. Monocytes were simulated with B. abortus (10^8 organisms/ml), LPS-BA (3 μg/ml) or LPS-E. coli (3 μg/ml) for 12 (hatched bars) or 36 (open bars) hours, washed and stained with FITC-conjugated anti-ICAM-1 antibody followed by flow cytometry. Data are presented as the fold increase of mean fluorescence units compared to control monocytes cultured in medium alone.

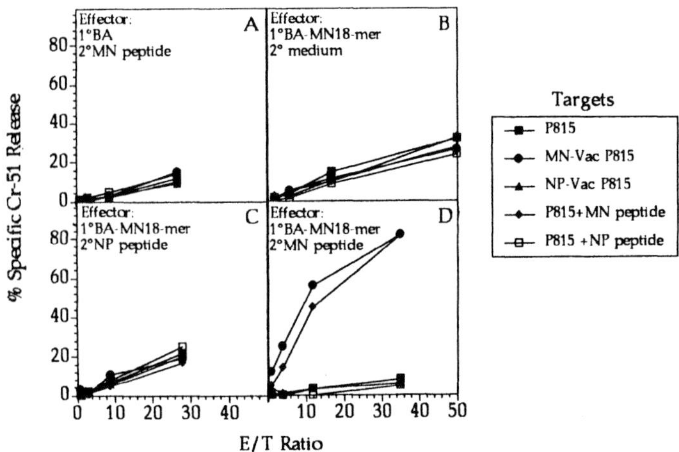

Figure 7. BA-conjugated MN 18mer induces a specific CTL response. Mice were immunized with BA (panels A), or BA-MN 18mer (panels B, C,D). Spleen cell suspensions were stimulated in vitro with medium (panel B), autologous cells + MN 18mer peptide (panels A, D), or NP peptide (panel C). These cells were used as effectors in a ^{51}Cr release assay against: P815 cells , P815 cells infected with MN-Vac, P815 cells infected with NP-Vac, P815 cells pulsed with MN 18mer (F), and P815 cells pulsed with NP peptide as indicated.

minimal H-2D^d-binding peptide from the HIV-1 (MN) V3 region of gp120 (BA-MN 18mer). Mice were immunized twice with 10^9 organisms. Since vaccinia virus has been shown to be a potent inducer of class I-restricted CTL responses (Bennink et al, 1984), a group of mice were immunized with a vaccinia recombinant expressing the entire gp160 envelope of HIV-1 MN as a positive control group. Single cell suspensions were prepared from spleens of primed mice and were cultured in vitro in either medium alone, or in the presence of autologous cells pulsed with the MN 18mer or with an irrelevant peptide derived from the influenza NP that has been shown to bind to H-2K^d (Table 1). The effectors generated in these cultures were tested for their ability to kill P815 targets that were either pulsed with the MN-18mer or NP peptides, infected with recombinant vaccinia expressing HIV-1 (MN) envelope or influenza NP, or incubated in medium alone. As can be seen in Fig. 7, mice immunized with BA alone, generated no CTL effectors, regardless of the in vitro stimulus. Spleen cells from mice primed with BA-MN18-mer, but cultured in vitro with medium alone or autologous cells pulsed with NP 18-mer peptide also exhibited no MN-specific cytotoxic activity. In contrast, spleen cells from mice primed with BA-MN18-mer, followed by in vitro restimulation with autologous cells pulsed with the MN18-mer, generated significant cytotoxic activity against P815 targets pulsed with the homologous, but not with irrelevant NP-derived, peptide. Importantly, the cytotoxic cells generated by in vivo priming with BA-MN18-mer followed by in vitro expansion with MN 18-mer peptide could also kill P815 cells infected with recombinant vaccinia that expressed MN envelope (but not control target cells infected with recombinant vaccinia that encodes influenza NP protein). Thus, they could recognize epitopes within the MN gp160 envelope protein which is endogenously expressed and processed. This is more similar to the processing and presentation of envelope protein in HIV-1 infected cells than the addition of exogenous peptide. In a separate experiment we determined that conjugation of the peptide to inactivated BA was absolutely required for in vivo generation of HIV-1-specific CTL (Lapham et al. 1996).

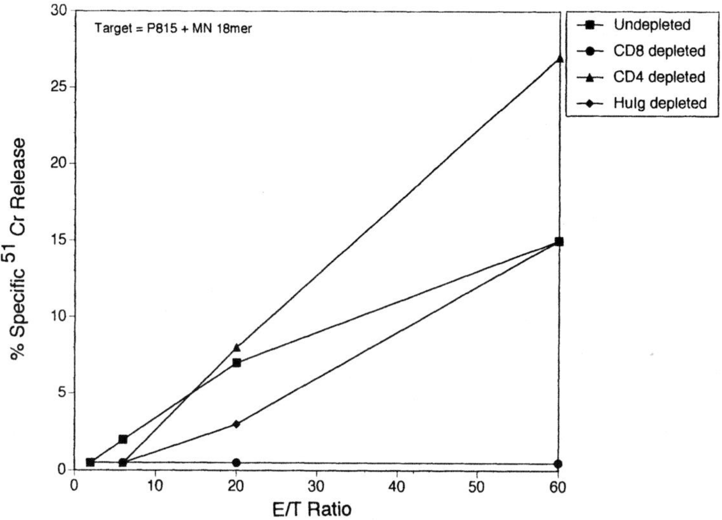

Figure 8. The CTL effectors induced by BA-MN 18mer are CD8$^+$. Mice were immunized with BA-MN 18mer and splenocytes were stimulated in vitro with autologous splenocytes pulsed with MN 18mer. Effector cells were depleted of CD4$^+$ or CD8$^+$ cells using a magnetic bead separation procedure. Unseparated or purified subsets were added to MN18mer-pulsed P815 targets at the indicated E/T ratios.

To determine the phenotype of the CTL effectors, CD4$^+$ or CD8$^+$ cells were negatively selected from the effector cell population at the end of culture prior to addition to the ^{51}Cr-labelled targets. Depletion of the appropriate populations ($\geq$ 90%) was verified using flow cytometric analysis (data not shown). In addition, nonspecific antibody against human immunoglobulin was used as a negative control to determine that the negative selection using magnetic beads did not have an adverse effect on the CTL assay. As seen in Fig. 8, depletion of CD8$^+$ cells completely removed the cytotoxic activity, while depletion of CD4$^+$ cells resulted in enhanced killing of the peptide pulsed targets. This enhancement may reflect the increased frequency of CD8$^+$ effectors. In separate experiments we confirmed that the cytotoxic activity measured was restricted to H-2D^d (Lapham et al. 1996). Together, these results suggest that all of the effectors generated in the cultures were CD8$^+$ cells and were restricted by MHC class I.

Generation of CTL in neonatal mice

As a potential prophylactic or therapeutic vaccine for individuals with HIV-1 infection, it was important to determine whether immunization of neonates is possible with this vaccine candidate. Newborn mice were immunized 1-3 days after birth, and were boosted once at 2 weeks. Their CTL response was evaluated 4 weeks later, and compared to CTL responses of adult mice similarly primed with BA-MN18-mer. A modest but significant CTL response was generated in the neonates compared to the adult mice (Fig. 9). It may reflect the immaturity of neonatal T cells in terms of cytokine production as previously described (Ehlers and Smith, 1991; Lewis et al, 1991).

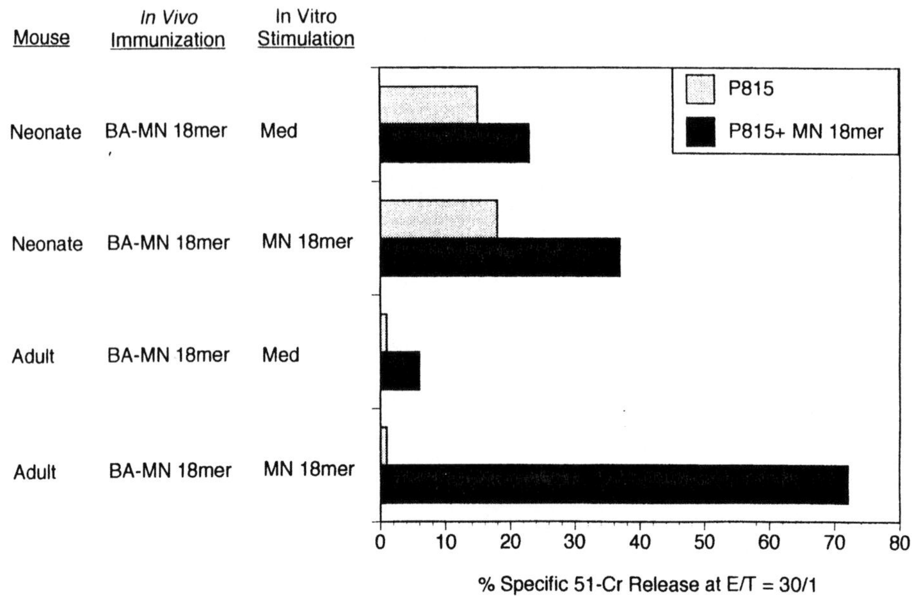

Figure 9. BA-conjugated peptides induce CTL activity in neonates. Neonates were immunized two days and two weeks after birth with BA-MN 18mer. Adults were immunized as previously described. Splenocytes were stimulated in vitro with MN 18mer peptide. Target cells: P815 cells and P815 cells pulsed with MN 18mer.

Effect of anti-L3T4 treatment on the induction of an anti-MN V3 CTL response

All the previous experiments were conducted in immunologically intact BALB/c mice. However, the potential target population for therapeutic HIV-1 vaccine is HIV-1-infected individuals with various degrees of $CD4^+$ T-helper cell dysfunction and/or depletion. The ability of a vaccine to reactivate virus-specific memory CTLs may be hampered by the lack of T cell help. However, in previous studies with a similar BA-peptide conjugate, we showed that it was possible to generate either primary or secondary antibody responses in mice depleted of CD4+ cells by chronic anti-L3T4 antibody treatment (Golding et al, 1995). Antibody titers were partially reduced in CD4-depleted mice, but the neutralization titers were only modestly reduced. It was important to determine if cytotoxic responses, which can also be dependent on helper cells, could also be induced in CD4-depleted mice by BA-MN18-mer. Mice were treated with GK1.5 (rat anti-L3T4 mAb) or with PBS on days -2, -1, and 0, and then once a week thereafter. Flow cytometry demonstrated that the anti-L3T4 treated mice were depleted of splenic $CD4^+$ T cells. As can be seen in Fig. 10, BA conjugated to MN 18mer induced very similar CTL responses in untreated mice (panel A) and in mice treated with anti-L3T4 antibodies (panel B). These data suggest that the BA-MN18-mer is capable of eliciting sufficient help from non-CD4+ cells to support priming of peptide-specific CTL. These findings support the use of Brucella abortus as a vaccine carrier for target populations with known CD4 T-helper cell immune.

DISCUSSION

A rational vaccine design must take into consideration the type of immune response likely to provide the best protective immunity against the pathogen, as well as the immunological

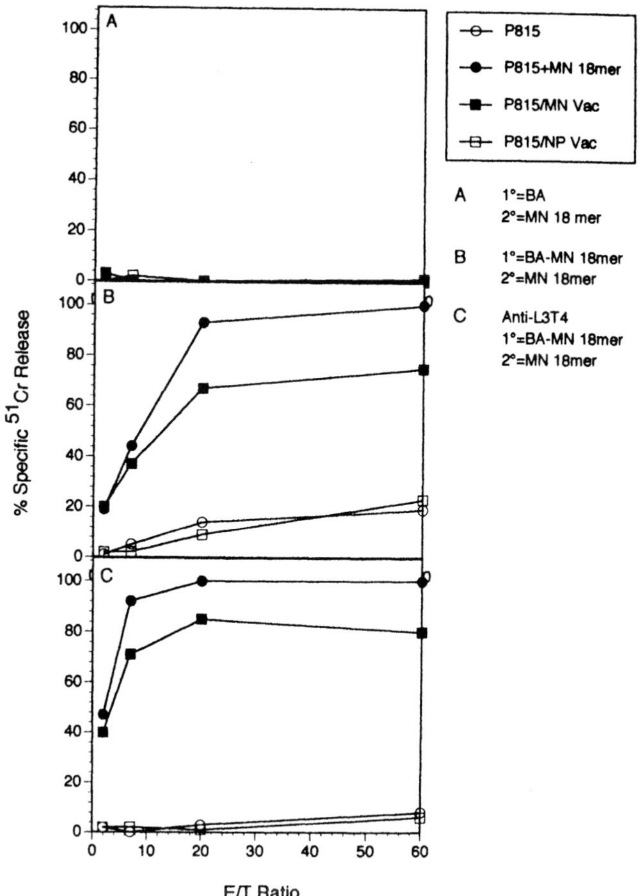

Figure 10. Anti-L3T4 treatment has little effect on the induction of a CTL response by BA-MN18mer. Control mice (Panel A) were immunized with BA. Normal BALB/c mice (panel B) or mice treated with anti-L3T4 (panel C) were immunized with BA-MN 18mer. After in vitro stimulation with MN 18mer-pulsed autologous splenocytes, these were tested in a ^{51}Cr-release assay against: P815 cells, P815 cells pulsed with MN 18mer, P815/MN-Vac, or P815/NP-Vac, as indicated

status of the target population. In the case of HIV-1 infection, it seems that strong cellular responses may be required to reduce the initial viral load (Koup et al, 1994), while both cellular and humoral responses act in concert to keep the chronic virus infection at bay. Since the virus infects and kills the pool of CD4$^+$ T helper cells, both arms of the immune response may eventually be effected. In addition, the funtion of macrophages as antigen presenting cells and as a source of cytokines required for TH1/TC1 differentiation may be reduced in HIV-1 infected individuals. In particular, infected individuals were found to have reduced IL-12 serum levels. Thus, a vaccine carrier/adjuvant that is capable of boosting APC function and elicit T cell help from non CD4$^+$ cells, may be particularly suitable for vaccination of high risk population for HIV-1 infection, as well as for other target populations with known immunodeficiencies.

Our studies focused on one such vaccine carrier candidate, heat-inactivated B. abortus. It was found that B. Abortus as well as LPS from B. abortus can activate human elutriated monocytes to secrete biologically active IL-12. IL-12 induction was followed at the transcriptional (mRNA) and translational (protein) levels using PCR primers and ELISA reagents specific for the p40 chain respectively. B. abortus induced p40 mRNA expression in elutriated monocytes within 4 hours and p40 protein was detected after 24 hours. To address the biological activity of the IL-12 p40/p35 heterodimer, we developed a bioassay which measured IFN-γ mRNA expression in pure T cells separated from the elutriated monocytes by a membrane with 0.1 μm pores. Using this approach it was demonstrated that monocytes stimulated with B. abortus induced IFN-γ mRNA expression in autologus T cells after 16 h. Futhermore, the induction of IFN-γ mRNA in the transwell system was blocked by an anti-IL-12 mAb. It is interesting to note, that in the same transwell cultures of T cells, the presence of IL-12 mAb resulted in a concomitant decrease in IFN-γ mRNA expression and an increase of IL-4 mRNA expression. These results are in agreement with the hypothesis that the target of IL-12 is the bipotential Th0 cell subset and IL-12 promotes the differentiation and selection of non-IL-4-producing cells (Manetti et al, 1994). In another system we demonstrated the ability of supernatant from B. abortus-activated monocytes to increase NK-mediated cytolysis.

Among the different accessory molecules expressed on antigen-presenting cells (APC), B7.1 and B7.2 molecules and ICAM-1 were found to play major roles in T cell activation by interacting with their counter-receptors CD28/CTLA4 and leukocyte function-associated antigen-1 (LFA-1) respectively (Gimmi et al, 1991; Linsley et al, 1991; Van Seventer et al, 1990). ICAM-1, which is constitutively expressed on all APC, is most efficient in costimulation of resting T cells (Damle et al, 1992). The importance of B7 in costimulation of $CD8^+$ cytotoxic T cells was also recently demonstrated (Guerder et al, 1995). In our study, it was found that heat-inactivated bacterium B. abortus rapidly induced B7.1 expression on resting human monocytes resulting in similar B7.1/B7.2 levels within 12 hours. At 36 hours, the ratios of B7.1 to B7.2 expression ranged between 1.5-3 in different experiments. Thus the effect of B. abortus on monocytes may be to facilitate costimulation of Th0/Tc0 cells via B7.1/B7.2 and together with IL-12 provide them with signals required to direct them to the Th1/Tc1 pathway. Productive T cell activation also requires interaction of LFA-1 and ICAM-1 molecules. In our study, we found that treatment of monocytes with B. abortus induced high levels of ICAM-1 expression. Thus, B. abortus may augment interactions of antigen-presenting cells with T cells via direct induction of ICAM-1 and B7.1/B7.2 on the APC, and indirectly, through IL-12 induced LFA-1 on T cells. The significance of cooperation between two independent signals one delivered through the B7/CD28 interaction and another through IL-12 for the maximal induction of proliferation and IFN-γ production by terminally differentiated Th1 clones was recently established (Murphy et al, 1994). Thus, the ability of B. abortus to upregulate costimulatory and adhesion molecules on APC, to induce IL-12 production by macrophages, and IFN-γ/IL-2 by $CD4^+$ and $CD8^+$ T cells (Zaitseva et al. 1995), clearly provide optimal conditions for the activation and propagation of antigen specific Th1/Tc1 type $CD4^+$ and $CD8^+$ cells as well as cytotoxic effector cells.

Together, these data support the potential use of B. abortus as a vaccine carrier or adjuvant when generation of a strong cellular response is favored. This idea was put to the test, using B. abortus chemically conjugated to a synthetic peptide derived from the V3 loop of HIV-1 (MN strain). Importantly, the cytokine pattern elicited by heat-inactivated B. abortus is maintained after its conjugation to a peptide or a protein (Scott et al., 1997) and is expected to facilitate the development of Th1/Tc1 antigen-specific cellular responses.

An 18 amino acid peptide from the V3 region of gp120 containing a B-cell and a CTL epitope (but no T-helper epitope) was conjugated to inactivated BA. This immunogen induced a strong CTL response in BALB/c mice. Targets pulsed with irrelevant peptide were not lysed. The cytotoxic T cells generated were therefore antigen specific. More importantly, they lysed targets that were either pulsed with the priming peptide or with cells that were infected with a recombinant vaccinia that expressed the intact HIV-1 (MN) envelope. The lysis of MN Vac-infected targets suggests that the effector CTLs that were induced by the peptide-BA priming will recognize the naturally processed endogenous envelope protein generated during in vivo HIV infection. Cell depletion experiments showed the CTL effectors to be $CD8^+$ and not $CD4^+$ lymphocytes. In addition, the use of vaccinia recombinants that express different murine class I antigens allowed us to determine that the cytolytic activity was restricted by $H\text{-}2D^d$. These results indicate that conjugation of a peptide to BA can induce an antigen-specific, MHC class I restricted CTL response. However, these experiments do not rule out the possibility that, if the appropriate MHC class II binding peptide were conjugated to BA, $CD4^+$ CTLs could also be induced. The mice were also tested for humoral responses. As in our previously published study, high IgG titers were generated with a predominant IgG2a component (Golding et al. 1994, Lapham et al. 1996). Our experiments identified an antigen dose (10^8 organisms) that is within the optimal ranges of both CTL and antibody responses.

For antigens to be processed and presented to T lymphocytes in the context of MHC class I, proteins usually must be produced intracellularly (as in the case of viruses) or introduced into the cytosol where peptides are thought to be produced. However, a few recent studies have shown that macrophages will process external particulate antigens (bacterial antigens, viruses, or proteins bound to silica beads) for presentation by pre-existing MHC class I molecules (Harding and Song, 1994; Ikonomidis et al, 1994; Kovacsovics-Bankowski et al, 1993; Pfeifer et al, 1993). Thus, for the induction of a $CD8^+$, MHC class I - restricted CTL response, conjugation of proteins to a particulate vaccine carrier such as BA may obviate the need for endogenous expression of the antigen.

Importantly, we demonstrated that the induction of $CD8^+$ MHC class I - restricted cytotoxic cells can take place not only in animals with an intact immune system, but also in animals with an immature immune system (neonates), and in animals depleted of peripheral $CD4^+$ T cells. The ability of BA conjugates to generate potent anti-viral humoral and cytotoxic reponses, even under conditions of limited $CD4^+$ T-cell function, makes it a very attractive candidate for a vaccine carrier to treat individuals with T-cell immunodeficiency. Thus, BA may be suitable as a carrier in therapeutic vaccines for patients already infected with the HIV-1/HIV-2 viruses as well as for prophylactic vaccines.

REFERENCES

Afonso, L., Scharton, T.M., Vieira, L.Q., Wysocka, M., Trinchieri, G. and Scott, P. 1994. The adjuvant effect of interleukin-12 in a vaccine against Leishmania major. Science, 263:235.

Bennink, J. R., Yewdell, J.W., Smith, G.L., Moller, C. and Moss, B. 1984. Recombinant vaccina virus primes and stimulates influenza haemagglutinin-specific cytotoxic T cells. Nature, 1:578.

Bertagnolli, M.M., Lin, B.Y., Young, D. and Hermann, S.H. 1992. IL-12 augments antigen-dependent proliferation of activated T lymphocytes. J. Immunol., 149:3778.

Bloom, E.T. and Horvath, J.A. 1994. Cellular and molecular mechanisms of the IL-12-induced increase in allospecific murine cytolytic T cell activity. Implications for the age-related decline in CTL. J. Immunol., 152:4242.

Chizzonite, R., Truitt, T., Desai, B.B., Nunes, P., Podlaski, F.J., Stern, A.S. and Gately, M.K . 1992. IL-12 receptor. I. Characterization of the receptor on phytohemagglutin-activated human lymphoblasts. J. Immunol., 148:3117.

Chouaib, S., Chehimi, J., Bani, L., Genetet, N., Tursz, T., Gay, F., Trinchieri, G. and Mami-Choaib, F. 1994. Interleukin 12 induces the differentiation of major histocompatibility complex class I-primed cytotoxic T lymphocyte precursors into allospecific cytotoxic effectors. Proc. Natl. Acad. Sci. USA, 91:12659.

Croft, M., Carter, L., Swain, S.L. and Dutton, R.W. 1994. Generation of polarized antigen-specific CD8 effector populations: reciprocal action of interleukin (IL)-4 and IL-12 in promoting type 2 versus type 1 cytokine profile. J. Exp. Med., 180: 1715.

Damle, N.K., Klussman, K., Linsley, P.S., Aruffo, A. and Ledbetter, J.A. 1992. Differential regulatory effects of intracellular adhesion molecule-1 on costimulation by the CD28 counter receptor B7.J.Immunol., 149:2541.

D'Andrea, A., Rengaraju, M., Valiante, N.M., Chehimi, J., Kubin, M., Aste-Amezaga, M., Chan, S.H.,

Kobayashi, M., Yong, D., Nickbarg, E., Chizzonite, R., Wolf, S.F. and Trinchieri, G. 1992. Production of natural killer stimulatory factor (NKSF/IL-12) by peripheral blood mononuclear cells. J.Exp. Med., 176:1387.

D'Andrea, A., Aste-Amezaga, M., Valiante, N.M., Ma, X., Kubin, M. and Trinchieri, G. 1993. Interleukin 10 inhibits human lymphocyte IFN-γ production by suppressing natural killer stimulatory factor/ interleukin-12 synthesis in accessory cells. J. Exp. Med., 178:1041.

Ehlers, S. and Smith, K.A.. 1991. Differentiation of T cell lymphokine gene expression: the in vitro acquisition of T cell memory. J. Exp. Med., 173:25.

Finkelman, F.D., Katona, I.M., Mosmann, T.R. and Coffman, R.L. 1988. IFN-γ regulate the isotypes of Ig secreted during in vivo humoral immune responses. J. Immunol.,140:1022.

Gately, M.K., Desai, B.B., Wolitzky, A.G., Quinn, P.M., Dwyer, C.M., Podlaski, F.J., Familletti, P.C., Sinigaglia, F., Chizonnite, R., Gubler, U. and Stern, A.S. 1991. Regulation of human lymphocyte proliferation by a heterodimeric cytokine, IL-12 (cytotoxic maturation factor). J. Immunol., 147:874.

Gimmi, C.D., Freeman, G.J., Gribben, J.G., Sugita, K., Freedman, A.S., Morimoto, C. and Nadler, L.M. 1991. B-cell surface antigen B7 provides a costimulatory signal that induces T-cells to proliferate and secrete interleukin-2. Proc. Natl. Acad. Sci. USA, 1991. 88:6575.

Golding, B., Golding, H., Preston, S., Hernandez, D., Beining, P.R., Manischewitz, J., Harvath, L., Blackburn, R., Lizzio, E. and Hoffman, T. 1991. Production of a novel antigen by conjugation of HIV-1 to Brucella abortus: studies of immunogenicity, isotype analysis, T-cell dependency and syncytia inhibition. AIDS Res. Hum. Retroviruses, 7:471.

Golding, B., Inmann, J., Highet, P., Blackburn, R., Manischewitz, J., Blyveis, N., Angus, R.D. and Golding, H. 1995. Brucella abortus conjugated with a gp120 or V3 loop peptide derived from human immuno-deficiency virus (HIV) type 1 induces neutralizing anti-HIV antibodies, and the V3-B. abortus conjugate is effective even after $CD4^+$ T-cell depletion. J. Virol., 69:3299.

Goldstein, J., Hoffman, T. Frasch, C., Lizzio, C.L., Beining, P.R., Hochstein, D., Lee, Y.L., Angus, R.D. and Golding, B. 1992. Lipopolysaccharide (LPS) from Brucella abortus is less toxic than lipopoly-saccharide from Escherichia coli, suggesting the possilble use of B. abortus or LPS from B. abortus as a carrier in vaccines. Infect. Immun., 60:1385.

Guerder, S., Carding, S.R. and Flavell, R.A. 1995. B7 costimulation is necessary for the activation of the lytic function in cytotoxic T lymphocyte precursors. J. Immunol., 155:5167.

Harding, C.V. and Song, R. 1994. Phagocytic processing of exogenous particulate antigens by macrophages for presentation by class I MHC molecules. J. Immunol., 153:4925.

Ikonomidis, G., Paterson, Y., Kos, F.J. and Portnoy, D.A.. 1994. Delivery of a viral antigen to the class I processing and presentation pathway by Listeria monocytogenes.J. Exp.Med., 180:2209.

Kobayashi, M., Fitz, L., Ryan, M., Hewick, R.M., Clark, S.C., Chan, S., Loudon, R., Sherman, F., Perussia, B. and Trinchieri, G. 1989. Identification and purification of natural killer cell stimulatory factor (NKSF). A cytokine with multiple biologic effects on human lymphocytes. J. Exp. Med., 170:827.

Koup, R.A., Safrit, J.T., Cao, Y., Andrews, C.A., McLeod, G., Borkowsky,W., Farthing, C. and Ho, D.D. 1994. Temporal association of cellular immune responses with the initial control of viremia in primary human immunodeficiency virus type 1 syndrome. J. Virol., 68:4650.

Kovacsovics-Bankowski, M., Clark, K., Benacerraf, B. and Rock, K.L.. 1993. Efficient major histo-compatibility complex class I presentation of exogenous antigen upon phagocytosis by macrophages. PNAS, 90:4942.

Lazdins, J. K., Woods-Cook, K., Walker, M. and Alteri, E. 1990. The lipophilic muramyl peptide MTO-PE is a potent inhibitor of HIV replication. AIDS Reserch and Human Retroviruses, 10:1157.

Lewis, D. B., Yu, C.C., Meyer, J., English, B.K., Kahn, S.J. and Wilson, C.B. 1991. Cellular and molecular mechanisms for reduced interleukin 4 and interferon-g production by neonatal T cells. J. Clin. Invest., 87:194.

Linsley, P.S., Brady, W., Grossmaire, L., Aruffo, A., Damle,N.K. and Ledbetter, J.A..1991. Binding of the B cell activation antigen B7 to CD28 costimulates T-cell proliferation and intracellular messenger RNA accumulation. J. Exp. Med., 173:721.

Manetti, R., Parronchi, P., Giudizi, M.G., Piccini, M.-P., Maggi, E., Trinchieri, G. and Romagnani, S. 1993. Natural killer cell stimulatory factor (interleukin 12 [IL-12] induces T helper type 1 (Th1)-specific immune responses and inhibits the development of IL-4-producing Th cells. J. Exp. Med., 177:1199.

Manetti, R., Gerosa, F., Giudizi, M.G., Biagiotti, R., Parrochi, P., Piccini, M-P., Sampognaro, S., Maggi, E., Romagnani, S. and Trinchieri, G. 1994. Interleukin 12 induces stable priming for IFN-γ production during differentiation of human T helper (Th) cells and transient IFN-γ production in established Th2 cell clones. J. Exp. Med., 179:1273.

Murphy, E.E., Terres, G., Macatonia, S.E., Hsieh, C.-S., Mattson, J., Lanier, L., Wysocka, M., Trinchieri, G., Murphy, K. and O'Garra, A. 1994. B7 and interleukin 12 cooperate for proliferation and interferon γ production by mouse T helper clones that are unresponsive to B7 stimulation. J. Exp. Med., 180:223.

O'Garra, A. and Murphy, K. 1994. Role of cytokines in determining T-lymphocyte function. Curr. Opinion in Immunol., 6:458.

Perussia, B., Chan, S.H., D'Andrea, A., Tsuji, K., Santoli, D., Pospisil, M., Young, D., Wolf, S.F. and Trinchieri, G. 1992. Natural killer (NK) cells stimulatory factor or IL-12 has differential effects on the proliferation of TcR alpha-beta^{+}, TcR gamma delta^{+} lymphocytes-T, and NK cells. J. Immunol., 149: 3495.

Pfeifer, J. D., Wick, M.J., Roberts, R.L., Findlay, K., Normark, S.J. and Harding, C.V. 1993. Phagocytic processing of bacterial antigens for class I MHC presentation to T cells. Nature, 361:359.

Romani, L., Mencacci, A., Tonnetti, L., Spaccapelo, R., Cenci, E., Wolf, S., Puccetti, P. and Bistoni, F. 1992. Interleukin-12 but not interferon-γ production correlates with induction of T helper type1phenotype in murine candidiasis. Eur. J. Immunol., 24:909.

Scott, D.E., Agranovich, I., Inman, J., Gober, M. and Golding, B., 1997. Inhibition of primary and recall allergen-specific T helper cell type2-mediated responses by a T helper type 1 stimulus. J.Immunol., 159, in press

Sedegah, M., Finkelman, F. and Hoffman, S.L.. 1994. Interleukin 12 induction of interferon γ-dependentp protection against malaria. Proc. Natl. Acad. Sci. USA, 91:10700.

Shirai, M., Pendleton, C.D., Ahlers, J., Takeshita, T., Newman, N. and Berzofsky, J.A. 1994. Helper-cytotoxic T lymphocyte (CTL) determinant linkage required for priming of anti-HIV CD8+ CTL in vivo with peptide vaccine constructs. J. Immunol.,152:549.

Snapper, C.M., Peschel, C. and Paul, P. 1988. IFN-gamma stimulates IgG2a secretion by murine B cells stimulated with bacterial lipopolysaccharide. J. Immunol., 140:2121.

Stern, A.S., Podlaski, F.J., Hulmes, J.D., Pan, Y.-C., Quinn, P.M., Wolitzky, A.G., Familleti, P.C., Stremlo, D.L., Truitt, T., Chizonite, R. and Gately, M.K. 1990. Purification to homogeneity and partial characterization of cytotoxic lymphocyte maturation factor from human B-lymphoblastoid cells. Proc. Natl. Acad. Sci. USA, 87:6808.

Svetic, A., Jian, Y.C., Lu, P., Finkelman, F.D. and Gause, W.C. 1993. Brucella abortus induces a novel cytokine expression pattern characterized by elevated IL-10 and IFN-γ in CD4^{+} T cells. Int. Immunol., 8:877.

Tripp, C.S., Gately, M.K., Hakimi, J., Ling, P. and Unanue, E. 1994. Neutralization of IL-12 decreases resistance to Listeria in SCID and C.B17 mice. J. Immunol., 154:1883.

Van Seventer, G.A., Shimizu, Y., Horgan, K.J. and Shaw, S. 1990. The LFA-1 ligand ICAM-1 provides an important costimulatory signal for T-cell receptor mediated activation of resting T-cells. J. Immunol., 144:4579.

Wolf, S.F., Temple, P.A., Kobayashi, M., Young, D., Dicig, M., Lowe, L., Dzialo, R., Fitz, L., Ferenz, C., Hewick, R.M., Kelleher, K., Herrmann, S.H., Clark, S.C., Azzoni, L., Chan, S.H., Trinchieri, G. and Perussia, B. 1991. Cloning of cDNA from natural killer cell stimulatory factor, a heterodimeric cytokine with multiple biologic effects on T-cells and natural killer cells. J. Immunol., 146:3074.

Wynn, T.A., Cheever, A.W., Jankovic, D., Poindexter, R.W., Caspar, P., Lewis, F. and Sher, A. 1995. An IL-12 based vaccination method for preventing fibrosis induced by schistosome infection. Nature, 376:594.

Yamauchi, A. and Bloom, E. 1993. Requirement of thiol compounds as reducing agents for IL-2-mediated induction of LAK activity and proliferation of human NK cells. J. Immunol., 151:1.

Zaitseva, M., Golding, H., Betts, M., Yamauchi, A., Bloom, E.T., Butler, L.E., Steven, L. and Golding, B. 1995. Human peripheral blood CD4^{+} and CD8^{+} T cells express Th1-like cytokine mRNA and protein following in vitro stimulation with heat-inactivated Brucella abortus. Infect. Immun., 63:2720.

Zaitseva, M., Golding, H., Manischewitz, J., Webb, D. and Golding, B. 1996. Brucella abortus as a potential vaccine carrier: Induction of interleukin-12 secretion and enhanced B7.1 and B7.2 and intercellular adhesion molecule 1 surface expression in elutriated human monocytes stimulated by heat-inactivated B. abortus. Infect. Immun., 64:3109.

Zhang, M., Gately, M., Wang, E., Gong, J., Wolf, S.F., Lu, S., Modlin, R. and Barnes, P. 1994. Interleukin 12 at the site of disease in tuberculosis. J. Clin. Invest., 93:1733.

THE POTENTIAL USE OF DIFFERENT VACCINATION PROTOCOLS TO TAILOR CYTOKINE PROFILES

Emmanuel Comoy, André Capron and Georges Thyphronitis

INSERM U167, Institut Pasteur de Lille, 1, rue du Pr. Calmette,
Lille, France

INTRODUCTION

Helper CD4+ T cells, through the production of cytokines, play a central role in the regulation of immune responses. In vitro studies with murine T cell clones have shown the existence of two types of Th cells that could be distinguished on the basis of their cytokine production (Mosmann et al., 1986; Mosmann and Coffman, 1989). The Th1 subset secretes IL-2 and IFN-γ, and preferentially promotes cell-mediated immunity and IgG2a production by B lymphocytes whereas the Th2 subset produces IL-4, IL-5, IL-10 and IL-13, and induces humoral immunity and IgG1 and IgE isotypes production (Snapper and Paul 1987; Coffman et al., 1986; Thyphronitis et al., 1989; Cocks et al., 1993). In vivo studies revealed that in some infections, these cytokine profiles determine the outcome of the disease, demonstrating that this dichotomy is physiologically relevant (Heinzel et al., 1989; Mielke et al., 1993; Yamamura et al., 1991; Flesch and Kaufmann 1987). In general Th1 responses are more effective against some intracellular pathogens (Heinzel et al., 1989; Hsieh et al., 1993), whereas Th2 responses are more appropriate in helminth parasitoses (Sher and Coffman 1992; Urban et al., 1991). Using animal models, it has been shown that in some diseases, the expression of the inappropriate profile can be deleterious and enhance pathology. This is best illustrated with the mouse leishmaniasis model. Animals that in response to infection, develop a Th1 type response, spontaneously heal, as opposed to mice that develop a Th2 response and succumb to the infection (Heinzel et al., 1989). Evolution of several other infectious diseases including T. muris infection in mice (Else et al., 1994), M. leprae infections in humans (Yamamura et al., 1991) and others have been shown to be dependent or associated with the one or the other type of Th responses.

Subsequently, it is of major importance to employ a type of vaccination, that will prepare the organism to fight an infection, in the context of the appropriate immune response. In that respect, two questions seemed essential to us. The first question concerns the use of appropriate antigens for vaccination, in association with different adjuvants, to generate characteristically oriented immune responses. The second question is to determine if polarized immune responses induced by immunizations will persist, especially after natural infection. Depending on the answers to these questions, one may adapt appropriate vaccination strategies, in order to obtain maximum protection.

Concerning the first question, the possibility that the antigen itself, depending on its proper nature, may play a significant role in polarization has been suggested in several studies, especially for allergens and parasite antigens, which have been proposed to induce Th2 type responses (Mahanty et al., 1993; Grzych et al., 1991; Parronchi et al., 1991; Wierenga et al., 1990). This assumption is supported by studies showing that T cells from patients with allergic diseases or helminth infections produce type 2 cytokines upon in vitro stimulation with the appropriate antigen(s). However, since in vivo primed memory T cells were used in these studies, it is possible that different factors, other than the antigen itself, were responsible for the initial polarization of the immune response. Concerning the second question, it is well established that in vitro generated T cell clones keep their polarized profile indefinitely. However, T cell clones are generated and proliferate in vitro under standard stable conditions. By contrast, in vivo, the immune milieu is subject to constant changes. Especially, it is possible that infectious agents by creating an appropriate immune milieu, are capable of modifying the orientation of an preestablished profile. Few studies have examined this question. In one study, antigen specific polarized T cells clones generated in vitro have been injected in mice, and the animals have been challenged with the antigen. In this study, the in vivo response strictly matched the profile of the T cell clones (Swain 1995).

In the present study, we examined whether two protein antigens of different origins (parasitic and bacterial) have the innate property of generating characteristic immune responses.

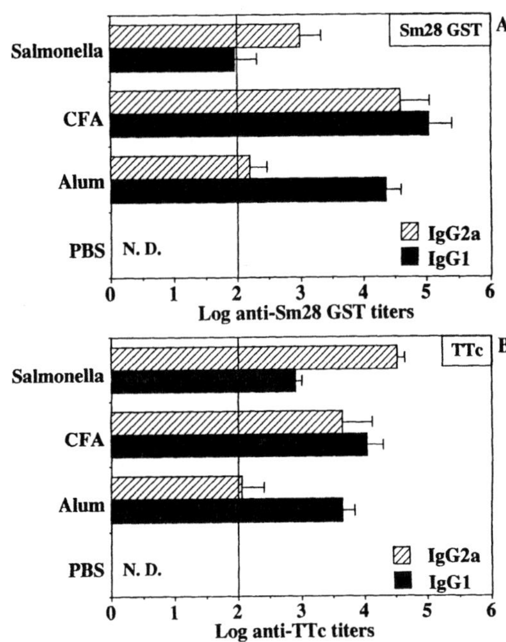

Figure 1. Specific anti-Sm28-GST and anti-Ttc IgG1 and IgG2a responses after immunization using different protocols. Mice (5 per group) were single-dose immunized subcutaneously with either Sm28 GST or recombinant Ttc (100 µg/mouse) in alum, CFA or PBS, or intravenously with rS. typhimurium (10^7 cfu/mouse) expressing the Ttc-Sm28 GST fusion protein. Sera were collected 28 days after immunizations. Results (Mean +/- Standard error) are expressed as logarithm of sera titers for Sm28 GST (A) or Ttc (B). The bar shows the first sera dilution that was tested by ELISA. One representative experiment out of 6 is shown. N.D.: Not detectable.

Glutathione-S-transferase of Schistosoma mansoni (Sm28-GST) (Balloul et al., 1987) is a major parasite protein representing approximately 3% of the total parasite protein, and a potent vaccine candidate against schistosomiasis (Balloul et al., 1987; Boulanger et al., 1991). In parallel, we examined whether the tetanus toxin fragment C (Ttc) had the capacity to polarize the immune response. In these experiments, mice were immunized against these two protein antigens in different adjuvants, or with recombinant S. typhimurium (Anjam-Khan et al., 1994) expressing these antigens as a fusion protein. Depending on the adjuvant formulation, cytokine and specific antibody Ig isotype responses ranged across the Th1/Th2 dichotomy for both antigens. Based on these results, we concluded that adjuvants, and not the nature of the protein antigen, played a crucial role in polarizing the immune response.

We are presently using this polarization model to study the second question. Mice that have developed a type 1 or 2 response against the Sm28 GST after primo-immunization, are subsequently challenged with the protein in alum or with rS. typhimurium, or with the protein alone and the evolution of the response will be determined. These experiments will allow us to estimate the persistence of polarized immune profiles under different challenge conditions.

RESULTS

Isotypic responses against Sm28 GST and Ttc are determined by the adjuvant

We first examined if different adjuvants induced characteristic isotypic responses against Sm28-GST and Ttc. Mice were immunized subcutaneously with antigens in aluminum hydroxide (alum) or in CFA, and rS. typhimurium was injected intravenously. IgG1 and IgG2a responses were examined, because these isotypes are regulated by the Th2 and Th1 products IL4 and IFN-γ respectively. Twenty eight days after immunizations, with either antigen in alum, a specific IgG1 response, and low to undetectable levels of IgG2a were observed. In contrast, rS. typhimurium induced low titers of specific IgG1, and a strong IgG2a response. When Sm28-GST or Ttc was administered in CFA, high titers of both specific IgG1 and IgG2a were observed, greater than those observed after immunization with alum and rS. typhimurium respectively (figure 1). The same isotypic profile persisted from day 7 up to 4 months after immunization (data not shown). Because IgE production, similar to IgG1, is stimulated by IL4,

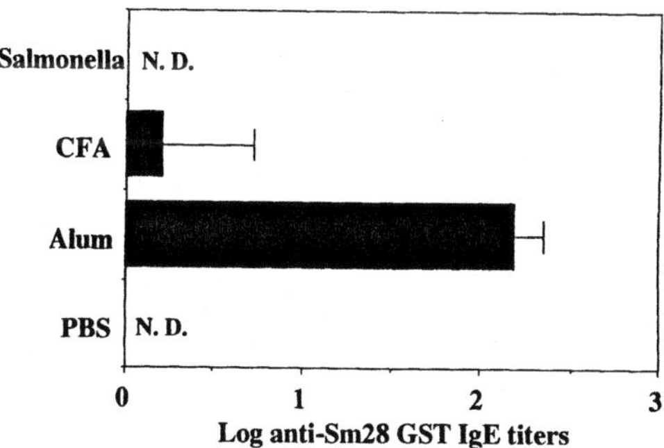

Figure 2. Specific anti-Sm28-GST IgE response after single-dose immunization. Mice (5 per group) were single-dose immunized subcutaneously with Sm28 GST (100 μg/mouse) in alum, CFA or PBS, or intravenously with recombinant Sm28-GST-expressing rS. typhimurium (10^7 cfu/mouse). Sera were collected 4 months after immunizations. Results (Mean +/- Standard error) are expressed as logarithm of sera titers. One representative experiment out of 2 is shown. N. D.: Not Detectable.

we next examined whether IgE specific antibodies were produced against Sm28-GST. As a result of a single dose immunization, specific IgE antibodies did not appear until day 70 and continued to rise until day 130. As shown in figure 2, high IgE titers were observed in alum-immunized animals, a weak IgE response with CFA, and no detectable levels after immunization with rS. typhimurium.

We next examined the possibility that the observed differences were due to the use of different routes of immunization for rS. typhimurium (i.v.), and the adjuvants (s.c.). This possibility was eliminated since mice immunized intraperitoneally with Sm28-GST in alum or CFA (intravenously administrations of these formulations are lethal), demonstrate similar responses to those that were produced by subcutaneous immunization (data not shown).

Together, these results suggested that the different adjuvant formulations used generated distinct Th responses, that stimulate the expression of different isotype profiles against the same antigen.

Similar isotype profiles are observed against immunodominant peptides of the Sm28-GST

A possible explanation for the different isotypic profiles is that different antigen epitopes became immunodominant depending on the adjuvant. These epitopes may induce different

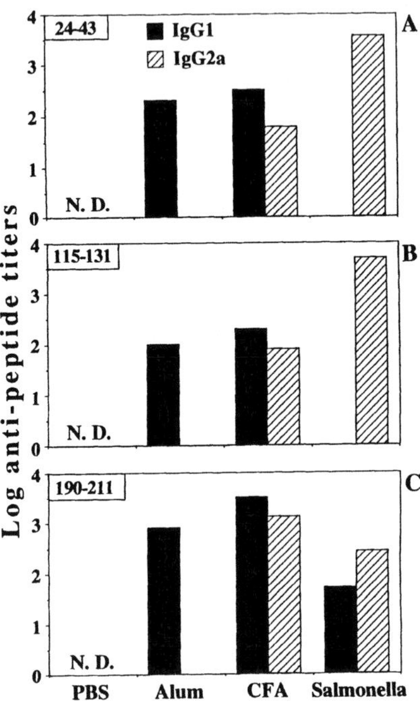

Figure 3. IgG1 and IgG2a responses against Sm28-GST peptides after immunization using different protocols. Mice (5 per group) were single-dose immunized subcutaneously with Sm28-GST (100 μg/mouse) in alum, CFA or PBS, or intravenously with recombinant Sm28-GST-expressing rS. typhimurium (10^7 cfu/mouse). Sera were collected 28 days after immunization. Specific IgG1 and IgG2a against peptides 24-43 (A), 115-131 (B) and 190-211 (C) of Sm28 GST were measured in these sera. Results (Mean +/- Standard error) are expressed as logarithm of sera titers. One representative experiment out of 3 is shown. N. D.: Not detectable.

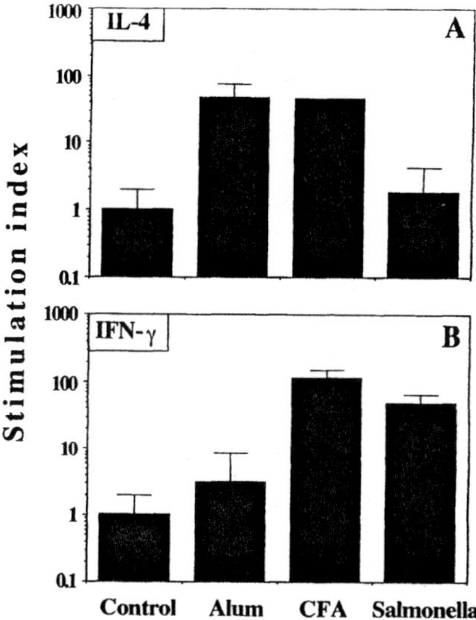

Figure 4. Levels of IL-4 and IFN-γ mRNA after immunization using different protocols. Mice (4 per group) were single-dose immunized subcutaneously with Sm28 GST (100 μg/mouse) in alum or CFA, or intravenously with Sm28-GST-expressing rS. typhimurium (10^7 cfu/ mouse). Six days after immunization, mice were sacrificed and RNA from inguinal lymph nodes (immunization with alum or CFA) and spleens (administration of rS. typhimurium) were assessed by semi-quantitative RT-PCR for IL-4 (A) and IFN-γ (B) mRNA expression. Results are expressed as index of stimulation, over control mice injected with 0.9% NaCl, arbitrarily considered as 1 (See Materials and Methods section). One representative experiment out of 3 is shown.

types of Th responses, that in turn generate different isotypic profiles. To address this question, sera from mice immunized against the Sm28-GST using the three different protocols, were tested for specific IgG1 and IgG2a antibody titers against the three immunodominant peptides of the Sm28-GST, that contain both T and B epitopes: peptides 24-43, 115-131 and 190-211 (Xu et al., 1993; Wolowczuk et al., 1991).

The results presented in figure 3 show that antibody responses against all peptides were generated. The isotypic profiles were determined by the adjuvant formulation, and were similar to those observed against the entire protein.

Cytokine expression in vivo correlates with isotype profiles

We next examined, using semi-quantitative RT-PCR, if the observed isotype profiles correlate with the expression of IL4 and IFN-γ, in lymphoid organs draining the sites of immunizations (inguinal lymph nodes for s.c. immunizations, spleens for i.v. administration). An increase of mRNA coding for IL4 was observed in the draining lymphoid organs, six days after mice immunization with alum (x 47) and with CFA (x 44), while no significant modification, compared to the controls, was observed when rS. typhimurium was administrated (figure 4). In contrast, levels of mRNA coding for IFN-γ increased when mice were immunized with rS. typhimurium (x 50) or Sm28-GST in CFA (x 110), while a minimal increase, in comparison to the control mice, was observed in mice immunized with the antigen in alum. Similar results were observed 10 days after immunization, and were confirmed in separate experiments (data not shown). When immunizations with alum or CFA were performed intraperitoneally, IL4 and IFN-γ mRNA expression in the spleen was similar to that observed in lymph nodes after subcutaneous administration of the antigen (data not shown). These results show that specific antibody isotypes, IgG1 and IgG2a, strictly correlate with IL4 and IFN-γ expression respectively.

Cytokine production after specific antigen stimulation in vitro

To determine if cytokine profiles produced after specific antigen stimulation, are similar to those observed after ex-vivo RT-PCR analysis, draining lymphoid organs (inguinal lymph nodes and spleens) were removed from mice, 7 days after immunization, and the cells were tested for their ability to produce IL4 and IFN-γ after stimulation with antigen. As shown in figure 5, spleen cells of mice immunized with rS. typhimurium produced significant levels of IFN-γ, when stimulated with either Ttc or Sm28-GST, and no detectable levels of IL4, while cells of lymph nodes did not produce detectable levels of either cytokines. In CFA-immunized mice, lymph node cells produced significant amounts of both IL4 and IFN-γ. For alum-immunized mice, we also observed production of both cytokines, but more IL4 and less IFN-γ than for CFA. It is of interest, that spleen cells from mice immunized s.c, produced similar cytokines profile when stimulated with antigen in vitro. These results further confirm that different type Th responses are induced when immunizing with the same antigen in different adjuvant formulations.

Does immune response polarization persist?

Experiments were designed to examine whether polarized cytokine profiles induced by immunization in alum (type 2) or with rS. typhimurium (type 1), will persist if recall immunizations were done in the absence of adjuvant, using the same adjuvant or the adjuvant promoting the opposite profile. In preliminary experiments, we examined whether the Th2

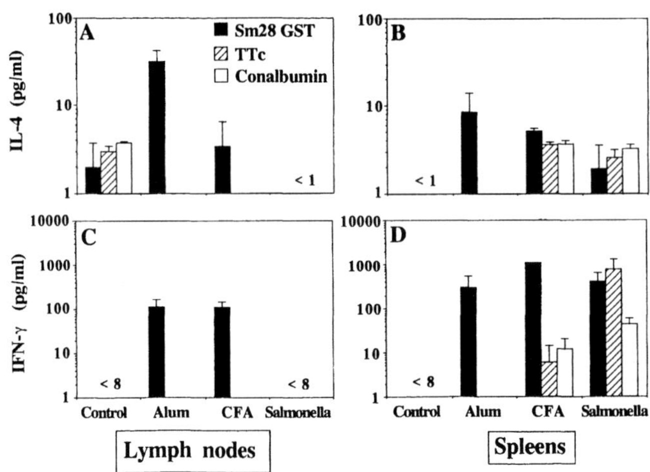

Figure 5. Production of IL-4 and IFN-γ after antigen specific stimulation in vitro. Mice (3 per group) were single-dose immunized subcutaneously with Sm28 GST (100 μg/mouse) in alum or CFA, or intravenously with recombinant Sm28-GST-expressing rS. typhimurium (10^7 cfu/mouse). Seven days after immunizations, mice were sacrificed and inguinal lymph node cells (A and C) and spleen cells (B and D) were stimulated in triplicate in vitro (5.10^6 cells/ml) with either Sm28 GST (20 μg/ml), Ttc (20 μg/ml), and Conalbumin (20 μg/ml) as irrelevant protein. Supernatants were assessed for IL-4 (A and B) and for IFN-γ (C and D). Results are expressed as the mean of triplicates. IFN-γ and IL4 production, in control stimulated cultures with 5μg/ml of ConA, was approximately 1500 pg/ml and 30 pg/mln respectively. One representative experiment out of 3 is shown.

profile will persist if recall immunizations were done in alum 3 months after primary immunization. T cell responses 7 days after a recall immunization were evaluated by antigen specific stimulation in vitro. As shown in figure 6, lymph node cells from non-boosted animals still produce relatively high IL4 and significant IFN-γ levels after in vitro antigen stimulation. When animals were boosted with Sm28-GST in alum, noticeably higher IL4 levels were induced, while IFN-γ production decrease significantly in comparison to the non-boosted animals. It is of interest that IFN-γ levels were lower in alum-boosted than in non-boosted mice, suggesting that the presence of alum exercises a negative effect on IFN-γ production.

DISCUSSION

The discovery that T helper cells may polarize their cytokine production to distinct profiles, brought a new insight in the regulation of immune responses. It is now clear that immune response polarization may greatly influence disease outcome in several infectious and allergic conditions (Heinzel et al., 1989; Yamamura et al., 1991; Wierenga et al., 1990; Finkelman and Urban, 1992). Therefore for vaccination and immunotherapy it is important to determine first which type of response is beneficial, and then to design protocols that will induce this type of response. This approach will certainly help us to design better immunotherapy and vaccination protocols. However, the basic mechanisms implicated in polarization are not yet well understood. Important questions should be addressed, before attempting to modulate immune responses for prophylactic or therapeutic reasons. How would the choice of the antigen or of the adjuvant influence the outcome of the vaccination? Would the cytokine profile established by vaccination persist during exposure to the corresponding infectious agent? These are, to our opinion, some of the important questions that should be answered.

The first question was examined by immunizing mice with the Sm28-GST, a trematode parasite antigen, and Ttc, a bacterial antigen, in different adjuvant formulations. Sm28-GST is of particular interest to us, because as it has been shown in our laboratory, it is a major S. mansoni antigen, and a promising vaccine candidate (Balloul et al., 1987; Boulanger et al., 1991; Xu et al., 1991). The results show that both antigens do not demonstrate any polarizing capacity. In contrast, depending on the adjuvant, responses ranged from mixed to Th1 or Th2. How may adjuvants promote the development of different types of immune responses? The possibility that, depending on the adjuvant, different Th1 or Th2 epitopes were presented seems unlikely, since the Ig isotype profiles against all three immunodominant epitopes of the Sm28-GST (Xu et al., 1993; Wolowczuk et al., 1991), were similar to the ones observed against the whole protein. Another possibility is that different APC are recruited, which by early cytokine production promote distinct Th responses. In that respect, it has been proposed that dendritic cells, by producing IL12, induce Th1-like responses (Caux et al., 1995; Macatonia et al., 1995). Conversely, macrophages may preferentially induce type 2 responses (Schmitz and Radbruch 1992; De Becker et al., 1994). This hypothesis does not explain our results, since after s.c. immunization, where dendritic cells are the main APC (Caux et al., 1995; Austyn 1996), we observed Th2 or mixed responses. Furthermore, i.p. administration of the Sm28-GST in AH, where peritoneal macrophages are mainly involved in presentation, generated responses similar to the ones observed after s.c. immunizations. Also, like others, we have found that S. typhimurium, that invades macrophages in the spleen, promotes a Th1 response (Chong et al., 1996; Thatte et al., 1993; Karem et al., 1995). Thus according to our results, there exists the possibility that, when alum is administered s.c., other types of APC, in addition to dendritic cells, are recruited, creating the appropriate milieu for Th2 development. Alternatively, it is also possible that depending on the stimuli, the same APC produce different sets of early cytokines that drive the immune response towards a Th1 or Th2 profile. In addition, independently of the

APC, different types of inflammatory cells may be recruited at the site of the injection, depending on the adjuvant. These cells may be capable of inducing characteristic early cytokine environments, necessary for Th polarization. In that regard, recent interesting findings showed that mast cells, basophils and eosinophils are capable of producing immunoregulatory cytokines such as IL4, IL10, and IFN-γ (Seder et al., 1991; Brunner et al., 1993; Lamkhioued et al., 1995; Moqbel et al., 1995). These cells may be responsible for the observed, early IL4 and IFN-γ mRNA expression, after immunizations in alum or with rS. typhimurium respectively (data not shown). Indeed, a substantial increase in IFN-γ mRNA expression was observed, as early as 2 hours after immunization. This rapid IFN-γ expression suggests that, rS. typhimurium directly stimulates, NK cells or other cell types to produce IFN-γ, in an IL12 independent way (Trinchieri 1989). The early IL4 mRNA expression in alum immunized mice, may also becoming from cell types other than antigen specific Th cells. In this regard, NK1.1$^+$ CD4$^+$ T cells or mast cells are possible candidates (Gollob et al., 1994; Yoshimoto and Paul 1994). Early IL4 production may be important for the establishment of a Th2 type of response, by inhibiting IFN-γ expression. This hypothesis is supported by the observation that early IL12 mRNA expression in the alum protocol was not followed by increased IFN-γ mRNA expression (data not shown). Alternatively, alum may exerts a direct negative effect on IFN-γ production. This is supported by experiments showing, that cells from animals immunized 3 months earlier, produce more IFN-γ, upon in vitro antigen stimulation, than their counterparts that received a booster immunization in alum, seven days earlier. In contrast, this later group produce significantly more IL4 than the non-boosted animals. We are presently examining these possibilities.

In the present study, we extend previous observations, made in polyclonally activated systems, demonstrating that IL4 induces IgG1 and IgE, and IFN-γ IgG2a (Snapper and Paul 1987), by showing that antigen specific isotypic responses are also regulated by these cytokines. The different cytokine profiles that were elicited by the three protocols are not as clear-cut as they have been first defined (Mosmann et al., 1986; Mosmann et al., 1989). Type 1 and type 2 cytokines were expressed in all protocols, and the final outcome of the response was determined by the balance between the opposing cytokines. Thus, low in vivo mRNA expression and significant in vitro IFN-γ production was observed by stimulation of lymph nodes from alum immunized animals. However, this IFN-γ was accompanied by high IL4

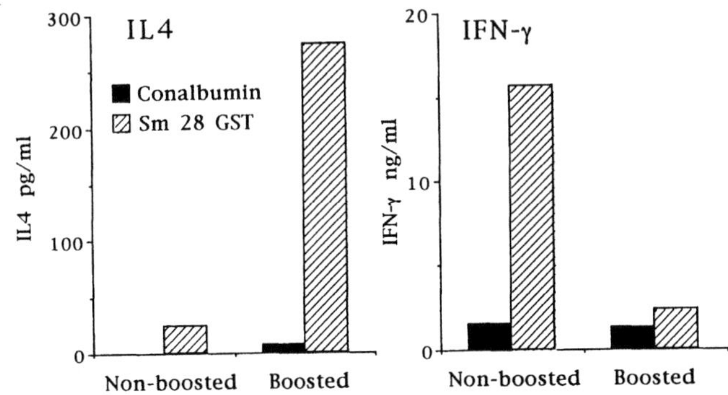

Figure 6. Production of IL4 and IFN-γ after recall immunization. Mice (3 per group) were immunized subcutaneously with Sm28 GST (100 μg/mouse) in alum. Three months later, mice received a recall immunization in alum or only PBS. Seven days after recall immunizations, mice were sacrificed and inguinal lymph node cells were stimulated in triplicate in vitro (5.10^6 cells/ml) with either Sm28 GST (20 μg/ml), or Conalbumin (20 μg/ml) as irrelevant protein. Supernatants were assessed for IL-4 (left panel) and for IFN-γ (right panel). Results are expressed as the mean of triplicates.

production (significantly higher than the one observed in the two other protocols) that dominates over IFN-γ and leads to the IgG1 and IgE production. It is of interest that, in response to CFA immunization, high levels of both IL4 and IFN-γ were expressed, and both IgG1 and IgG2a were produced. It will be interesting to determine whether or not different sets of Th cells are producing these cytokines. Moreover, it will be interesting to know if this mixed profile will persist after challenge immunization. The results presented here imply that, by choosing the appropriate adjuvant, different types of immune responses could be induced. However, whether this is true for all antigens has to be proven. Several additional questions have to be examined in this context. For example, it is important to determine if adjuvants induce similar type of responses in mice having a different genetic background. Also, it is important to determine if the antigen dose and multiple immunizations would modulate the polarizing capacities of adjuvants. Another important question, that we are presently studying, is the persistence of polarized profile after recall immunization. Not surprisingly, preliminary results show that cytokine profiles persist 3 months after immunization, in both non-boosted and animals boosted using the same protocol. However, additional work is needed to answer the most important question in this respect: what will happen if the adjuvant promoting the opposite cytokine profile, is used in recall immunizations?. In conclusion the results presented in this paper futher stress the need for developing new adjuvants with well characterized properties for human use.

Acknowledgments

This work was supported by the Institut National de la Santé et de la Recherche Médicale (INSERM). The authors would like to acknowledge Drs. C. Anjam Khan, C. Hormaeche, A. O'Garra, J-M. Grzych, F. Finkelman, J.-P. Kusnierz, R. Pierce, H. Salvelkoul and A. Tartar for generous gifts of reagents. We would like also to acknowledge A. Caron, J. Fontaine and C. Vendeville for expert technical assistance.

REFERENCES

Anjam Khan, C. M., Villarreal-Ramos, B., Pierce, R. J., Riveau, G., Demarco de Hormaeche, R., Mc Neill, H., Ali, T., Fairweather, N., Chatfield, S., Capron, A., Dougan, G. and Hormaeche, C. E., 1994. Construction, expression, and immunogenicity of the Schistosoma mansoni P28 Glutathione S-transferase as a genetic fusion to tetanus toxin fragment C in a live Aro attenuated vaccine strain of Salmonella. Proc. Natl. Acad. Sci. USA, 91:11261.

Austyn, J. M., 1996. New insights into the mobilization and phagocytic activity of dendritic cells. J. Exp. Med., 183:1287.

Balloul, J.-M., Sondermeyer, P., Dreyer, D., Capron, M., Grzych, J.-M., Pierce, R. J., Carvallo, D., Lecocq, J.-P. and Capron, A., 1987. Molecular cloning of a protective antigen of schistosomes. Nature, 326:149.

Balloul, J.-M., Grzych, J.-M., Pierce, R. J. and Capron, A., 1987. A purified 28.000 Dalton protein from Schistosoma mansoni adult worms protects rats and mice against experimental schistosomiasis. J. Immunol., 138:3448.

Boulanger, D., Reid, G. D., Sturrock, R. F., Wolwczuk, I., Balloul, J.-M., Grezel, D., Pierce, R. J., Otieno, M.F., Guerret, S., Grimaud, J. A., Butterworth, A. E. and Capron, A., 1991. Immunization of mice and baboons with the recombinant Sm28 GST affects both worm viability and fecundity after experimental infection with Schistosoma mansoni. Parasite Immunol., 13:473.

Brunner, T., Heusser, C.H. and Dahinden, C.A., 1993. Human peripheral blood basophils primed by interleukin 3 (IL-3) produce IL-4 in response to immunoglobulin E receptor stimulation. J. Exp. Med. 177: 605.

Caux, C., Liu, Y.-J. and Banchereau, J. 1995. Recent advances in the study of dendritic cells and follicular dendritic cells. Immunol. Today, 16:2.

Chong, C., Bost, K. L. and Clements, J. D. 1996. Differential production of interleukin-12 mRNA by murine macrophages in response to viable or killed Salmonella spp. Infect. Immun., 64:1154.

Cocks, B.G., de Waal Malefyt, R., Galizzi, J-P., de Vries, J.E. and Aversa, G., 1993. IL-13 induces proliferation and differentiation of human B cells activated by the CD40 ligand. Int. Immunol., 5:657.

Coffman, R. L., Ohara, J., Bond, M.W., Carty, J., Zlotnik, A. and Paul, W.E., 1986. B cell stimulatory factor-1 enhances the IgE response of lipopolysaccharide-activated B cells. J. Immunol., 136:4538.

De Becker, G., Sornasse, T., Nabavi, N., Bazin, H., Tielemans, F., Urbain, J., Leo, O. and Moser, M., 1994. Immunoglobulin isotype regulation by antigen-presenting cells in vivo. Eur.J.Immunol., 24:1523.

Else, K.J., Finkelman, F.D., Maliszwewski, C.R. and Grencis, R.K., 1994, Cytokine-mediated regulation of chronic intestinal helminth infection. J.Exp.Med., 179:347.

Finkelman, F.D. and Urban Jr, J.F., 1992. Cytokines: making the right choice. Parasitol.Today., 8:311.

Flesch, I. and Kaufmann, S.H.E., 1987. Mycobacterial growth inhibition by interferon-γ-activated bone marrow macrophages and differential susceptibility among strains of Mycobacterium tuberculosis. J. Immunol., 138:4408.

Gollob, K.J. and Coffman, R.L., 1994. A minority subpopulation of CD4+ T cells directs the development of naive CD4+ T cells into IL-4-secreting cells. J. Immunol., 152:5180.

Grzych, J.-M., Pearce, E., Cheever, A., Caulada, Z., Caspar, P., Hieny, S., Lewis, F. and Sher, A., 1991.Egg deposition is the major stimulus for the production of TH2 cytokines in murine Schistosomiasis mansoni. J. Immunol., 146:1322.

Heinzel, F.P., Sadick, M.D., Holaday, B.J., Coffman, R.L. and Locksley, R.M., 1989. Reciprocal expression of interferon or IL-4 during the resolution or progression of murine leishmaniasis. J. Exp. Med., 169:59.

Hsieh, C.-S., Macatonia, S.E., Tripp, C.S., Wolf, S.F., O'Garra, A. and Murphy, K.M., 1993. Development of TH1 CD4+ T cells through IL-12 produced by listeria-induced macrophages. Science, 260:547.

Karem, K.L., Chatfield, S., Kuklin, N. and Rouse, B.T., 1995. Differential induction of carrier antigen-specific immunity by Salmonella typhimurium live-vaccine strains after single mucosal or intravenous immunization of BALB/c mice. Infect. Immun., 63:4557.

Lamkhioued, B., Aldebert, D., Gounni, A.S., Goldman, M., Capron, A. and Capron, M., 1995. Synthesis of cytokines by eosinophils and their regulation. Int. Arch. Allergy Immunol., 107:122.

Macatonia, S.E., Hosken, N.A., Litton, M., Vieira, P., Hsieh, C.S., Culpepper, J.A., Wysocka, M., Trinchieri, G., Murphy, K.M. and O'Garra, A., 1995. Dendritic cells produce IL-12 and direct the development of TH1 cells from naive CD4+ T cells. J. Immunol., 154:5071.

Mahanty, S., King, C.L., Kumaraswami, V., Regunathan, J., Maya, A., Jayaraman, K., Abrams, J.S., Ottesen, E.A. and Nutman, T.B., 1993. IL-4 and IL-5-secreting lymphocyte populations are preferentially stimulated by parasite-derived antigens in human tissue invasive nematode infections. J. Immunol., 151:3704.

Mielke, M.E., Ehlers, S. and Hahn, H., 1993. The role of cytokines in experimental listeriosis. Immunobiol., 189: 285.

Moqbel, R., Ying, S., Barkans, J., Newman, T.M., Kimmitt, P., Wakelin, M., Taborda-Barata, L., Meng, Q., Corrigan, C.J., Durham, S.R. and Kay, B., 1995. Identification of messenger RNA for IL-4 in human eosinophils with granule localization and release of the translated product. J. Immunol., 155:4939.

Mosmann, T.R., Cherwinski, H., Bond, M.W., Giedlin, M.A. and Coffmann, R.L., 1986. Two types of murine helper T cell clone. I. Definition according to profiles of lymphokine activities and secreted proteins. J. Immunol., 136:2348.

Mosmann, T.R., and Coffman, R.L., 1989. TH1 and TH2 cells: Different patterns of lymphokine secretion lead to different functional properties. Ann. Rev. Immunol., 7:145.

Parronchi, P., Macchia, D., Piccinni, M-P., Biswas, P., Simonelli, C., Maggi, E., Ricci, M., Ansari, A.A. and Romagnani, S., 1991. Allergen- and bacterial antigen-specific T-cell clones established from atopic donors show a different profile of cytokine production. Proc. Natl. Acad. Sci. USA, 88:4538.

Seder, R.A., Plaut, M., Barbieri, S., Urban, J., Finkelman, F.D. and Paul, W.E., 1991. Mouse splenic and bone marrow cell populations that express high-affinity Fcε receptors and produce interleukin 4 are highly enriched in basophils. Proc. Natl. Acad. Sci. USA, 88: 2835.

Schmitz, J. and Radbruch, A., 1992. Distinct antigen presenting cell-derived signals induce Th cell proliferation and expression of effector cytokines. Intern. Immunol., 4:43.

Sher, A. and Coffman, R.L., 1992. Regulation of immunity to parasites by T cells and T cell-derived cytokines. Annu. Rev. Immunol., 10:385.

Snapper, C.M. and Paul, W.E., 1987. Interferon-γ and B Cell stimulatory factor-1 reciprocally regulate Ig isotype production. Science, 236:944.

Swain, S.L., 1995. Generation and in vivo persistence of polarized Th1 and Th2 memory cells. Immunity, 1:543.

Thatte, J., Rath, S. and Bal, V., 1993. Immunization with live versus killed Salmonella typhimurium leads to the generation of an IFN-γ-dominant versus an IL-4-dominant immune response. Int. Immunol., 5:1431.

Thyphronitis, G., Tsokos, G.C., June, C., Levine, A.D. and Finkelman, F.D., 1989. IgE secretion by Epstein-Barr virus-infected purified human B lymphocytes is stimulated by interleukin 4 and suppressed by interferon-γ. Proc. Natl. Acad. Sci. USA, 86:5580.

Trinchieri, G., 1989. Biology of natural killer cells. Adv. Immunol., 47:187.

Urban, J.F., Jr., Katona, I.M., Paul, W.E. and Finkelman, F.D., 1991. Interleukin 4 is important in protective immunity to a gastrointestinal nematode infection in mice. Proc. Natl. Acad. Sci. USA, 88:5513.

Wierenga, E.A., Snoek, M., de Groot, C., Chretien, I., Bos, J.D., Jansen, H.M. and Kapsenberg, M.L., 1990. Evidence for compartmentalization of functional subsets of CD4+ T lymphocytes in atopic patients. J. Immunol., 144:4651.

Wolowczuk, I., Auriault, C., Bossus, M., Boulanger, D., Gras-Masse, H., Mazingue, C., Pierce, R.J., Grezel, D., Reid, G.D., Tartar, A. and Capron, A., 1991. Antigenicity and immunogenicity of a multiple peptidic construction of the Schistosoma mansoni Sm-28 GST antigen in rat, mouse and monkey. J. Immunol., 146:1987.

Xu, C.B., Verwaerde, C., Grzych, J.-M., Fontaine, J. and Capron, A., 1991. A monoclonal antibody blocking the Schistosoma mansoni 28 kDa glutathione-S-transferase activity reduces female worm fecundity and egg viability. Eur. J. Immunol., 21:1801.

Xu, C.-B., Verwaerde, C., Gras-Masse, H., Fontaine, J., Bossus, M., Trottein, F., Wolowczuk, I., Tartar, A. and Capron, A., 1993. Schistosoma mansoni 28-kDa glutathione S-transferase and immunity against parasite fecundity and egg viability. J. Immunol., 150:940.

Yamamura, M., Uyemura, K., Deans, R.J., Weinberg, K, Rea, T.H., Bloom, B.R. and Modlin, R.L., 1991. Defining protective responses to pathogens: cytokine profiles in leprosy lesions. Science, 254:277.

Yoshimoto, T. and Paul, W.E., 1994. CD4pos, NK1.1pos T cells promptly produce interleukin 4 in response to in vivo challenge with anti-CD3. J. Exp. Med., 179:1285.

MODULATION OF CYTOKINE RESPONSES BY ISCOMS AND ISCOM-MATRIX

Maria Villacres-Eriksson, Shahriar Behboudi,
Karin Lövgren-Bengtsson and Bror Morein

Swedish University of Agricultural Sciences, Section of Virology,
Biomedical Centre, Uppsala, Sweden

INTRODUCTION

ISCOM AND MATRIX

The immunomodulating complex (iscom) is a formulation in which protein antigens are coincorporated with glycosylated triterpenoids possessing adjuvant activity in the same particle (Morein et al, 1984). In electron microscopy, the iscoms appear as organized cage-like structures of 30-40 nm in diameter (Özel et al, 1989). Chemically, iscoms consist of glycosylated triterpenoids from Quillaja saponaria Molina, cholesterol, phospholipids and amphipathic protein antigens (Lövgren and Morein, 1988a). Complexes prepared without protein are called iscom-matrix (matrix) and have the same electron microscopic morphology as iscoms (Özel et al, 1989). The basic concept of the iscom is to deliver the adjuvant and the protein antigen in the same particle, assuring optimal activation of antigen-presenting cells (APC).

IMMUNOENHANCING CAPACITY OF ISCOMS AND MATRIX

Iscoms markedly enhance the immunogenicity of the incorporated antigen, both in terms of antibody and cell-mediated immune responses (reviewed in Morein et al, 1995). Typically, the antibody response to iscom-borne antigens encompasses mainly the IgG1 and IgG2a subclasses, although other subclasses are also enhanced (Lövgren 1988b). The cytokine profile of polyclonal response after in vitro restimulation of iscom-primed splenocytes indicates a preferential stimulation of Th1 cytokines (Villacres-Eriksson et al, 1992, Villacres-Eriksson, 1995). A particular feature of iscoms is their prominent capacity to elicit CTL responses as demonstrated with a variety of antigens (Jones et al, 1988, Takahashi et al, 1990, Mowat et al, 1991, 1993, Trudel et al, 1992, Van Binnendijk et al, 1992). Induction of CTL responses

Vaccine Design: The Role of Cytokine Networks
Edited by Gregoriadis *et al.*, Plenum Press, New York, 1997

implicates access of iscom-borne antigens to the cytosol of APC for processing and loading onto MHC class I and II molecules. Interestingly, iscom-borne antigens evoke strong immune responses also after intranasal (Lövgren, 1988b, Ben Ahmeida et al, 1992, Sundquist et al, 1988) or oral immunization (Mowat et al, 1991, 1993). Recent data show that immunization of juvenile animals with iscoms results in clear-cut responses even in the presence of maternal antibodies (Nordengrahn et al, 1996).

The iscom-matrix is a particulate complex with composition, shape and appearance identical to the iscom, but lacking incorporated antigens (Lövgren and Morein, 1988a, Rönnberg, et al, 1995). Since the iscom-matrix contains adjuvant active Quil A it can be used as an adjuvant simply added to antigens. Less information is available concerning the adjuvant activity of iscom-matrix (Snodgrass et al, 1995, Sjölander et al, 1996, Jones et al, 1995) especially in comparison to iscoms (Lövgren et al, 1996). Iscom-matrix is a potent adjuvant for particulate antigens and shares some but not all of the characteristics of iscoms.

PROTECTIVE IMMUNITY ELICITED BY ISCOM-BORNE ANTIGENS

Iscoms have been shown to elicit protective immunity against various infectious agents such as influenza virus (Jones et al, 1988), rabies virus (Fekadu et al, 1992), Epstein-Barr virus (Morgan et al, 1988), simian immunodeficiency virus (Osterhaus et al, 1992a,b), measles virus (De Vries et al, 1988a), canine distemper virus (CDV) (De Vries et al, 1988b), and Trypanosoma cruzi (Araujo and Morein, 1991).

Table 1. Examples of micro-organism against which protective immunity has been mediated by iscoms

Miro-organism	Route	Species	Reference
Influenza virus	s.c/i.n/i.m	mouse	Lövgren (1988), Ben Ahmeida et al. (1992)
Measles virus	i.m	mouse	De Vries (1988a)
CDV	i.m	dog/seal	De Vries (1988b), Visser et al. (1989)
HSV1	s.c	mouse	Erturk et al (1989, 1992)
BHV1	s.c/i.m	rabbit/calf	Trudel et al (1987, 1988)
Pseudorabies virus	i.m	pig/mouse	Tsuda et al (1991)
EBV	s.c	tamarin	Morgan et al (1988)
Rabies virus	i.p	mouse/dog	Fekadu et al (1992)
FeLV	i.m	cat	Osterhaus et al (1985, 1989)
SIV	i.m	monkey	Osterhaus et al (1992a,b)
BVDV	s.c/i.m	sheep	Carlson et al (1991)
EHV-2	i.m	foal	Nordengrahn et al (1996)
Toxoplasma Gondii	s.c	mouse	Lunden, A., et al. (1993)
Trypanozoma. Cruzi	s.c	mouse	Araujo, F. and Morein (1991)
Mycoplasma g.	i.m	chicken	Sundquist, B. et al (1996)

POSSIBLE MECHANISMS OF IMMUNOGENICITY MEDIATED BY ISCOMS

In vitro studies indicate that iscom-borne antigens are taken up with high efficiency by APC (Villacres-Eriksson et al, submitted). The simultaneous delivery of antigen and adjuvant in the same particle enhances the targeting of both these components to the same APC, which results in increased activation of the presenting cell. In fact, influenza virus iscoms have been shown to stimulate the secretion of IL-1 (Villacres-Eriksson et al, 1993, Behboudi et al, 1996), IL-6 (Behboudi et al, 1997) and IL-12 (Villacres-Eriksson et al, 1997). Interestingly, matrix can elicit IL-1 and IL-6 secretion in the absence of antigen (Villacres-Eriksson et al, 1993, Behboudi et al, 1996, Behboudi et al, 1997), indicating that the capacity of the immune complex to stimulate cytokine secretion is to a great extent guided by the adjuvant component. However, the protein antigen may play a role in this respect by facilitating the uptake of the complexes or by its intrinsic capacity to stimulate cytokines. The proper activation of APC is most likely pivotal in initiating a response that leads to T cell activation.

Table 2. Factors important for the immunogenicity of iscoms

1. Enhanced internalization by APC
2. Access of iscom-borne antigen to the cytosol in APC
3. Production of proinflammatory cytokines by APC
4. Stimulation of Th1 cytokine responses

The role of iscoms in stimulating the expression of costimulatory molecules is presently under investigation, although early studies have already shown increased expression of MHC Class II molecules mediated by influenza virus iscoms both in vitro and in vivo (Watson et al, 1992, Bergstrom-Mollaoglu et al, 1992).

STIMULATION OF PROINFLAMMATORY CYTOKINES BY ISCOMS AND MATRIX

Iscoms carrying influenza virus envelope proteins stimulate secretion of IL-1 and IL-6 by murine resident peritoneal cells (Villacres-Eriksson et al, 1993, Behboudi et al, 1996, Behboudi et al, 1997) and by adherent splenocytes (Villacres-Eriksson et al, 1993). Iscoms containing rabies virus glycoproteins also elicit secretion of IL-1 by murine resident peritoneal cells (Villacres-Eriksson, unpublished observations). In vivo, the influenza virus iscoms elicit the production of IL-12 in mice (Villacres-Eriksson et al, 1997).

The matrix of the iscom also stimulates secretion of IL-1 and IL-6, although less efficiently than iscoms (Villacres-Eriksson et al, 1993, Behboudi et al, 1996, Behboudi et al, 1997). In vivo experiments using antibodies neutralizing IL-12 indicate that this cytokine is also stimulated by matrix (Villacres-Eriksson et al, 1997). As with IL-1 and IL-6, the matrix

Table 3. Activation of antigen-presenting cells by iscoms or matrix (spikoside formulation)

	In vitro		In vivo	
	iscom	matrix	iscom	matrix
secreted IL-1α	+	+	-	-
IL-6	+	+	+	+
IL-12	-	-	+	(+)
TNF α	-	-	-	-

stimulates IL-12 less efficiently than iscoms (Villacres-Eriksson et al, 1997). There is evidence that IL-6 and IL-12 are important for the generation of CTL responses (Gajewski et al, 1995). Also IL-1 may cooperate in the differentiation of $CD8^+$ lymphocytes into CTL effectors (Renauld et al, 1989). Therefore, the capacity of iscoms and matrix to stimulate these cytokines is likely to be relevant for the generation and/or expansion of CTL.

The capacity of glycosylated triterpenoid adjuvants incorporated into matrix to stimulate cytokine production has recently been explored as a parameter to predict the immunoenhancing capacity of new adjuvant formulations (Behboudi et al, 1997). The matrix 7.0.3 (70 % QH-A, 0 % QH-B and 30 % QH-C Quil A components) was the formulation which elicited the production of IL-1 and IL-6 most efficiently (Behboudi et al, 1996, Behboudi et al, 1997). The level of antigen-presenting cell activation reflected by the cytokine response correlates with the magnitude of the antibody response, i.e. matrix 7.0.3 evoked the highest antigen-specific antibody response.

STIMULATION OF T-CELL CYTOKINES BY ISCOM AND MATRIX

Splenocytes from mice immunized with iscoms carrying influenza virus envelope proteins preferentially secrete IL-2 and IFNγ (Fossum et al, 1990, Villacres-Eriksson et al, 1992, Villacres-Eriksson, 1995). In this system, the capacity to secrete IL-4 was similar for splenocytes from mice primed either with iscoms or with protein micelles (Villacres-Eriksson, 1995), whereas the IL-10 response was clearly downregulated in mice primed with iscoms (Villacres-Eriksson, 1995) (Table 4). For recombinant EBV gp340 incorporated into iscoms, the IL-2 and IFNγ responses were enhanced, IL-10 was downregulated and IL-4 was undetectable (Dotsika et al, 1997). It was shown in this study that the cytokine response correlated with the dose of Quillaja adjuvant used for immunization. Proteins from a flagellar fraction of <u>Trypanosoma cruzi</u> incorporated in iscoms resulted in enhanced secretion of IL-2 and downregulation of IL-10, whereas IL-4 and IFNγ were undetectable. Common observations from these studies were the enhanced production of IL-2 and the diminished production of IL-10 after immunization with iscom-borne antigens.

Table 4. Summary of cytokine production by iscom-primed murine splenocytes

Iscoms carrying:	IL-2	IL-4	IL-10	IFNγ
Influenza virus glycoproteins	+	=	-	+
Recombinant EBV gp340	+	ud	-	+
<u>T. cruzi</u> - flagellar fraction	+	ud	-	ud

+, enhanced; -, diminished; =, not changed; ud, undetectable.

The influence of the intrinsic biological activity of the antigen on the capacity to secrete T-cell cytokines is reflected by the lack of IL-4 detected in splenocyte supernatants from mice immunized with <u>Trypanosoma cruzi</u> iscoms or EBV gp340 iscoms compared to those immunized with influenza virus iscoms. In spite of the enhanced IL-2 response, the <u>Trypanosoma cruzi</u> flagellar fraction iscoms do not elicit protective immunity in mice, which correlates with the lack of IFNγ production in splenocyte supernatants of immunized mice (Carlomagno et al, submitted). Interestingly, the <u>Trypanosoma cruzi</u> flagellar fraction contains a polypeptide component which is a potent inducer of TGFβ (Hansen et al, 1997 in press), again strongly indicating that the intrinsic activity of the protein antigen is a critical factor to consider in the design of efficient vaccines. These data also suggest that the modulatory effects of the adjuvant/immunomodulator are not neccessarily able to completely overrun the biological effects mediated by the protein antigen.

INTRACELLULAR DISTRIBUTION OF ISCOM-BORNE ANTIGENS

APC pulsed with biotinylated iscom-borne antigens were analyzed by immuno electron microscopy. Cells pulsed with influenza virus envelope proteins in iscoms presented a broad distribution of antigen, including labelling of the cell membrane, clear and dense vesicles, and scattered labelling of membrane-free intracellular space (Villacres-Eriksson et al, submitted). The results were confirmed by immunoassay of cell lysates after fractionation by differential centrifugation. These studies also showed that several APC populations such as peritoneal cells, splenic dendritic cells and splenic B cells take up antigens incorporated in iscoms with high efficiency. Iscoms carrying ovalbumin were internalized with a 50-fold lower efficiency compared to influenza virus iscoms, suggesting that the nature of the protein antigen influences the capacity of APC to take up iscoms. In conclusion, these studies provide evidence that antigens incorporated into iscoms indeed reach the cytosolic space in APC. Although more research is required for further elucidation of this mechanism, the electron microscopy analysis suggests that the bulk of iscom pulse is taken up by the endosomal route. After endosomic uptake the iscom may integrate into the endosomal membrane but also into the outer plasma membrane, exposing the antigen to both sides of the membrane. The access of iscom components, adjuvant and antigen, to the cytosol is likely to be a relevant factor influencing the immunoenhancing properties of the complexes. In this context, it is also possible that the stimulation of proinflammatory cytokines by iscoms and matrix results from the access of glycosylated triterpenoid adjuvant components to the cytosol.

FUTURE DIRECTIONS FOR THE ISCOM TECHNOLOGY

One major area for research is the development of iscoms as a delivery system for mucosal administration of various antigens. Ongoing experiments show that administration of iscoms intranasaly evoke strong antibody responses in the respiratory tract as well as at the remote mucosa of the genital tract.

REFERENCES

Araujo, F and Morein, B. 1991 Immunization with Trypanozoma cruzi epimastigote antigens incorporated into iscoms protects against lethal challenge in mice. Inf. Immun., 59, 2909.

Behboudi, S., Morein, B. and Villacres-Eriksson, M. 1996, In vitro activation of antigen-presenting cells (APC) by defined composition of Quillaja saponaria Molina triterpenoids. Clin. Exp. Immunol., 105, 26.

Behboudi, S., Morein, B. and Villacres-Eriksson, M. 1997, In vivo and in vitro induction of IL-6 by Quillaja saponaria Molina triterpenoid formulations. Cytokine, in press.

Ben Ahmeida, E.T.S., Jennings, R., Erturk, M., and Potter, C.W., 1992, The IgA and subclass IgG responses and protection in mice immunised with influenza antigens administered as iscoms, with FCA, ALH or as infectious virus, Arch Virol., 125:71.

Bergström-Mollaoglu, M., Lövgren, K., Åkerblom, L., Fossum, C.K. and Morein, B. 1992, Antigen-specific increases in the number of splenocytes expressing MHC class II molecules following restimulation with antigen in various physical forms. Scand.J. Immunol., 36, 565.

Carlomagno, M., Hansen, D., Åkerblom, L., Esteva, M.I., Villacres-Eriksson, M.,Segura, E., and Morein, B.

Stimulation of IL-2 by immunization without concominant stimulation of IFN-γ does not provide protection against Trypanosoma cruzi infection. Submitted Manuscript.

Carlson, U., Alenius, S., and Sudquist, B., 1991, Protective effect of an iscom bovine virus diarrhoea virus (BVDV) vaccine against an experimental BVDV infection in vaccinated and non-vaccinated pregnant ewes, Vaccine, 9:577.

De Vries, P., Van Binnendijk, R.S., Van der Marel, P., Van Wezel, A.L., Voorma, H.O., Sundquist, B., UytdeHaag, F.G.C.M. and Osterhaus, A.D.M.E., 1988a, Measles virus fusion protein presented in an immune stimulating complex (iscom) induces haemolysis- inhibiting and fusion inhibiting antibodies, virus-specific T cells and protection in mice. J. Gen. Virol., 69:549.

De Vries, P., UytdeHaag, F.G.C.M., and Osterhaus, A.D.M.E., 1988b, Canine distemper virus (CDV) immunestimulating complex (iscom), but not measles virus iscoms, protects dogs against CDV infection, J.Gen.Virol., 69:2071.

Dotsika, E., Karagouni, E., Sundquist, B., Morein, B., Morgan, A. and Villacres-Eriksson, M., 1997, Influence of Quillaja saponaria triterpenoid content on the immunomodulatory capacity of Epstein-Barr virus (EBV) iscoms. Scand.J.Immunol., 45:261.

Erturk, M., Jennings, R., Hockley, D., and Potter, C.W., 1989, Antibody response and protection in mice immunized with herpes simplex virus type I antigen immuno-stimulating complex preparations. J.Gen.Virol., 70:2149.

Erturk, M., Hill, T.J., Shimeld, C. and Jennings, R., 1992, Acute and latent infection of mice immunized with HSV-1 iscom vaccine. Arch. Virol., 125:87.

Fekadu, M., Shaddock, J.H., Ekström, J., Osterhaus, A.D.M.E., Sanderlin, D.W., Sundquist, B. and Morein, B. 1992, An immune stimulating complex subunit rabies virus vaccine protects mice and dogs against street rabies challenge, Vaccine, 10, 192.

Fossum, C., Bergström, M., Lövgren, K., Watson, D.L. and Morein, B. 1990, Effect of iscom and/or their adjuvant moiety (matrix) on the initial proliferation and IL-2 responses in vitro. Comparison of spleen cells from mice inoculated with iscoms and/or matrix. Cell. Immunol., 129, 414.

Gajewski, T.F., Renauld, J.C., Pel, A.V. and Boon, T. 1995, Costimulation with B7-1, IL-6 and IL-12 is sufficient for primary generation of murine antitumor cytolytic T lymphocytes in vitro. J. Immunol., 154, 5637.

Hansen, D., Villacres-Eriksson, M., Åkerblom, L., Hellman, U., Segura, E., Carlomagno, M. and Morein, B. 1997, An immunoaffinity purified Trypanosoma cruzi antigen supresses cellular proliferation through a TGF-β-mediated mechanism. Scand. J. Immunol., in press.

Jones, P.D., Tha Hla, R., Morein, B., Lövgren, K. and Ada, G.L., 1988, Cellular immune responses in the murine lung to local immunization with influenza A virus glycoproteins in micelles and immunostimulatory complexes (iscoms), Scand. J. Immunol., 27:645.

Jones, G.E., Jones, K.A., Machell, J., Brebner, J., Anderson, I.E. and How, S. 1995, Efficacy trials with tissue-culture grown, inactivated vaccines against chamydial abortion in sheep. Vaccine, 13, 715.

Lövgren, K. and Morein, B., 1988a. The requirement of lipids for the formation of immuno-stimulating complexes (iscoms). Biotechnol. Appl. Biochem., 10:161.

Lövgren, K. 1988b, The serum antibody response distributed in subclasses and isotypes after intranasal and subcutaneous immunization with influenza virus immunostimulating complexes. Scand. J. Immunol., 27:241.

Lövgren, K., Kåberg, H. and Morein, B., 1990, An experimental subunit vaccine (iscom) induced portective immunity to influenza virus infection in mice after a single intranasal administration. Clin. Exp. Immunol., 82:435.

Lövgren Bengtsson, K. and Sjölander, A. 1996, Adjuvant activities of iscoms and iscom matrix; two different formulations of Quillaja saponin and antigen. Vaccine, 14:753.

Lunden, A., Lövgren, K., Uggla, A. and Araujo, F.G. 1993, Immune response and resistance to Toxoplasma gondii in mice immunized with antigens of parasite incorporated into imunostimulating complexes. Infect. Immun., 6:2639.

Morein, B., Sundquist, B., Höglund, S., Dalsgaard, K. and Osterhaus, A., 1984. Iscom, a novel structure for antigenic presentation of membrane proteins from enveloped viruses . Nature, 308:457.

Morein, B., Lövgren, K., Rönnberg, B., Sjölander, A. and Villacres-Eriksson, M. 1995, Immunostimulating complex: Clinical potential in vaccine development. Clin. Immunother., 6 :461.

Morgan, A.J., Finerty, S., Lövgren, K., Scullion, F.T. and Morein, B. 1988, Protection of Epstein-Barr (EB) virus-induced lymphoma in cottontop tamarins by vaccinations with the EB virus envelope glycoprotein gp340 incorporated into immunostimulating complexes,J. Gen. virol., 69:2093.

Mowat, A.M., Donachie, A.M., Reid, G. and Jarret, O., 1991, Immune-stimulating complexes containing Quil A and protein antigen prime class I MHC restricted T lymphocytes in vivo and are immunogenic by the oral route, Immunology, 72: 317-322.

Mowat, A. M., Maloy, K. J., Donachie, A. M., 1993, Immune-stimulating complexes as adjuvants for inducing local and systemic immunity after oral imunization with protein antigen. Immunology, 80:527.

Nordengrahn, A., Rusvai, M., Merza, M., Ekström, J., Morein, B. and Belak, S., 1996, Equine herpes virus type 2 (EHV-2) as a predisposing factor for Rhodococcus equi pneumonia in foals: prevention of the bifactorial disease with EHV-2 immunostimulating complexes. Vet. Microbiol., 51:55.

Osterhaus, A.D.M.E., Weijer, K., UytdeHaage, F.G.C.M., Knell, P., Jarret, O., Sundquist, B., and Morein, B., 1985, Induction of protective immune response in cats by vaccination with feline leukaemia virus iscoms. J. Immunol., 135:591.

Osterhaus, A.D.M.E., Weijer, K., UytdeHaage, F.G.C.M., Knell, P., Jarret, O. and Morein, B., 1989, Serological response in cats vaccinated with FeLV iscom and an inactivated FeLV vaccine, Vaccine, 7:137.

Osterhaus, A.D.M.E., De Vries, P., and Heeney, J. 1992a, AIDS vaccine developments, Nature, 355:684.

Osterhaus, A.D.M.E., De Vries, P., Morein, B., Åkerblom, L. and Heeney, J. 1992b, Comparison of protection afforded by whole virus iscom versus MDP-adjuvanted formalin inactivated SIV vaccines from iv cell-free or cell associated homologous challenge, AIDS Res. Hum. Retroviruses, 8:1507.

Özel, M., Höglund, S., Gelderblom, H.R. and Morein, B., 1989. Quaternary structure of the immuno-stimulating complex (iscom). J. Ultrastructure Mol. Structure Res., 102:240.

Renauld, J. C., Vink, A. and Snick, J. 1989, Accessory signals in murine cytolytic T cell responses. Dual requirement for IL-1 and IL-6. J. Immunol., 15:143 (6) 1894.

Rönnberg, B., Fekadu, M. and Morein, B., 1995. Adjuvant activity of non toxic Quillaja saponaria Molina components for use in iscom-matrix. Vaccine, 13:1375

Sjölander, S., Hansen, J.E., Lövgren Bengtsson, K., Åkerblom, L. and Morein, B. 1996 Induction of homologous virus neutralizing antibodies in guinea-pigs immunized with two human immuno-deficiency virus type 1 glycoprotein gp 120-iscom preparations. A comparison with other adjuvant systems. Vaccine, 14:344.

Snodgrass, D.R., Campbell, I., Mwenda, J.M., Chege, G., Seleman, M.A., Morein, B., and Hart, C.A. 1995, Stimulation of rotavirus IgA, IgG and neutralising antibodies in baboon milk by parenteral vaccination. Vaccine, 13:408.

Sundquist, B., Lövgren,K., and Morein, B., 1988, Influenza virus iscoms: Antibody response in animals, Vaccine, 6:49.

Sundquist, B., Czifra, Gy. and Stipkovits, L. 1996, Protective immunity induced in chicken by a single immunization with mycoplasma gallisepticum immunostimulating complexes (ISCOMS). Vaccine, 9:892.

Takahashi, H., Takeshita, T., Morein, B., Putney, S., Germain, R.N. and Berzofsky, J.A., 1990, Induction of $CD8^+$ cytotoxic T cells by immunization with purified HIV-1 envelope protein in iscoms, Nature, 344:873.

Trudel, M., Nadon, F., Seguin, C., Boulay, G. and Lussier, G., 1987, Vaccination of rabbits with a bovine herpes type I subunit vaccine: Adjuvant effect of iscoms, Vaccine, 5:239.

Trudel, M., Boulay, G., Seguin, C., Nadon, F. and Lussier, G., 1988, Control of infectious bovine rhinotracheitis in calves with a BHV-1 subunit iscom vaccine, Vaccine, 5:525.

Trudel, M., Nadon, F., Seguin, C. and Brault, S., Lusignan, Y., and Lemieux, S., 1992, Initiation of cytotoxic T cell response and protection of BALB/c mice by vaccination with an experimental iscoms respiratory syncytial virus subunit vaccine. Vaccine, 10:107.

Tsuda, T., Sugimura, T. and Murakami, Y., 1991, Evaluation of glycoprotein gII iscom subunit vaccine for pseudorabies in pig. Vaccine, 9:648.

Van Binnendijk, R.S., Van Baalen, C.A., Poelen, M.C.M., De Vries, P., Boes, J., Cerundolo, V., Osterhaus, A.D.M.E. and UytdeHaag, F.G.C.M., 1992, Measles virus trans-membrane fusion protein synthesized de novo or presented in iscom is endogenously processed for HLA class I and class II restricted cytotoxic T cell recognition. J. Exp. Med., 176:119.

Villacres-Eriksson, M., Bergström-Mollaoglu, M., Kåberg, H. and Morein, B. 1992, Involvement of interleukin-2 and interferon-gamma in the immune response induced by influenza virus iscoms. Scand. J. Immunol., 36:421.

Villacres-Eriksson, M., Bergström-Mollaoglu, M., Kåberg, H., Lövgren, K. and Morein, B. 1993, The induction of cell-associated and secreted IL-1 by iscoms, matrix and micelles in murine splenic cells. Clin. Exp. Immunol., 93,120.

Villacres-Eriksson, M. 1995, Antigen presentation by naive macrophages, dendritic cells and B cells to primed T lymphocytes and their cytokine production following exposure to immunostimulating complexes. Clin. Exp. Immunol., 102:46.

Villacres-Eriksson, M., Behboudi, S., Morgan, A. J., Trinchieri, G., Morein, B. 1997, Immunomodulation by Quillaja saponaria adjuvant formulations: in vivo stimulation of interleukin-12 and its effects on the antibody response. Cytokine, 9:73.

Villacres-Eriksson, M., Nikkilä, T., Lövgren-Bengtsson, K. and Morein, B. Internalization of iscom-borne antigens and intracellular distribution in antigen-presenting cells. Submitted Manuscript.

Visser, I.K.G., Van de Bildt, M.W.G., Brugge, H.N., Reijnders, P.J.M., Vedder, E.J., Kuiper, J., De Vries, P., Groen, J., Walvoort, H.C., UytdeHaag, F.G.C.M., and Osterhaus, A.D.M.E., 1989, Vaccination of harbour seals (Phoca vitulina) against phocid distemper with two different inactivated canine distemper virus (CDV) vaccines, Vaccine, 7:521.

Watson, D.L., Watson, N.A., Fossum, C., Lövgren, K. and Morein, B. 1992, Interactions between immune-stimulating complexes (iscoms) and peritoneal mononuclear leucocytes. Microbiol. Immunol., 36: 119.

VACCINES AND VACCINE DELIVERY SYSTEMS: EXPERIENCE WITH HSV, INFLUENZA AND MUCOSAL ROUTES OF IMMUNISATION

R. Jennings, D. Ní Challanáin, H.O. Ghazi and C.S. McLean*

Department of Medical Microbiology, University of Sheffield Medical School, Beech Hill Road, Sheffield S10 2RX, *Cantab Pharmaceuticals Research Ltd., 184 Science Park, Milton Road, Cambridge CB4 4GN, UK

INTRODUCTION

The primary route of entry into the body for many viruses, including herpes simplex virus type 2 (HSV-2) and the influenza virus, is via mucosal surfaces. It follows that, depending on the numbers of virions deposited on such surfaces, their infectious quality and distribution over the mucosal surface, the existence or early mobilisation of specific defence mechanisms at the time of this contact, supplementing or enhancing any non-specific resistance mechanisms already operating at these sites may tip the balance in favour of the host and result in elimination of the invading virus before it can become established in the tissues and produce disease symptoms.

It is possible to envisage a number of specific immune defence factors operative in this initial viral contact with the host's mucosal surface. Secretory IgA (s-IgA) and IgG antibodies, the plasma cells producing these antibodies, cell cytotoxicity mediated by cytotoxic T lymphocytes (CTLs), and antibody-dependent cell cytotoxicity (ADCC), together with appropriate $CD4^+$ helper T lymphocytes (Th cells), may all, if present at the mucosal surface when this is impregnated with an invading virus, contribute to its elimination at this stage of infection. The realisation of the potential of these activities has resulted in considerable recent interest (McGhee and Kiyono, 1993; Walker, 1994) in defining procedures whereby such specific immune defences may most effectively be stimulated, and there have been many studies undertaken in recent years aimed at promoting these defences at mucosal surfaces through immunisation. For both HSV-2(Bowen et al, 1992; Byars et al, 1994; Gallichan and Rosenthal, 1995; Hazama et al, 1993; McBride et al, 1988;, McDermott et al, 1990; Thapar et al, 1990) and influenza viruses (Asanuma et al, 1995; de Haan et al, 1995; Ghazi et al, 1995b; Jones et al, 1988; Meitin et al, 1991; Moldoveanu et al, 1993; Pang et al, 1992) innumerable studies have explored both the route of immunisation and the nature and form of the immunising agent most effective in promoting immune defences, usually antibody, at the mucosal surface, and protecting against subsequent live challenge virus infection.

Although it is likely that more than one specific immune mechanism is active in protection against viral infections at mucosal surfaces, recent passive transfer studies have highlighted a role for local antibodies in both HSV-2 (Eis-Hubinger et al, 1993; Whaley et al, 1994) and influenza (Renegar and Small, 1991) infections. The paucity of information on the value of cellular immune responses to viral infections, especially the relative importance of effector CTL activity at the mucosal surface probably reflects the inherent difficulties in assessing such responses at these sites particularly with respect to HSV infections. However, specific CTLs at the intestinal mucosal surface have been reported following rotavirus infection in mice, and recent studies have indicated a long-lived CTL memory response specific for HSV glycoprotein B, in mucosal tissues providing the initial route of immunisation was also via the mucosal surface (Gallichan and Rosenthal, 1996; Offit and Dudzik, 1989).

The present work focuses on two major parameters influencing the immune responses at mucosal surfaces following vaccination, namely the immunising route used and the form of presentation of the viral antigen(s) to the immune system, employing two experimental animal model systems, the female guinea-pig for studies with HSV-2 and the mouse for studies involving the influenza virus.

IMMUNISATION OF THE FEMALE GUINEA-PIG WITH A DISABLED INFECTIOUS SINGLE CYCLE HSV-2 VIRUS VACCINE

It has been suggested that effective immunisation against virus diseases may best be achieved by use of live vaccines and it is possible to cite the live, attenuated poliovirus vaccine as an example of such a preparation that has, through its immunological success and widespread use, virtually eliminated the wild-type poliovirus from the Western World, although reversions to neurovirulence can (rarely) occur with poliovirus vaccine strains. However, by the application of modern molecular biology and genetic engineering techniques it is now possible to produce genetically-disabled viruses and the disabled, infectious single cycle (DISC) herpes

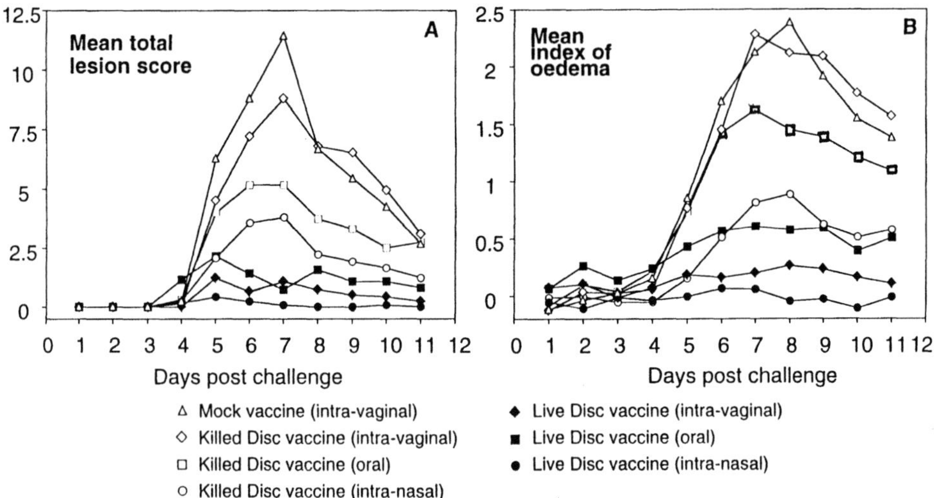

Figure 1. Mean total lesion score (A) and index of oedema (N), per day in groups of guinea-pigs immunised with live or killed DISC HSV-1 vaccine and subsequently challenged with HSV-2.

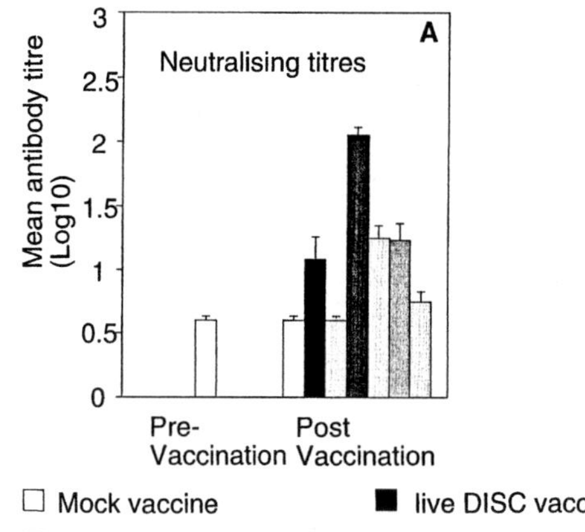

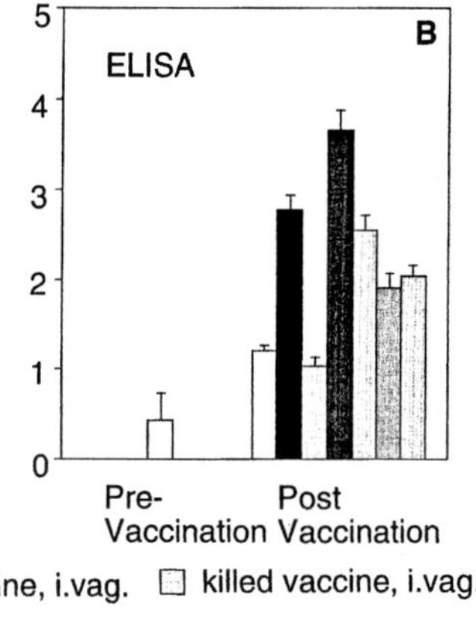

Figure 2. Neutralising (A) and ELISA (B) antibody titres against HSV-1 in sera pre- and post-vaccination of animals with live or killed DISC HSV-1 vaccine given by different routes.

simplex virus (Farrell et al, 1994) which lacks the coding potential for one of its essential glycoproteins (gH), can complete only one round of replication, and therefore lacks the ability to spread in the host, is the first such virus to be evaluated in humans as a vaccine. Extensive testing of DISC virus in mice and guinea-pigs (Farrell et al, 1994; McLean et al, 1994; McLean et al, 1996) has indicated that this virus provides effective protection against wild-type HSV challenge infection.

Furthermore, studies with HSV virus in the female guinea-pig model of genital herpes (Erturk et al, 1991; Thornton et al, 1984) have shown the influence of both the route of immunisation and the form of the virus (live or inactivated) in eliciting local, vaginal immune responses and protection against wild-type challenge infection. In the current work, using either inactivated or live DISC HSV-1 virus, groups of 12 female Dunkin-Hartley guinea-pigs were inoculated with two doses, 18 days apart, each of 8 x 10^6 pfu via one of three mucosal routes, intranasal (i.n.), intravaginal (i.vag.) or oral, while one further group received mock vaccine by the i.vag. route. Seventeen days following the second immunisation, all guinea-pigs were challenged i.vag. with $10^{5.2}$ pfu of HSV-2 (strain MS), and monitored for local, clinical disease over the subsequent 11 days. The results (Figure 1A and B), show that compared to the mock-immunised animals, and to a lesser extent to those given inactivated virus by the oral or i.vag. routes, guinea-pigs immunised with live DISC vaccine via the oral, i.vag. or i.n. routes were significantly more protected against HSV-2 challenge.

In addition, although the differences were not significant, the i.n. route of immunisation provided the greatest degree of protection against challenge when comparing the different routes used for administration of live DISC vaccine or inactiveted preparations separately (Figure A and B). These findings of a high level of protection against heterologous HSV-2 challenge infection following immunisation by the i.n. route with live DISC HSV-1, were accompanied by significantly higher NT and ELISA antibody levels in these animals compared to those recorded post-vaccination in animals immunised by i.vag. or oral routes or using inactivated DISC HSV-1 (Figure 2A and B).

In addition to the correlation observed between clinical symptoms and circulatory antibody levels to HSV-1 in guinea-pigs immunised with live DISC HSV-1 by the i.n. route,

Table 1. Post-Immunisation Levels of HSV-Specific IgG and IgA Antibodies in Guinea- pig Vaginal Washes Samples

Vaccine Preparation	Route of Inoculation	ELISA IgG Absorbance Values (Mean ± S.E.)	ELISA IgA Absorbance Values (Mean ± S.E.)
Mock	Intravaginal	0.06 (± 0.02)	0.01 (± 0.01)
Live DISC	Intravaginal	0.16 (± 0.07)	0.04 (± 0.04)
Killed DISC	Intravaginal	0.07 (± 0.04)	0.003 (±0.002)
Live DISC	Intranasal	0.64 (± 0.08)	0.12 (± 0.02)
Killed DISC	Intranasal	0.17 (± 0.05)	0.003 (± 0.01)
Live DISC	Oral	0.07 (± 0.02)	0.002 (± 0.02)
Killed DISC	Oral	0.09 (±0.03)	0.03 (± 0.02)

S.E. = Standard Error

a correlation was also noted between the IgG and IgA antibody levels detected in vaginal washes collected 15 days subsequent to the second immunisation with DISC HSV-1 (48 h prior to HSV-2 challenge infection), and clinical symptoms. Thus (Table 1), IgA was only detectable by ELISA in vaginal washings from guinea-pigs immunised with live DISC HSV-1 intranasally, while this same group also had significantly higher levels of vaginal IgG detectable by ELISA than all other groups (Table 1).

The above experiments were carried out using a heterologous system, immunisation using HSV-1 and challenge with HSV-2. In further experiments to evaluate both live DISC HSV vaccine and the optimum route of immunisation, the homologous system was employed to compare the i.vag. with the subcutaneous (s.c.) routes of immunisation. Figure 3 (A and B) shows that although a high level of protection against HSV-2 challenge was afforded to guinea-pigs immunised twice by the i.vag. route with live DISC HSV-2 vaccine preparation at a dosage of either $10^{6.0}$ or $10^{7.0}$ pfu, immunisation via the s.c. route with 2 x $10^{6.0}$ or 2 x $10^{7.0}$ live DISC HSV-2 completely eliminated disease symptoms on challenge of these animals with $10^{5.2}$ pfu of the MS strain of HSV-2 (Figure 3A and B).

There was also a marked reduction in challenge virus replication in those animals given $10^{6.0}$ or $10^{7.0}$ pfu of live DISC HSV-2 by the s.c. route compared to animals given mock vaccine (Figure 3D). In the former group, virus was cleared from the vagina to below detectable levels by day 5 post-infection, and the virus titres reduced by 100-fold from days 2 to 7 compared to the mock-immunised animals. Ten of twelve mock-immunised animals still showed vaginal virus presence on day 5, and virus did not become undetectable in this group until day 9 post-infection (Figure 3D). In contrast, immunisation with a similar dose regime of live DISC HSV-2 via the i.vag. route induced reductions of only about 10-fold in virus titre compared to the mock-vaccinated animals (Figure 3C).

IMMUNISATION OF MICE WITH INFLUENZA ISCOM VACCINE

It is increasingly being recognised that one of the most potent adjuvant/carriers for

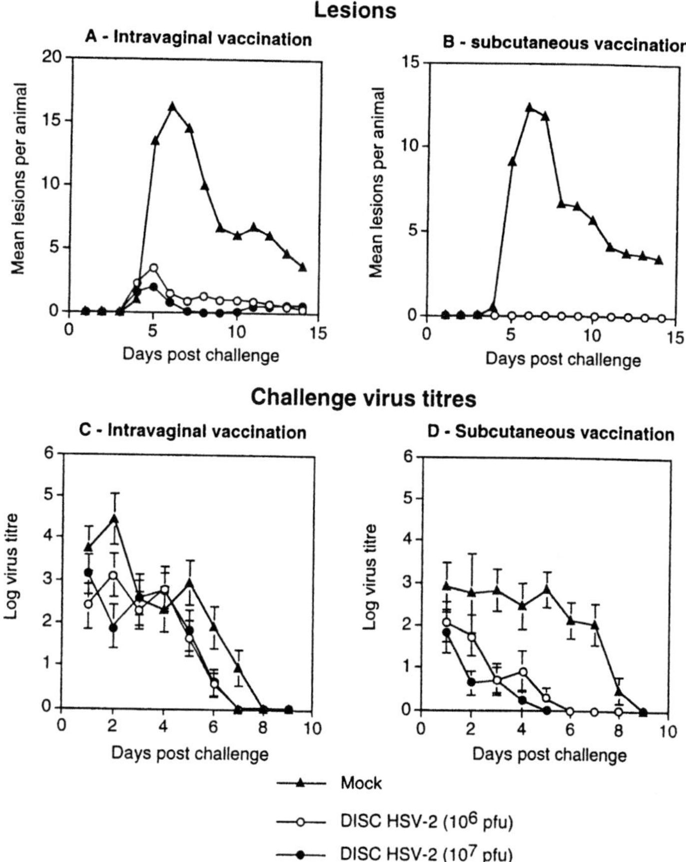

Figure 3. Effect of immunisation on HSV-2-induced primary disease. A and B, mean number of lesions per animal. C and D, mean titres of HSV-2 challenge virus. Animals were immunised intravaginally (A and C0 or subcutaneously (B and D) with 106 or 107 pfu of DISC HSV-2 vaccine or a mock preparation.

maximising the immune potential of microbial glycoproteins is the immunostimulatory complex or ISCOM, (Barr and Mitchell, 1996; Morein et al, 1984) and in a number of studies carried out in our laboratories using both influenza and herpes simplex virus antigens (Ben-Ahmeida et al, 1992; Ben-Ahmeida et al, 1993; Erturk et al, 1989; Erturk et al, 1991; Erturk et al, 1991; Erturk et al, 1992; Ghazi et al, 1995a; Hassan et al, 1996) several parameters, including route of immunisation, have been investigated to ascertain factors influencing ISCOM immunogenicity.

ISCOMs formulated with the influenza virus surface haemagglutinin (HA) and neuraminidase (NA) glycoproteins were assessed for their capability to induce immune responses and protection in mice following administration by either the oral or intramuscular (i.m.) routes.

Table 2 shows that seven weeks following immunisation with either one or two doses of an influenza ISCOM vaccine to mice by oral gavage, the levels of circulating antibody as measured by ELISA were considerably lower than those induced following immunisation using similar regimes, but employing the i.m. route. Indeed, the immune response following two doses of influenza A/Sichuan/2/87 subunit antigen ISCOMs administered orally was significantly lower than that elicited following a single dose given by the same route, and in addition lower than those levels achieved following two doses of A/Sichuan subunit antigen preparation given via the i.m. route (Table 2). From Table 2 it can also been seen that the protection afforded to mice against homologous influenza virus challenge, in terms of the incidence of virus recovery in nasal washings or lung suspensions collected three days after challenge infection, was lower in animals given two doses of influenza antigen ISCOMs by the oral route compared to those given two doses intramuscularly. However, this difference was not apparent seven weeks post-immunisation with one dose of vaccine (Table 2).

DISCUSSION AND CONCLUSIONS

It is possible to envisage that in response to deposition of a number of infectious virions on a mucosal surface, there will be a rapid mobilization of any available, specific defence mechanisms to supplement or combine with existing non-specific defences at the site of infection in the immunocompetent host. Classical immunological principles state that in responding to a second contact with the invading virus a higher and more rapid mobilization of these specific defences takes place than is seen following initial contact (Roitt et al, 1996). However, the availability of the mediators of specific defence mechanisms at the actual mucosal surface at the time of the infection, or the time lapsing before such specific defences reach the mucosal surface in a second contact with antigen, remains uncertain. Current theory hypothesizes that delivering viral antigens to a mucosal surface is likely to stimulate high, local immune responses, and that such responses will be relatively higher and able to access the local site more rapidly on subsequent contact with the viral antigen at that same site; such responses would be enhanced over those obtained under similar circumstances had the initial contact (immunisation) with antigen been via a non-mucosal route.

The work described in the present paper using experimental HSV-2 and influenza virus in vivo model systems, does not entirely support this hypothesis. Both HSV-2 and influenza viruses are natural pathogens at mucosal surfaces, yet administration of live DISC HSV-2

Table 2. Antibody Responses and Protection of Balb/c Mice Immunised by Oral or Intramuscular Routes with Influenza A/Sichuan ISCOM or Subunit Antigen Preparations

Antigen Preparation (0.25μg HA in 0.5ml)	Route of Inoculation	Seven Weeks Following One Immunisation				Seven Weeks Following Two Immunisations			
		No. of Mice	Mean ELISA Absorbance Values (SD)	No. of Infections after Challenge/Total		No. of Mice	Mean ELISA Absorbance Values (SD)	No. of Infections after Challenge/Total	
				Nasal Washes	Lung Suspensions			Nasal Washes	Lung Suspensions
A/Sichuan ISCOMS	Oral	5	1.59 (0.05)	2/5	0/5	12	0.84 (0.31)	3/9	2/9
A/Sichuan Subunits	Oral	4	0.48 (0.16)	3/4	2/4	10	0.75 (0.44)	5/8	3/8
A/Sichuan ISCOMs	I/M	5	2.15 (0.13)	2/5	0/5	10	2.62 (0.05)	0/9	0/9
A/Sichuan Subunits	I/M	4	1.37 (0.28)	2/4	1/4	10	2.00 (0.21)	4/8	2/8
PBS	I/M	5	0.16 (0.02)	5/5	5/5	5	0.28 (0.04)	5/5	5/5

PBS = phosphate buffered saline; I/M = 3 intramuscular; SD = standard deviation.

vaccine to guinea-pigs via the i.vag. route failed to induce as effective immune responses (data not shown) and protection against local, clinical HSV-2 disease or virus replication, as could be achieved following subcutaneous inoculation with the same preparation at an equivalent dosage. Using a subunit glycoprotein HSV-1 vaccine, other workers have reported similar results (Bowen et al, 1992). In addition, administration of live HSV-1 DISC vaccine to guinea-pigs by the i.n. route elicited superior local and systemic immune responses and levels of protection against clinical disease following i.vag. HSV-2 challenge infection (although not inducing better protection against virus growth), than was observed following equivalent doses of the same preparation via the i.vag. (or oral) routes. Similarly, the current studies show that immunisation of mice via the oral route induces lower immune humoral responses and less effective protection against viral replication following mucosal surface challenge than when the influenza ISCOM vaccine is given via the i.m. route.

These results must pose questions as to the value of mucosal administration of viral antigens in inducing the required level and form of specific immunity to combat a subsequent viral infection at these sites. While it is accepted that immunisation via the oral route may represent a special case involving acidic and proteolytic barriers (Walker, 1994) oral tolerance (Mowat, 1987), preferential induction of Th-2 lymphocyte responses (McGhee and Kiyono, 1993) and the requirement for high or repeated dosages of antigen (Farag et al, 1988; Mowat et al, 1991; Mowat et al, 1993), the relatively poor performance of different forms of vaccines, discussed in this paper when administered via mucosal routes in in vivo systems raises concern regarding the validity of this approach. Furthermore, although i.n. inoculation of mice with influenza virus vaccines was not carried out in the present studies, other workers (Meitin et al, 1991) have reported that inactivated influenza virus given parenterally induces high circulating IgG antibodies together with protection of mouse lungs, but not murine nasal passages, against homologous influenza virus challenge infection. In contrast, i.n. immunisation using a vaccinia virus recombinant containing the influenza HA gene protected murine nasal passages but not lungs (Meitin et al, 1991).

The work reported here suggests that high levels of protection may be achieved at mucosal surfaces following parenteral immunisation.

REFERENCES

Asanuma, H., Koide, F., Suzuki, Y., Nagamine, T., Aizawa, C., Kurata, T and Tamura, S., 1995,Cross-protection against influenza virus infection in mice vaccinated by combined nasal/subcutaneous administration. Vaccine, 13, 3.

Barr, I.G. and Mitchell, G.F., 1996, ISCOMs (immunostimulating complexes): The first decade. Immunology and Cell Biology, 74, 8.

Ben-Ahmeida, E.T.S., Jennings, R., Erturk, M. and Potter, C.W., 1992, The IgA and subclass IgG responses and protection in mice immunised with influenza antigens administered as ISCOMs, with FCA, ALH or as infectious virus. Archives of Virology, 125, 71.

Ben-Ahmeida, E.T.S., Gregoriadis, G., Potter, C.W. and Jennings, R., 1993, Immuno-potentiation of local and systemic humoral immune responses by ISCOMs, liposomes and FCA: role in protection against influenza A in mice. Vaccine, 11, 1302.

Bowen, J.C., Alpar, H.O., Phillpotts, R. and Brown, M.R.W., 1992, Mucosal delivery of herpes simplex virus vaccine. Research in Virology, 143, 269.

Byars, N.E., Fraser-Smith, E.B., Pecyk, R.A., 1994, Vaccinating guinea-pigs with recombinant glycoprotein D of herpes simplex virus in an efficacious adjuvant formulation elicits protection against vaginal infection. Vaccine, 12, 200.

de Haan, A., Renegar, K.B., Small, P.A. Jr. and Wilschutt, J., 1995, Induction of a secretory IgA response in the murine female urogenital tract by immunisation of the lungs with liposome-supplemented viral subunit antigen.Vaccine, 13, 613.

Eis-Hubinger, A.M., Schmidt, D.S. and Schneweis, K.E., 1993, Anti-glycoprotein B mono-clonal antibody protects T-cell depleted mice against herpes simplex virus infection by inhibition of virus replication at the inoculated mucous membranes. Journal of General Virology, 74, 379-385.

Erturk, M., Jennings, R., Hockley, D. and Potter, C.W., 1989, Antibody responses and protection in mice immunised with herpes simplex type 1 antigen immune-stimulating complex preparations. Journal of General Virology, 70, 2149.

Erturk, M., Jennings, R., Phillpotts, R.J. and Potter, C.W., 1991, Biochemical characterisation of herpes simplex type 1 immunostimulating complexes (ISCOMs): A multiglyco- protein structure. Vaccine, 9, 668.

Erturk, M., Phillpotts, R.J. Welch, M.J. and Jennings, R., 1991, Efficacy of HSV-ISCOM vaccine in the guinea- pig model of HSV-2 infection. Vaccine, 9, 728.

Erturk, M., Hill, T.J., Shimeld, C. and Jennings, R., 1992, Acute and latent infection of mice immunised with HSV-1 ISCOM vaccine. Archives of Virology, 125, 87.

Farag, I.F., Phili, R.W., Rosborough, J.P. and Six, H.R., 1988, Immunogenicity and efficacy of orally administered inactivated influenza virus vaccine in mice. Vaccine, 6, 262.

Farrell, H., McLean, C.S., Harley, C., Efstathiou, S., Inglis, S.C. and Minson, A.C., 1994,Vaccine potential of a herpes simplex virus type 1 mutant with an essential glyco- protein deleted. Journal of Virology, 68, 927.

Gallichan, W.S. and Rosenthal, K.L., 1995, Specific secretory immune responses in the female genital tract following intranasal immunisation with a recombinant adenovirus expressing glycoprotein B of herpes simplex virus. Vaccine, 13,1589.

Gallichan, W.S. and Rosenthal, K.L., 1996, Long-lived cytotoxic T lymphocyte memory in mucosal tissues after mucosal but not systemic immunisation. Journal of Experimental Medicine, 184, 1879.

Ghazi, H.O., Potter, C.W., Smith, T.L. and Jennings, R., 1995a, Comparative antibody responses and protection in mice immunised by oral or parenteral routes with influenza virus subunit antigens in aqueous form or incorporated into ISCOMs. Journal of Medical Microbiology, 42, 53.

Ghazi, H.O., Erturk, M., Stannard, L.M., Faulkner, M., Potter, C.W. and Jennings, R., 1995b, Immunogenicity of influenza and HSV-1 mixed antigen ISCOMs in mice. Archives of Virology, 140, 1015.

Hassan, Y., Brewer, J.M., Alexander, J. and Jennings, R., 1996, Immune responses in mice induced by HSV-1glycoprotein presented with ISCOMs or NISV delivery systems. Vaccine, In press.

Hazama, M., Mayumi-Aono, A., Miyazaki, T., Hinuma, S. and Fujisawa, Y., 1993, Intranasal immunisation against herpes simplex virus infection by using a recombinant glyco- protein D fused with immuno-modulating proteins, the B subunit of Escherichia coli heat-labile enterotoxin and interleukin-2. Immunology, 78, 643.

Jones, P.D., Tha-Hla, R., Morein, B., Lovgren, K. and Ada, G.L., 1988, Cellular immune responses in the murine lung to local immunisation with influenza A virus glyco- proteins in micelles and immuno-stimulatory complexes. Scandinavian Journal of Immunology, 27, 645.

McBride, B.W., Ridgeway, P., Phillpotts, R. and Newell, D.G., 1988, Mucosal antibody response to vaginal infection with herpes simplex virus in pre-vaccinated guinea-pigs. Vaccine, 6, 414.

McDermott, M.R., Brais, L.J and Evelegh, M.J., 1990, Mucosal and systemic antiviral antibodies in mice inoculated intravaginally with herpes simplex virus type 2. Journal of General Virology, 71, 1497.

McGhee, J.R. and Kiyono, H., 1993, New perspectives in vaccine development: Mucosal immunity to infections. Infectious Agents and Disease, 2, 55.

McLean, C.S., Erturk, M., Jennings, R., Ni Challanain, D., Minson, A.C., Duncan, I. Bournsell, M.E.G. and Inglis, S.C., 1994, Protective vaccination against primary and recurrent disease caused by herpes simplex virus (HSV) type 2 using a genetically disabled HSV-1. Journal of Infectious Diseases, 170,100.

McLean, C.S., Ni Challanain, D., Duncan, I., Bournsell, M.E.G., Jennings, R. and Inglis, S.C., 1996, Induction of a protective immune response by mucosal immunisation with a DISC HSV-1 vaccine. Vaccine, 14, 987.

Meitin, C.A., Bender, B.S. and Small, P.A. Jr., 1991, Influenza immunisation: intranasal live vaccinia recombinant contrasted with parenteral inactivated vaccine. Vaccine, 9, 751.

Moldoveanu, Z., Novak, M., Huang, W-Q, Gilley, R.M., Staas, J.K., Schafer,D., Compans, R.W. and Mestecky, J., 1993, Oral immunisation with influenza virus in biodegradable microspheres. Journal of Infectious Diseases, 167, 84.

Moldoveanu, Z., Clements, M.L., Prince, S.J., Murphy, B.R. and Mestecky, J., 1995, Human immune responses to influenza virus vaccines administered by systemic or mucosal routes. Vaccine, 13, 1006.

Morein, B., Sundquist, B., Hoglund, S., Dalsgaard, K. and Osterhaus, A., 1984, ISCOM, a novel structure for antigenic presentation of membrane proteins from enveloped viruses. Nature, 308, 457.

Mowat, A. McI., 1987, The regulation of immune responses to dietary protein antigens. Immunology Today, 8, 93.

Mowat, A.McI., Donachie, A.M., Reid, G. and Jarrett, O., 1991, Immune-stimulating complexes containing Quil A and protein antigen prime class I MHC-restricted T lymphocytes in vivo and are immunogenic by the oral route. Immunology, 72, 317.

Mowat, A.McI., Maloy, K.J. and Donachie, A.M., 1993, Immune stimulating complexes (ISCOMs) are unique adjuvants for oral immunisation with protein antigens. Immunology, 80, 661.

Offit, P.A. and Dudzik, K.I., 1989, Rotavirus-specific cytotoxic T lymphocytes appear at the intestinal mucosal surface after rotavirus infection. Journal of Virology, 63, 3507.

Pang, G.T., Clancy, R.L., O'Reilly, S.E. and Cripps, A.W., 1992, A novel particulate influenza vaccine induces long-term and broad-based immunity in mice after oral immunisation. Journal of Virology, 66, 1162.

Renegar, K.B. and Small, P.A. Jr., 1991, Passive transfer of local immunity to influenza virus infections by IgA antibody. Journal of Immunology, 146, 1972.

Roitt, I., Brostoff, J. and Male, D., eds., 1996, Vaccination, In: "Immunology", Chapter 19; p.191. 4th Edition, Published by Mosby.

Thapar, M.A., Parr, E.L. and Parr, M.B., 1990, The effect of adjuvants on antibody titres in mouse vaginal fluid after intravaginal immunisation. Journal of Reproductive Immunology, 17, 207.

Thornton, B., Baskerville, A., Bailey, N.E., Melling, J.M. and Hambleton, P., 1984, Herpes simplex virus genital infection of the female guinea-pig as a model for evaluation of an experimental vaccine. Vaccine, 2, 141.

Walker, R.L., 1994, New strategies for using mucosal vaccination to achieve more effective immunisation. Vaccine, 12, 387.

Whaley, K.J., Zeitlin, L., Barratt, R.A., Hoen, T.E. and Cone, R.A., 1994, Passive immunisation of the vagina protects mice against vaginal transmission of genital herpes infections. Journal of Infectious Diseases, 169, 647.

ACTIVE IMMUNOTHERAPY FOR SOLID TUMOURS

A. Maraveyas and A.G. Dalgleish

Division of Oncology, St George's Hospital Medical School
Cranmer Terrace, London SW17 0RE, UK

INTRODUCTION

Although the concept of treating human cancer with vaccines has been explored for several decades, it is only in the last 10-15 years that a concerted effort has started to be made to prove or disprove the possibility that "therapeutic vaccines" may have more than just anecdotal efficacy against cancer. The recognition that the immune system could be stimulated into rejecting established tumour came from the work of Coley (1893/1894) who refined earlier observations of a number of workers, such as Fehleisen (1882) and Bruns (1887-1888), that infectious empyemas occasionally led to the resolution of an established tumour. This led him to develop a heat-killed pool of bacteria that came to be known as Coley's toxins. Therapy with tumour cell vaccines per se was first described in 1902 by von Leyden and Blumenthal (1902). From the start however similar procedures were to yield conflicting results at the hands of different researchers; for example Coca and colleagues reported tumour regression in some patients while Risley found no response in his cancer patients using Coca's "vaccine emulsion" (Coca et al, 1912; Coca and Gilman, 1909; Risley, 1911). Both researchers administered autologous or allogeneic tumour cell extracts at 14 day intervals. Experimentation continued for example with intraperitoneal administration of tumour extracts by Vaughan (1914) or the investigation of combination treatments with radiotherapy by Graham and Graham (1962) who reported that the administration of a tumour cell vaccine to patients from whom tumour had been removed appeared to radiosensitize the residual disease. These therapeutic "blends" with or without live bacteria fell into disuse and disrepute following the discovery of mustard based chemotherapy and radiotherapy which became popular after the 2nd world war. Cause and effect in the form of dose response were easier concepts to transfer to the clinic, due to the fact that pharmacokinetic, pharmacodynamic and response end-points could be measured. Nevertheless, the work of these early pioneers helped establish the basic principles of immunotherapy such as the need for minimal residual disease and the need for an immune response from the host.

Several observations support the potential value of active specific immunotherapy for the treatment of cancer including (1) vaccine-induced immunity against cancer in animal models, (2) the regression and eradication of tumours injected directly with immuno-stimulants, (3)

Vaccine Design: The Role of Cytokine Networks
Edited by Gregoriadis *et al.*, Plenum Press, New York, 1997

occasional regression of non-injected tumours after the intralesional injection of bacillus Calmette-Guerin (BCG) mostly noted in melanoma, a tumour where spontaneous regression is a well described phenomenon (Morton et al. 1974) and 4) the development of anti-tumour antibodies by the host (Livingstone, 1993a).

The continuing disparity between promising therapeutic results in animal models and the lack of efficacy in the clinic does not only afflict vaccine treatments but many other forms of cancer treatments. On the one hand transition of cytotoxic treatments, based on the ability of chemotoxic agents or high dose radiotherapy to kill cells and eradicate tumours also, from animals to human studies has been relatively successful. On the other hand however, understanding the more complex pathways such as blocking drug resistance, gene products or channels (i.e.cyclosporine), modifying tumour blood flow and tumour cell oxygenation and achieving directed meaningful immunostimulation or immunosuppression have been less reliable. Moreover the general scepticism of the scientific community and that of the traditional cancer therapists have not helped in tumour immunology and therapeutic vaccines achieving a more widespread research base. Nevertheless, our increasing ability to dissect the immune response both in vitro and in vivo in the clinic is now generating a new interest in the concept of using immunotherapy to achieve surrogate endpoints (measurable) i.e. a Th1 or a DTH response and then correlating this with a clinical response. The clinical responses of some cancer types to cytokines, such as IFN and IL-2 has led to a greater interest in this field with the re-emergence of cancer immunotherapy and cancer vaccines in particular. The pervading feeling of the researchers in the field at the present time is that minimal residual disease is and should remain, the primary target for these treatments.

Prior to the development of what now is coined active specific immunotherapy a large number of molecules including BCG have been used as non-specific immuno-stimulants which despite early promise have now mostly been abandoned as single agents (Table 1). They do however appear as adjuvants in composite "specific" vaccines as will be reviewed later.

The recognised goals of active immunotherapy with cancer vaccines are 1) to overcome the immunosuppression produced by tumour derived factors/milieu 2) to stimulate specific/selective immunological processes (e.g. T-cell, antibody response or NK-cell response) that will destroy tumour cells and 3) to focus the immune response against antigens born by the host's tumour by enhancing the immunogenicity/ presentation of relevant tumour-associated antigens. This review will centre on the concepts of immunostimulation through active specific immunotherapy as designed and used at present and then the evidence of clinical efficacy or otherwise against solid tumours will be summarised.

ADJUVANTS

Although currently a number of therapeutic vaccines have been developed and it is clearly not possible to discuss the rationale of each and every one, the majority contain an immunostimulatory/immunopotentiating component (adjuvant) combined with an antigen in the hope of inducing an immune response against the host's tumour.

Immunostimulation - adjuvants/immunopotentiators

Repeated efforts have been made to increase the immunogenicity of tumour vaccines by adding an adjuvant. Adjuvants used in clinical trials have included live vaccinia virus, Salmonella extracts, viable BCG and BCG derivatives such as cell wall cytoskeleton, trehalose dimycolate, muramyl dipeptide and glycolipids (Table 1). Data obtained in clinical trials and in animal models (Hanna et al. 1991) underline the importance of the ratio of tumour cells to

Table 1. Non-specific host defences stimulants

CATEGORY	EXAMPLE	NOTES
Intact micro-organisms	Viable: BCG Viable incativated: OK-432 (Picibanil). Non-viable: C. *parvum*	
Microbial cell wall	BCG cell-wall skeleton. *Nocardia* cell-wall skeleton. Methanol extraction residue of BCG.	
Glucans	Glucan (yeast) and fungal derivatives.	Reported as effective in Japan. Not pursued by others.
Protein-bound polysaccharide	PSK (Krestin) (fungal).	
Microbial glycopriteins	*Klebsiella* glycopritein (Biostim).	
Purified or synthetic components	Peptidoglycans. Muramyl dipeptide (MDP). MDP derivatives of BCG Trehalose dimycolate (P_3). Endotoxins (lipopolysaccharide) to reduce systemic modified endotoxins (detoxified) toxicity.	 Active component. Used in liposomes.
Interferon inducers polynucleotides	Poly IC. } Poly IC-LC. } Poly AU. }	Early promise.
Pyran copolymers.	Ampligen. } MVE-2. }	Not confirmed.
Low molecular weight inducers.	Prymidinones (ABPP, AIPP).	

adjuvant as well as the sequence and site of administration of the tumour cell preparation and the adjuvant.

Protein adjuvants

Addition of a highly antigenic carrier protein to an otherwise nonantigenic substance can often evoke an immune response. The antibodies formed against the complex are specifically directed against the previously nonantigenic substance as well as against the foreign protein in the complex. Early reports using rabbit gamma globulin attached to proteins of autologous tumour cells reported some therapeutic benefit (Cunningham et al, 1969; Czajkowski et al, 1967) but the efficacy of this type of treatment has not been confirmed.

Viral adjuvants

There is convincing evidence in animal models that infection of tumour cells with viruses augments the immunogenicity of tumour antigens (Cassel et al. 1983; Wallack and Michaelides

1984). Based on animal models, randomised clinical trials have been undertaken with viral oncolysates allogeneic or autologous tumour cells infected with Newcastle disease virus, vesicular stomatitis virus (Livingstone et al. 1985) and vaccinia virus in patients with melanoma and osteosarcoma.

Bacterial adjuvants

Immunologic adjuvants such as BCG (Morton et al. 1992), extract from Salmonella Minnesota (Livingstone et al. 1987), C. parvum (Livingstone et al. 1985), methanol extractable residue of the tubercle bacillus (Mitchell et al. 1988) and Freund's complete adjuvant (Hollinshead et al. 1982) are potent immunostimulants in animal systems capable of enhancing the humoral and cellular immune response to a variety of antigens.

Chemical adjuvants

Tumour associated differentiating antigens (TADA) in human tumour cells can also be modified in a variety of ways by chemicals such as iodoacetate and cholesteryl hemisuccinate, which increase the immunogenicity of tumour cells (Seigler et al. 1972). Certain enzymes such as neuraminidase, enhance the immunoresponse to neoplasms by chemically altering the surface glyco-conjugates (Simmons and Rios 1971). Repeated intradermal immunisation with neuraminidase-treated allogeneic acute myeloid leukemic cells prolonged disease-free survival in patients treated with chemotherapy.

IMMUNOFOCUSING MOLECULES (TUMOUR ANTIGENS)

The main problem in designing tumour antigen vaccines is to identify tumour antigens that are truly tumour specific and also immunogenic. Although tumour cells do express potentially immunogenic molecules these are often found in normal tissues at much lower concentrations therefore they are commonly referred to as tumour associated antigens (TADAs). TADAs can be broadly grouped into four categories. The first includes oncofetal antigens that are not expressed by any normal tissues but may be expressed on fetal tissues at some point of embryonic development (Carney, 1988) a classical example of which is alpha-fetoprotein. A second group of TADAs include neoantigens that are usually not expressed by the normal cells from which the cancer cells are derived, but that can be found in other normal tissues e.g. the human melanoma associated ganglioside GD2, which is expressed on the surface of human melanomas but not normal melanocytes, can be found in human brain and spinal cord (Volk et al. 1975). The third group consists of cell surface molecules that are commonly abundant but have antigenic epitopes "unmasked" due to aberrant metabolism of the tumour cell, e.g. core protein of regular mucins (Burchell et al. 1989; Gendler et al. 1988). Finally, a small group of antigens appear to be tumour specific antigens in that they are not found in normal adult or foetal tissues an example of which is the truncated c-erb-b3 receptor on glioblastomas (Hills et al. 1995). Under appropriate conditions, antigens of all three groups can serve as targets for active immunotherapy with cancer vaccines. If one assumes sequential steps in tumourigenesis, it is very likely that during the cell's life-events, leading to the completely transformed immortal cell with malignant potential, novel mutated proteins/ products of mutated genes will be expressed (Vogelstein et al. 1988).

TUMOUR ASSOCIATED IMMUNOSUPPRESSION

The question remains of how immunosurveillance is evaded. A number of theories have been advanced and experimental evidence exists pointing to many mechanisms being operative.

(a) Heterogeneity enables subsets of the tumour cell population to evade the host's immune response as well as to resist chemical, physical and biological therapies (Heppner, 1984; Nowell, 1986).Melanoma ganglioside profile changes in parallel with the increase in radial dimension of the tumour (Ravindranath and Irie, 1988). This is consistent with the possibility that antigenic variants are being selected for their ability to escape from immune surveillance.

(b) The density of the antigen on a cell may be lower than a threshold level required for recognition by the immune system (Welt et al. 1987). The pattern of a surface distribution of the antigen may differ between normal and tumour cells. Sialylated TADAs are only weakly immunogenic. Removal of sialic acid with neuraminidase can enhance immune recognition and tumour cell destruction (Takita et al. 1978).

(c) The host immune system may be overwhelmed by an overload of continuously shed TADAs with a net result of induction of tolerance. This would be proportionate to the tumour's size offering one explanation of the progressive deterioration of the immune status of the host with progression of the cancer (Herlyn et al. 1985). Such suppression may be reversed by removing the growing neoplasm. It has also been shown that circulating TADA-antibody complexes may reduce the ability of circulating antibodies to mediate complement dependant ADCC (Gupta et al. 1979).

(d) T-cells can be stimulated only if they encounter the relevant antigen presented by APC's. Activated T-cells can home in on cancer cells only if expression of MHC-I on the tumour cells is present. Furthermore the expression of co-stimulatory molecules such as B7 is mandatory for T-cell activation (Townsend et al. 1993). Many tumour cells evolve into states where these molecules are either deficient or non-existent (Freeman et al. 1993). It is thought that this immunoselection occurs from the continuing pressure of an initially immunocompetent host defence. One of the most common findings is a defect in the β2-microglobulin or TAP gene. Of great interest also is the observation that if antigen is presented without the co-stimulatory molecules a state of anergy can be induced, reviewed by Dalgleish (1996).

(e) Humoral effects of tumour milieu on the T-cell population; tumour infiltrating lymphocytes proliferate less readily in response to IL-2 or mitogens, yet CD4 T-cells are more abundant in TIL subpopulations possibly furthering immunosuppression through propagation of local Th2 response cytokines. Cell-suspensions from melanomas derived from patients have been shown to manufacture immunosuppressant cytokines e.g IL-10 (Sato et al. 1996). Even more interestingly VEGF (Gabrilovich et al. 1996) a growth factor ubiquitously expressed by cancer cells has been shown to have a profound immunosuppressant effect on APC's, perturbing adequate antigen presentation.

(f) Ability of tumours to induce apoptosis of activated T-cells through a FasL-Fas mediated pathway was recently demonstrated in metastatic melanoma (Hahne et al 1996). The interesting finding was that the melanoma cells had lost expression of the Fas receptor and consequently were protected from apoptosis through this mechanism.

Although some characterisation of the immunosuppressive substances produced by tumours has taken place the evidence points to a multitude of mechanisms many of which are still to be clarified, working both at the level of the tumour milieu and at the level of the hosts immune system. These processes are not mutually exclusive and probably operate at one time or another as the tumour progresses through the different stages.

STRATEGIES IN DESIGNING VACCINES

Choice of the appropriate antigen is crucially important. Unfortunately the procedures are empirical, subject to the bias of each researcher and to date only anecdotally effective. On the one hand there is the clean-cut approach of using a purified antigenic tumour peptide for example. This is scientifically optimal, as it is much easier to control and standardise and decreases the worrying aspect of introducing a multitude of unknown latent harmful molecules into the host, and would potentially circumvent, in the long term, many of the licensing/ethical issues that may be associated with cellular approaches. However this does not cater for the well known tumour-antigen heterogeneity and host variability. It is highly unlikely that all remaining tumour cells even following maximal debulking will be even remotely antigenically similar and will express the necessary peptide in a relevant conformation for such an approach to be effective. However proponents of peptide vaccine strategies believe that a carefully selected peptide cocktail relevant for the host's HLA profile should not suffer from such a drawback. The argument is mathematical; selection through CTL pressure against a given antigen is thought to lead to the emergence of an antigen-loss variant cell population at the level of the genome. If CTL pressure is raised simultaneously against many unconnected melanoma antigens on the same tumour cell, an escape variant would have to lose or dampen the expression of several independent genes simultaneously. If one reasons with data from immunoselection experiments in vitro where antigen-loss variants for a single gene arise at a frequency of about 10^{-7}, one double loss variant would be present among 10^{14} tumour cells. This corresponds to a tumour burden of 100 kg (Coulie, 1996). This line of reasoning however obviously assumes competent MHC molecules and disregards evidence that a first genetic event may induce genomic instability and precipitate further mutations at accelerated rates.

Another approach is to administer a multi-immunogenic cell line or a mixture of cell lines which may be more likely to succeed but also involves the above initiators. It also generates the further issue of whether to use allogeneic, autologous or even xenogeneic challenges for maximal effect.

COMPARING AUTOLOGOUS AND ALLOGENEIC VACCINES

Autologous cells can be used in two ways: either a cell line can be raised from excised tissue or a cell suspension can be reintroduced into the host with the appropriate adjuvant. Since autologous tumour cells express the same blood group and histocompatibility antigens as the host, they are considered ideal for tumour cell vaccines. However, the availability of autologous tumour tissue is limited and hence the amount of vaccine and thus, the number of immunizations possible is restricted. Moreover, antigen expression may vary from site to site and a vaccine prepared from autologous cells isolated from any particular nodules may not have the same TADA profile as tumour at another metastatic site. Cell line production is also fraught with problems e.g. infection of cultures, failure of cultures, lengthy procedure and culturing a dominant clone that isn't representative of the actual initial tumour.

Allogeneic tumour cell cultures can provide a sufficient number of cells for multiple injections. Mixtures of cells from different tumours can provide a spectrum of TADAs. Similarly however, passage of tumour cells in culture may introduce contaminants and favour the growth of subpopulations that diverge from the antigenic phenotype of the original cancer. Tumour cells grown in culture may also undergo antigenic alterations similar to those documented for ganglioside profiles of human melanoma and glioma. In some cases, these alterations have been used to advantage by mixing different cell lines with increased TADA expression to prepare allogeneic tumour cell vaccines.

CLINICAL TRIALS OF ACTIVE SPECIFIC IMMUNOTHERAPY IN CANCER

A massive amount of research has been invested in melanoma immunotherapy. This stems from the early observations on the pathology of melanoma by Handley (1907) which established this tumour as the archetype of an immune-dependant tumour. It is not therefore by chance that more tumour-associated antigens have been detected for melanoma than for any other tumour and that more immunotherapy strategies have been employed to treat melanoma than all the other tumour types put together. The uniquely variable clinical course of this malignancy (Bodenham, 1968) both entices further research but also draws criticism of achieved clinical results. The work by Morton et al (1974) who studied a non-specific immunotherapy protocol using BCG intralesionally, rekindled interest in this field; they demonstrated complete regression of metastatic tumour nodules after intralesional injection of BCG in 90% of 184 melanoma metastases in 8 patients. Many subsequent clinical trials confirmed this observation. Earlier work (Finney et al. 1960) had demonstrated at least antibody responses in patients with a variety of malignant tumours where tumour cell antigens were administered as a tumour cell homogenate admixed with complete Freund's adjuvant intramuscularly. The stage for specific immunotherapy vaccines was set. It is therefore appropriate to look more closely at the evidence from existing specific immunotherapy in melanoma before reviewing the state of experience with the other solid malignancies.

Malignant Melanoma

There is intense debate between researchers advocating a whole living cell vaccine and those who advocate highly purified tumour antigens and/or peptides. There is no evidence from any randomised trial to indicate that either of these procedures is superior. Most of the existing evidence is based on Phase II trials comparing achieved results to historical controls. Scepticism is compounded by the experience of two extremely promising vaccine procedures having failed to exhibit efficacy in Phase III studies (Helling et al. 1994; Livingstone et al. 1987; Wallack et al. 1986; Wallack et al. 1995) or by the fact that very promising results (Morton et al. 1992; Morton et al. 1993) have yet to be put through the rigorous test of a Phase III randomised trial.

Cell-based Vaccines

Autologous cell vaccines. Several trials using unmodified autologous melanoma cells have been reported. Cells were administered ± BCG adjuvant and some modification procedures of the tumour cells or host were also variably undertaken e.g. treatment of cells with neuraminidase or cholesterol enrichment procedures. Results from these trials have not been promising enough for any Phase III study to be justified (Ikonopisov et al. 1970; Oettgen et al. 1991; Oettgen and Old 1991; Seigler et al. 1972; Van Den Brenk, 1969)

Hapten-attached cell vaccines. Based on the understanding that a strong T-cell response to adjuvant/hapten modified antigen may be accompanied by a response to unmodified antigen which otherwise would not have arisen researchers have attached hapten (DNP) to autologous melanoma cells (Berd et al. 1986; Berd et al. 1990; Berd and Mastrangelo, 1987; Berd and Mastrangelo, 1988a; Berd and Mastrangelo 1988b). An ingenious treatment protocol involving cutaneous priming of the host with the hapten to ensure a DTH and administering low-dose cyclophosphamide designed to suppress a Th2 response was followed by 4-weekly administration of the modified irradiated melanoma cells mixed with BCG in 64 patients with advanced stage malignant melanoma. Eight cycles were given and DTH responses, CD8+ infiltrate of tumour nodules was documented. Response of tumour nodules was reported and increased survival of disease-free patients was claimed; however the number of patients is small and the comparison has been made to a historical control group treated with the non-hapten modified vaccine, a Phase III randomised trial is definitely required.

Cell lysate vaccines. Although a number of oncolysates have been introduced into clinical trials (Savage et al. 1986) the principal examples in this field is the viral melanoma oncolysate (VMO) using vaccinia virus and the DETOX-melanoma cell lysate, known as Theracine, where DETOX is an adjuvant mixture of cell-wall skeletons of Mycobacterium phlei in squalene oil and Tween-80 and lipid A from Salmonella Minnesota. Melanoma cells are procured from allogeneic melanoma cell lines in culture and they are rendered nucleus-free. Ongoing work since the late seventies (Wallack et al. 1977) demonstrated antibody and CTL responses in melanoma patients correlating with therapeutic efficacy (Kan-Mitchell et al. 1993; Mitchell et al. 1993; Wallack et al. 1986; Wallack and Michaelides, 1984; Wallack and Sivanandham, 1993) in limited Phase I/II studies. Phase III double-blind randomised trials (Wallack et al. 1995) have been initiated but have failed to verify the optimistic preliminary results for both preparations (Dore et al. 1990; Elliott et al. 1992; Hersey et al. 1987; Mitchell et al. 1993; Wallack et al. 1986; Wallack and Sivanandham, 1993). Marginal if any efficacy of the VMO-vaccinia preparation has been found (Wallack et al. 1995) while no activity of DETOX is anticipated although the final trial analysis has not been published to date.

Allogenic polyvalent cell vaccines. This vaccine strategy employs allogeneic melanoma cells harvested from cell lines established and maintained for their immunogenicity (Jones et al. 1981). A number of trials have been undertaken where patients with melanoma are treated with these cell lines administered intradermally with contemporaneous priming with BCG. Over a period of 15 years survival and immunological data have been compiled on numerous patients receiving this treatment with or without other immunomodulatory treatment e.g. cimetidine, cyclophosphamide, indomethacine or low dose interferon/IL-2. The main observation, apart from establishing the minimal toxicity of these procedures, was that efficacy is associated with a reaction by the host. This concurs with data from other contemporary trials but, other than qualifying the response, does not offer an advance on the primary observation made 83 years by Vaughan (1914) who thought that minimal disease and a leukocyte reaction to the administration of the vaccine equated to a more hopeful outcome. Indicators of efficacy are a positive DTH (Morton et al. 1992; Morton et al. 1993), increase in IgM antiganglioside antibodies (Ravindranath et al. 1989) and a positive mixed lymphocyte tumour reaction (Morton et al. 1992; Morton et al. 1993) and ability to minimise tumour load even by extensive surgical intervention. A 2-fold increase in survival for Stage IIIA and a three-fold increase in survival for Stage IV patients has been claimed (Morton et al. 1992). This however has not to date been put to the test of a randomised Phase III trial therefore the data can be only viewed as promising but speculative.

Soluble (protein/peptide) Vaccines

Advocates of the use of specific soluble antigen as a vaccine whether it is a peptide, supernatant or cloned protein believe that patients can and should be matched to the immunogen. As our capability to do so improves so should this method of vaccination become more effective. Eligibility criteria should include HLA typing and analysis of expression by the tumour of the genes encoding the available antigens for treatment (Radrizzani et al. 1991). The purified HLA-depleted vaccines include recombinant proteins/peptides, gangliosides, antiidiotypic antibodies and polyvalent shed antigen vaccines.

The category carrying a great deal of pharmaceutical potential is that of the recombinant peptides as they can be easily characterised, produced, purified, standardised, they are free of viral, DNA or other contaminants and study of responses in vivo are not confounded by allo- or xeno- responses. A long list of promising melanoma antigens has been cloned, all carrying the potential of being tumour immunogens (Demetrick et al 1992; Farzaneh et al 1991; Wollina et al. 1991). The best characterised is MAGE1 expressed in 40% of melanomas, presented by HLA-A1 and located on the X chromosome (Xq27-qter) (Carrel and Johnson, 1993; Oaks et al. 1994; Van Der Bruggen, 1991). Clinical trials with these reagents with or without adjuvants are in very early stages and no results are yet available.

Ganglioside vaccines on the other hand have entered clinical trials. In initial serological studies in melanoma patients immunised with whole cell vaccines the only clearly defined response was an occasional antibody response to GD2 and/or GM2. Based on this finding purified GM2 ganglioside was promoted for clinical studies (Livingstone 1993b; Livingstone et al. 1985). The results of a recent Phase III randomised trial randomising patients to receive GM2 with BCG or GM2 alone or BCG alone showed no "significant" advantage for GM2. However subset analysis showed significant survival benefit in patients responding serologically with high IgG anti-GM2 titres. A further randomised trial is under way using a more immunogenic ganglioside without BCG but coupled to KLH (Helling et al. 1994). Current studies are linking GM2 to a highly potent adjuvant QS-21 a Quail-A Saponine adjuvant.

Shed material purified from the supernatant of melanoma cell cultures comprises highly enriched cell surface macromolecules and antigens. A preparation of this form from 4 different melanoma cell lines (Bystryn et al. 1981) has shown activity in the clinic in Phase I and II trials in advanced melanoma (Stage III and IV) (Bystryn et al. 1992; Bystryn et al. 1991). Results have been promising when compared to historical controls but a randomised trial is pending. The problem is that the active ingredients although non-toxic contain xenogeneic material, as one of the original cell lines is of hamster origin!

Finally antiidiotypic antibodies, the binding sites of which resemble epitopes on tumour antigen, have been used as immunogens. Two such antibodies (MF11-30 and MK2-23) resembling epitopes on HMW-MAA have been used in the clinic in Phase I trials in advanced Stage IV melanoma (Ferrone, 1993; Ferrone and Tagashita, 1988; Mittelman et al. 1992). Adjuvants used have been either BCG or KLH. Minimal toxicity and some activity in 57 patients have been documented but the overall procedure has to be optimised and the results are not encouraging enough at this stage for a Phase III trial to be undertaken.

Lung Cancer

Treating patients after surgery in an adjuvant setting is generally thought to be the most optimal time due to the low residual tumour load. About a third of lung cancer patients undergoing pulmonary resection harbour residual tumour cells within the thorax or at distant sites, therefore trials of active specific immunotherapy as adjuvant therapy for lung cancer have been carried out. Post-surgery patients were treated intradermally with a vaccine composed of purified antigenic extracts from autologous lung cancer cells in combination with complete Freund's adjuvant (Stewart et al. 1982). Survival in Stage I patients treated with immunotherapy was superior to that in nonrandomized controls. The studies showed increases in cell-mediated immunity to antigenic tumour preparations when tested by DTH responses in the skin. In another study, patients were randomised after resection into three different groups (Takita et al. 1982); group 1 received no treatment, group 2 received tumour antigens admixed with Freund's adjuvant intradermally 3 times and group 3 received only Freund's adjuvant. Actuarial analysis yielded estimates of three-year survival of 34% for group 1, 84% for group 2, and 89% for group 3. The difference in survival rates between the control arm and each of the immunotherapy arms is statistically significant ($P<0.05$). These trials were forerunners of the most encouraging recent trials where an "ultrapure" preparation of allogeneic tumour-associated antigens from various cancer types was used. This was administered together with Freund's complete adjuvant to Stage I or II patients with SCC or adenocarcinoma of the lung (Hollinshead, 1991; Hollinshead et al. 1988). Although an increase in 5-year survival, especially amongst patients with good antibody responses to a number of antigenic determinants was noted amongst the first 64 patients studied, the true long term efficacy of this preparation will only be assessable when the results from the ongoing multi-centre randomised Phase III study are published.

In an earlier study (Perlin et al 1980; Reid et al. 1982) 45 Stage I and 6 Stage II patients with operable non-small cell lung cancer were randomised to receive a) no further therapy after resection b) BCG alone or c) BCG plus allogeneic tumour cells administered intradermally twice monthly for 2 years. Only a marginal benefit was documented for the patients on the immunotherapy arms. In patients with more advanced stage disease experience is limited. In 15 Stage III lung cancer patients treated with complete Freund's adjuvant in combination with antigens extracted from autologous tumour the survival rate increased to 63% at 2 years (Takita et al. 1978). In another trial where an autologous cell vaccine was used in combination with BCG in operable non-small cell carcinoma, no appreciable improvement in studied end-points was noted (Schulof et al. 1988).

Colorectal Cancer

Active specific immunotherapy for colorectal cancer has been in clinical trials since 1981 and a Phase III randomised trial was carried out (Hoover et al. 1985) in an adjuvant setting. Following standard surgical resection, patients who were at high risk for recurrence (Gunderson-Sosin stages B2, B3 and C1-3) were randomized to receive postoperative follow-up or active specific immunotherapy using 10^7 irradiated, autologous tumour cells mixed with 10^7 BCG organisms at weekly intervals for three weeks. DTH to the autologous tumour cells developed in 67% of patients following immunisation but in none of the controls. Of 24 vaccinated colon cancer patients there were 3 deaths and 5 recurrences; of 23 controls there were 7 deaths and 12 recurrences. However in rectal carcinoma patients there was no advantage to be seen in the vaccinated population. Trials with autologous cell vaccination incorporating levamisole with or without 5-FU are still ongoing. Two further trials shows cleared efficacy using monoclonal antibodies to gp70-72 MW antigens. One of these M17-1A showed a significant survival in Duke's C resected patients when given as an i.v. bolus compared to randomised controls. (Fagerberg et al 1995; Reithmuller et al 1994). Another MAb from Nottingham (personal communication) has increased survival when given as a vaccine in patients with liver metastases, compared to historical controls. Large Phase III trials for both have now commenced.

Breast Cancer

In contrast to some of the hopeful results in other adenocarcinomas, trials of vaccines for breast cancer have met with generally disappointing results, despite the fact that it has been one of the first solid tumours to be subjected to immunotherapeutic studies since 1951. Active immunotherapy using extracts of tumour tissue or freeze-thawed autologous lysates gave no responses (Stone, 1951). Although intralesional injection of BCG has produced regression of skin metastases from breast carcinoma (Smith et al. 1973), the administration of irradiated autologous tumour vaccine after radical mastectomy for breast carcinoma has showed no therapeutic benefit. BCG, levamisole and C. parvum have all been tried as adjuvants (Hubay et al. 1985; Treurniet-Donker et al. 1987). Several clinical trials have attempted combination immunotherapy and chemotherapy. Vaccines of allogeneic or autologous tumour cells combined with chemotherapy have similarly been ineffective (Aisner et al. 1987; Anderson et al. 1977; Anderson et al. 1974; Partridge et al 1979; Sparks et al. 1976). The most recent vaccination strategies are focusing on PEM-based immunogens. The further evidence that tumour associated mucins can activate T-cell cytotoxicty through a non-MHC restricted route has greatly increased both expectations and scientific interest in this area (Acres et al. 1993; Aisner et al. 1987; Barnd et al. 1989; Hareuveni et al. 1991; Maclean et al. 1993).

Renal Cell Carcinoma

The occurrence of documented spontaneous regressions in renal cell carcinoma has placed it second only to melanoma in the ongoing debate on whether these patients have a latent, potentially possible to manipulate, immune response to their tumour. This debate has been further fuelled by the evidence both from non-specific immunotherapy with IL-2 and from adoptive immunotherapy (LAK or TIL plus IL-2) trials which have shown an unequivocal if modest measure of success in treating this solid cancer (Rosenberg et al. 1993; Rosenberg et al. 1988). Active immunotherapy of renal cell carcinoma has also overall demonstrated low toxicity, a reasonable response rate and lengthening of overall, and disease- free survival. Only a few examples will be discussed as the bulk of the existing work is in the form of anecdotal evidence or Phase I/II trials.

A controlled study where patients with advanced Stage IV renal cell carcinoma undergoing palliative nephrectomy-debulking, was reported for the patients treated with a vaccine that contained autologous tumour polymerized with ethylchlorformate and PPD or Candida albicans (Tykka, 1981). Four further trials non-controlled (Neidhart et al. 1980; Prager et al. 1981; Sahasrabudhi et al. 1986; Tallberg et al. 1986), are worth mentioning where, similarly, autologous tumour cells were administered with differing adjuvants or other immunomodulatory procedures e.g. concomitant use of cyclophosphmide (Sahasrabudhi et al. 1986). Overall promising responses have been obtained but unfortunately the adage that these trials have been small and non-randomised holds; therefore no recommendations can be made. No randomised trial is pending in this area of active specific immunotherapy. The modest efficacy of IL-2 and the adoption of renal cell carcinoma as the tumour for further study using autologous transfected cells with IL-2 and GM-CSF as part of NIH-approved gene therapy protocols is an exciting project from which much is expected.

Other Solid Tumours

Small trials with similar to the above principles have been reported for soft tissue sarcomas (Eilber et al. 1975; Morton, 1972; Townsend et al. 1976), ovarian cancer (Hudson et al. 1976; Imperato et al. 1974), head and neck cancer (Taylor et al. 1977) and gliomas (Mahaley et al. 1983). Some responses have been claimed but most of the evidence remains anecdotal.

FUTURE DIRECTION

Clinical Studies

The success of the therapy in the hands of some and failure in the hands of others, requires that positive results be viewed with caution. Several factors may have influenced the outcome of different trials including the source of vaccine and adjuvant, method of preparation, and schedule of administration as well as the patients' tumour burdens prior to therapy. There is little doubt that reduction of the tumour burden would enhance the success rate of immunotherapy. The variable clinical phenotype of human cancer, especially of melanoma and renal cell carcinoma the quintessential immune-dependant malignancies, calls for precise definitions of the population of patients chosen to enter a clinical trial . The only appropriate method of discrimination is the randomised controlled trial with simple but well defined end-points. The problems of experimental design and performance of clinical trials for immunotherapy are not fundamentally different from those encountered more generally in cancer clinical trials. However the yardstick of follow-up decision making i.e. complete or partial response may not be as straightforward as with traditional chemotherapy-response assessment. The immunotherapist will often have to persevere at least over the first 3-4 months even in the face of progressive disease before abandoning a line of treatment. The mounting of a successful immune-response especially in studies involving advanced stage cancer may be prolonged and support by frequent debulking procedures may be warranted.

New Approaches/Strategies

Ultimate success of immunotherapy depends on a better understanding of a) the heterogeneity of TADAs on the cancer cell and b) the role of immunopotentiators and adjuvants in breaking tolerance and in rectifying the immunodeficiency encountered in patients with different kinds of cancer. In simple terms three fields seem to be the ones from where improvements in active specific immunotherapy are anticipated:

Adjuvants. Further directions in the active specific immunotherapy of cancer depend on understanding the *modus operandi* of adjuvants administered with tumour cell vaccines. While BCG has proven to be an excellent non-specific immunostimulant, regulation of T-cell responses, trafficking of cells within the immune system and paracrine cytokine "cross-talk" are not well understood. The role of various components of BCG and other mycobacteria, such as M.vaccae as well as, BCG cell walls, trehalose dimycolate, muramyl dipeptide and nontoxic derivatives from lipopolysaccharides of tumour-cell vaccines requires further study. New promising adjuvants need studying (Morrissey et al. 1987; Souberbielle et al. 1996), and the optimal route and timing of their use needs to be less empirical.

Antigens. Vaccine treatment in the future should be adjusted depending upon antigenic profile of biopsied tumour cells and MHC profile of the host. Different combinations of tumour cellular vaccines or pre-specified vaccine peptide "cocktails" may prove optimal for different groups of patients. Alternatively, the identification of non-MHC restricted TADA's and of alternative pathways of antigen presentation via the highly conserved HSP system allows cause for optimism for the development of novel vaccine preparations (Lukacs et al. 1993; Srivastava et al. 1994; Suto and Srivastava 1995; Udono et al. 1994). Recent evidence that large antigens can be presented as a 'DNA' vaccine requires that this mode of presentation be further studied.

In vitro gene transfer. Transfection of genes encoding different cytokines into autologous or allogeneic tumour cells should provide a novel approach to immunostimulation within vaccines. The advantage of using autologous cells is that all the potential antigens are present in the right HLA context for the host's CTLs. the disadvantages have already been addressed. Cytokine genes that have been transfected into tumour cells and have been shown to be very effective in animal experiments are IL-2, IL-4, IL-7, Ifn-γ, TNFα and GM-CSF (Asher et al. 1991; Dranoff et al. 1993; Fearon et al. 1990; Gansbacher et al. 1990; Hoch et al. 1991; Patel et al. 1993; Pordagor et al. 1992). A number of protocols following these successful animal experiments have been approved for human studies (Gansbacher, 1992; Patel et al. 1994). A final possibility is to engineer an APC to express a tumour specific antigen, e.g. MAGE1 for melanoma; these cells then would form the basis of a vaccine(Boon 1993). All these enticing possibilities are food for thought and hope for the future of successful active specific immunotherapy of cancer.

REFERENCES

Acres, R.B., Hareuveni, M., Balloul, J.-M. and Kieny, M.P. 1993. Vaccinia virus MUC1 immunisation of mice: immune response and protection against the growth of murine tumours bearing the MUC1 antigen. J.Immunother. 14:136.

Aisner, J., Weinberg, M., Perloff, M., Weiss, R., Perry, M., Korzum, A., Ginsberg, S. and Holland, J.F. 1987. Chemotherapy versus chemoimmunotherapy (CAF v CAFVP v CFM each +/- MER) for metastatic carcinoma of the breast: a CALGB study. J.Clin.Oncol. 5:1523.

Anderson, J.M., Kelly, F., Gettinby, G. and Wood, S.E. 1977. Prolonged survival after immunotherapy (irradiated cancer autografts) for mammary cancers assessed by a measure of therapeutic deficiency. Cancer. 40:30.

Anderson, J.M., Kelly, F., Wood, S.E. and Halnan, K.E. 1974. Stimulatory immunotherapy in mammary cancer. Br.J.Surg. 61:778.

Asher, A., Mule, J.J., Kasid, A., Restifo, N.P., Salo, J.C., Reichert, C.M., Jaffe, G., Frendly, B., Krieger, M. and Rosenberg, S.A. 1991. Murine tumor cells transduced with the gene for tumor necrosis factor-a. .Immunol. 146:3227.

Barnd, D. L., Lan, M.S., Metzgar, R.S. and Finn, O.J. 1989. Specific, major histocompatibility complex-unrestricted recognition of tumour-associated mucins by human cytotoxic T cells. Proc.Ntl.Acad.Sci. USA. 86:7159.

Berd, D., Maguire Jr. H.C. and Mastrangelo, M.J. 1986. Induction of cell-mediated immunity to autologous melanoma cells and regression of metastases after treatment with a melanoma cell vaccine preceded by cyclophosphamide. Cancer Res. 46:2572.

Berd, D., Maguire Jr. H.C., McCue, P. and Mastrangelo, M.J. 1990. Treatment of metastatic melanoma with an autologous tumor-cell vaccine: clinical and immunological results in 64 patients. J. Clin. Oncol. 8:1858.

Berd, D. and Mastrangelo, M.J. 1987. Effect of low dose cyclophosphamide on the immune system of cancer patients: Reduction of T suppressor function without depletion of the CD8+ subset. Cancer Res. 47:3317.

Berd, D and Mastrangelo, M.J. 1988a. Active immunotherapy of human melanoma exploiting the immuno-potentiating effects of cyclophosphamide. Cancer Invest. 6:335.

Berd, D. and Mastrangelo, M.J. 1988b. Effect of low dose cyclophosphamide on the immune system of cancer patients: Depletion of CD4+ 2H4+ suppressor-inducer T-cells. Cancer Res. 48:1671.

Bodenham, D.C. 1968. A study of 650 observed malignant melanomas in the South-West region. An. Royal Col.Surg.Engl., 43:218.

Boon, T. 1993. Tumor antigens recognized by cytolytic T lymphocytes: present perspectives for specific immunotherapy. Int.J.Cancer. 54:177.

Bruns, P. 1887-1888. Die Heilwirking des Erysipels auf Geschwulste. Beitr.Klin.Chir. 3:443.

Burchell, J., Taylor-Papadimitriou, J., Boshell, M., Gendler, S. and Duhig, T. 1989. A short sequence, within the amino acid tandem repeat of a cancer-associated mucin, contains immunodominant epitopes. Int.J.Cancer. 44:691.

Bystryn, J.-C., Tedholm, C.A. and Heaney-Kieras, J. 1981. Release of surface macromolecules by humane-lanoma and normal cells. Cancer Res. 41:91.

Bystryn, J.C., Oratz, R., Henn, M., Adler, A., Harris, M.N. and Roses, D.F. 1992. Relationship between immune response to melanoma vaccine and clinical outcome in stage II malignant melanoma. Cancer. 69:1157.

Bystryn, J.C., Oratz, R., Roses, D.F., Harris, M.N., Henn, M. and Lew, R. 1991. Improved survival of melanoma patients with delayed hypersensitivity response to melanoma vaccine immunization. Clin.Res. 39:503A.

Carney, W. 1988. Human tumor antigens and specific tumor therapy. Immunol. Today.9:363.

Carrel, S. and Johnson, J. 1993. Immunologic recognition of malignant melanoma by autologous lymphocytes. Curr.Opin.Oncol. 5:383.

Cassel, W. A., Murray, D.R. and Phillips, H.S. 1983. A phase II study on the post-surgical management of Stage II malignant melanoma with a Newcastle disease virus oncolysate. Cancer. 2:856.

Coca, A.F., Dorrance, G.M. and Lebredo, M.G. 1912. Vaccination in cancer: a report of the results of vaccination therapy as applied to seventy-nine cases of human cancer. Z.Immun. Exp.Ther. 13:543.

Coca, A.F. and Gilman, G. 1909. The specific treatment of carcinoma. Phil.J.Sci.Med. 4:381.

Coley, W.B., 1894. Treatment of inoperable malignant tumours with the toxins of erysipelas and the Bacillus prodigosus. Trans.Am.Surg.Assoc. 12:183.

Coulie, P.G. 1996. Human tumor antigens recognized by cytolytic T-lymphocytes. Tumor Immunology: Immunotherapy and Cancer Vaccines. Cambridge, University Press.

Cunningham, T.J., Olson, K.B., Laffin, R., Horton, J. and Sullivan, J. 1969. Treatment of advanced cancer with active immunization. Cancer. 24:932.

Czajkowski, N.P., Rosenblatt, M., Wolf, P.L. and Vasquez, J. 1967. A new method of active immunization to autologous human tumour tissue. Lancet. 2:905.

Dalgleish, A.G. 1996. Co-stimulatory molecules and their role in tumour immunity. In: "Tumor Immunology: Immunotherapy and Cancer Vaccines". Cambridge, University Press.

Demetrick, D.J., Herlyn, D., Tretiak, M., Creasey, D., Clevers, H., Donoso, L.A., Vennegoor, C.J., Dixon, W.T. and Jerry, L.M. 1992. ME491 melanoma-associated glycoprotein family: antigenic identity of ME491, NKI/C-3, neuroglandular antigen (NGA) and CD63 proteins. J.Natl.Cancer Inst. 84:422.

Dore, J. F., Portoukalian, J., Berthier-Vergnes, O., Jacubovich, R., Geneve, J., Bailly, M., Leftheriotis, E. and Weissbrod, A. 1990. Responses de malades atteints de melanome a l'immunisation par oncolysats de melanomes au virus de la vaccine. Bull. Cancer. 77:881.

Dranoff, G., Jaffee, E., Lazenby, A., Golumbek, P., Levitsky, H., Brose, K., Jackson, V., Hamada, H., Pardoll, D. and Mulligan, R.C. 1993. Vaccination with irradiated tumor cells engineered to secrete murine granulocyte-macrophege colony-stimulating factor stimulates potent, specific and long-lasting anti-tumor immunity. Proc.Natl.Acad. Sci. USA. 90:3539.

Eilber, F.R., Townsend Jr, C.M. and Morton, D.L. 1975. Osteosarcoma: Results of treatment employing adjuvant immunotherapy. Clin.Orthop.Rel.Res. 111:94.

Elliott, G.T., McLeod, R.A., Perez, J. and von Eschen, K.V. 1992. Results of phase II multicenter trial evaluating the activity of melacine melanoma theracine in the treatment of disseminated melanoma. Proc.Am.Assoc. Cancer Res. 33:332.

Fagerberg, J., Steinitz, M., Wigzell, H., Askelof, P., Mellstedt, H. 1995. Human antiidiotypic antibodies induced a humoral and cellular immune response against a colorectal carcinoma-associated antigen in patients. Proc.Nat.Acad.of Sci. 92(11): 4773.

Farzaneh, N.K., Walden, T.L., Hearing, V.J., Gersten and D.M. 1991. B700, an albumin-like melanoma-specific antigen, is a vitamin D binding protein. Eur.J. Cancer. 27:1158.

Fearon, E.R., Pardoll, D.M., Itaya, T., Golumbek, P., Levitsky, H.I., Simons, J.W., Karasuyama, H., Vogelstein, B. and Frost, P. 1990. Interleukin-2 production by tumor cells bypasses T-helper function in the generation of an anti-tumor response. Cell. 60:397.

Fehleisen, F. 1882. Uber die Zuchtung der Erysipel-Kokken auf kuntschlichen Nahrboden und die Ubertragbarkeit auf den Menschen. Deutsche Med. Wschr. 8:533.

Ferrone, S. 1993. Human tumor-associated antigen mimicry by anti-idiotypic antibodies. Immunogenicity and clinical trials in patients with solid tumors. Ann.N.Y.Acad.Sci. 690:214.

Ferrone, S. and Tagashita, T. 1988. Human high molecular weight melanoma-associated antigen as a target for active specific immunotherapy: a Phase I clinical trial with murine monoclonal antibodies. J.Dermatol. 15:457.

Finney, J.W., Byers, E.H. and Wilson, R.H. 1960. Studies in tumour auto-immunity. CancerRes. 20:351.

Freeman, G.J., Gribben, J.G., Boussiotis, V.A., Ng, J.W., Restivo, Jr.V.A., Lombard, L.A., Gray, G.S. and Nadler, L.M. 1993. Cloning of B7-2: a CTLA-4 counter receptor in B7-deficient mice. Science. 262:907.

Gabrilovich, D.I., Chen, H.L., Girgis, K.R., Cunningham, H.T., Meny, G.M., Nadaf, S., Kavanaugh, D. and Carbone, D.P. 1996. Production of vascular endothelial growth factor by human tumors inhibits the functional maturation of dendritic cells. Nature Med. 2:1096.

Gansbacher, B. 1992. A pilot study of immunization with HLA-A2 matched allogeneic melanoma cells that secrete interleukin-2 in patients with metastatic melanoma. Hum. Gene Ther. 3:677.

Gansbacher, B., Bannerji, R., Daniels, B., Zier, K., Cronin, K. and Gilboa, E. 1990. Retroviral vector-mediated γ-interferon gene transfer into tumor cells generates potent and long-lasting antitumor immunity. Cancer Res. 50:7820.

Gendler, S., Taylor-Papadimitriou, J., Duhig, T., Rothbard, J. and Burchell, J. 1988. A highly immunogenic region of a human polymorphic epithelial mucin expressed by carcinomas is made up of tandem repeats. The Journal of Biological Chemistry. 263: 12280.

Graham, J.B. and Graham, R.M. 1962. Autologous vaccine in cancer patients. Surg.Gynec.Obstet. 109:121.

Gupta, R.K., Golub, S.H. and Morton, D.L. 1979. Correlation between tumor burden and anticomplementary activity in sera from patients. Cancer Immunol. Immunother. 6:63.

Hahne, M., Rimoldi, D., Schröter, M., Romero, P., Schreier, M., French, L. E., Schneider, P., Bornand, T., Fontana, A., Lienard, D., Cerottini, J-C. and Tschopp, J. 1996. Melanoma cell expression of Fas (Apo-1/CD95) ligand: implications for tumour immune escape. Science 274:1363.

Handley, W.S. 1907. The pathology of melanotic growths. Lancet. 1:927.

Hanna, M., Peters, L.C. and Hoover, H.C. 1991. Immunotherapy by active specific immunization: basic principles and preclinical studies. In: "Biologic Therapy of Cancer". Philadelphia, Lippincott.

Hareuveni, M., Wreschner, D.H., Kieny, M.P., Dott, K., Gautier, C., Tomasetto, C., Keydar, I., Chambon, P.

and Lathe, R. 1991. Vaccinia recombinants expressing secreted and transmembrane forms of breast cancer-associated epithelial tumour antigen (ETA). Vaccine. 9:618.

Helling, F., Shang, A., Calves, M., Shang, A., Calves, M., Zhang, S., Ren, S., Yu, R.K., Oettgen, H.F. and Livinston, P.O. 1994. GD3 vaccines for melanoma: superior immunogenicity of keyhole limpet hemocyanin conjugate vaccines. Cancer Res. 54:197.

Heppner, G.H. 1984. Tumor heterogeneity. Cancer Res. 44:2259.

Herlyn, M., Thurin, J., Balaban, G., Bennicelli, J.L., Herlyn, D., Elder, D.E., Bondi, E., Guerry, D., Nowell, P., Clark, W.H. and Koprowski, H. 1985. Characteristics of human melanocytes isolated from different stages of tumor progression. Cancer Res. 45:5670.

Hersey, P., Edwards, A., Coates, A., Shaw, H., McCarthy, W.H. and Milton, G.W. 1987. Evidence that treatment with vaccinia melanoma cell lysates (VMCL) may improve survival of patients with stage II melanoma. Cancer Immunol. Immunother. 25:257.

Hills, D., Rowlinson-Busza, G. and Gullick, W.J. 1995. Specific targeting of a mutant, activated EGF receptor found in glioblastoma using a monoclonal antibody. Int.J.Cancer. 63:537.

Hoch, H., Dorsch, M., Diamantstein, T. and Blankenstein, T. 1991. Interleukin 7 induces CD4+ T cell-dependent tumor rejection. J.Exp.Med. 174:1291.

Hollinshead, A. 1991. Active specific immunotherapy and immunochemotherapy in the treatment of lung and colon cancer. Semin.Surg.Oncol. 7:199.

Hollinshead, A., Takita, H., Stewart, T. and Raman, S. 1988. Specific active lung cancer immunotherapy: immune correlates of clinical responses and an update of immunotherapy trials evaluations. Cancer. 62:1662.

Hollinshead, A., Arlen, M., Yonemoto, R., Cohen, M., Janner, K., Kundin, W.D. and Scherrer, J. 1982. Pilot studies using melanoma tumor-associated antigens (TAA) in specific active immunotherapy of malignant melanoma. Cancer. 49:1387.

Hoover, Jr. H.C., Surdyke, M.G., Dangel, M.G., Peters, L.C. and Hanna Jr. M.G. 1985. Prospectively randomised trial of adjuvant active-specific immunotherapy for human colorectal cancer. Cancer. 55:1236.

Hubay, C. A., Pearson, O.H., Manni, A., Gordon, N.H. and McGuire, W.L. 1985. Adjuvant endocrine therapy, cytotoxic chemotherapy and immunotherapy in Stage II breast cancer: 6-year result. III. Anti-estrogens in combination with chemotherapy in early breast cancer. J.SteroidBiochem. 23:1147.

Hudson, C.N., McHardy, J.E., Curling, O.M., English, P.E., Levin, L., Poulton, T.A., Crowther, M. and Leighton, M. 1976. Active specific immunotherapy for ovarian cancer. Lancet. 2:877.

Ikonopisov, R.L., Lewis, M.G., Hunter-Craig, I.D., Bodenham, D.C., Phillips, T.M., Cooling, C.I., Proctor, J., Fairley, G.H. and Alexander, P. 1970. Autoimmunization with irradiated tumour cells in human malignant melanoma. Br.Med.J. 2:752.

Imperato, S., Rossi, R., Ermiglia, G., De Marini , M. and Cassolino, A. 1974. Active specific immunotherapy with immunological monitoring in late stage ovarian cancers. Acta Eur.Fertil. 5:25.

Jones, P.C., Sze, L.L., Liu, P.Y., Morton, D.L. and Irie, R.F. 1981. Prolonged survival for melanoma patients with elevated IgM antibody to oncofetal antigen. J.Natl. Cancer Inst. 66:249.

Kan-Mitchell, J., Huang, X.Q., Steinamn, L., Oksenberg, J.R., Harel, W., Parker, J.W., Goedegebuure, P.S. and Darrow, T.L. 1993. Clonal analysis of in vivo activated CD8+ cytotoxic T Lymphocytes from melanoma patient responsive to active specific immunotherapy. Cancer Immunol. Immunother. 37:15.

Livingstone, P.O. 1993a. Approaches to augmenting the IgG antibody response to melanoma ganglioside vaccines. Ann. N. Y. Acad. Sci. 690:204.

Livingstone, P.O. 1993b. Approaches to augmenting the IgG antibody response to melanoma ganglioside vaccines. Ann.N.Y.Acad.Sci. 690:204.

Livingstone, P.O., Albino, A.P., Chung, T.J.C., Real, F.X., Houghton, A.N., Oettgen, H.F. and Old, L.H. 1985. Serological response of melanoma patients to vaccines prepared from VSV lysates of autologous and allogeneic cultured melanoma cells. Cancer. 55:713.

Livingstone, P.O., Calves, M.J. and Natoli, E.J. 1987. Approaches to augmenting the immunogenicity of the ganglioside GM2 is superior to whole cells. J.Immunol. 138: 1524.

Livingstone, P.O., Kaelin, K., Pinsky, C.M., Oettgen, H.R. and Old, L.J. 1985. The serological response of patients with stage II melanoma to allogeneic melnoma cell vaccines. Cancer. 56:713.

Livingstone, P.O., Natoli, E.J., Calves, M.J., Stockert, E., Oettgen, H.F. and Old, L.J. 1987. Vaccines containing purified GM2 ganglioside elicit GM2 antibodies in melanoma patients. Proc.Natl.Ac. Aci USA. 84:2911.

Lukacs, K.V., Lowrie, D.B., Stokes, R.W. and Colston, M.J. 1993. Tumor cells transfected with a bacterial heat-shock gene lose tumorigenicity and induce protection against tumors. J. Exp.Med. 178:343.

MacLean, G.D., Reddish, M., Koganty, R.R., Wong, T., Gandhi, S., Smolenski, M., Samuel, J., Nabholtz, J.M. and Longenecker, B.M. 1993. Immunization of breast cancer patients using a synthetic sialyl-

Tn glycoconjugate plus detox adjuvant. 36: 215-222.
Mahaley, Jr. M.S., Bigner, D.D., Dudka, L.F., Wilds, P.R., Williams, D.H., Bouldin, T.W., Whitaker, J.N. and Bynum, J.M. 1983. Immunobiology of primary intracranial tumors part 7: Active immunization of patients with anaplastic human glioma cells: a pilot study. J.Neurosurg. 59:201.
Mitchell, M. S., Harel, W., Kan-Mitchell, J., LeMay, L.G., Goedegebuure, P., Huang, X.Q., Hofman, F. and Groshen, S. 1993. Active specific immunotherapy of melanoma with allogeneic cell lysates. Rationale, results and possible mechanisms of action. Ann.N.Y.Acad.Sci. 690:153.
Mitchell, M. S., Kan-Mithcell, J., Kempf, R.A., Harel, W., Shau, H. and Lind, S. 1988. Active specific immunotherapy for melanoma : Phase I trial of allogeneic lysates and a novel adjuvant. Cancer Res. 48 5883.
Mittelman, A., Chen, Z.J., Yang, H., Wong, G.Y. and Ferrone, S. 1992. Human high molecular weight melanoma associated antigen (HMW-MAA) mimicry by mouse anti-idiotypic monoclonal antibody MK2-23: induction of humoral anti-HMW-MAA immunity and prolongation of survival in patients with Stage IV melanoma. Proc.Natl.Acad.Sci. USA. 89:466.
Morrissey, P. J., Bressler L., Park L. S., Alpert, A. and Gillis, S. 1987 Granulocyte-macrophage colony-stimulating factor augments the primary antibody response by enhancing the function of antigen-presenting cells. J.Immunol. 139:1113.
Morton, D.. L. 1972. Immunotherapy of human melanomas and sarcomas. J.Natl. Cancer Inst. 35:375.
Morton, D. L., Eilber, F.R., Holmes, E.C., Hunt, E.C., Ketcham, A.S., Silverstein, M.J. and Sparks, F.C. 1974. BCG immunotherapy of malignant melanoma: summary of a seven year experience. Ann.Surg. 180:635.
Morton, D. L., Foshag, L.J., Hoon, D.S.B., Nizze, J.A., Famatiga, E., Wanek, L.A., Chang, C., Davtyan, D.G., Gupta, R.K. and Elashoff, R. 1992. Prolongation of survival in metastatic melanoma after specific immunotherapy with a new polyvalent melanoma vaccine. Ann.Surg. 216:465.
Morton, D. L., Hoon, D.S.B., Nizze, J., Foshag, L.J., Famatiga, E., Wanek, L.A., Chang, C., Irie, R.F., Gupta, R.K. and Elashoff, R. 1993. Polyvalent melanoma vaccine improves survival of patients with metastatic melanoma. Ann.N.Y.Acad.Sci. 690:120.
Neidhart, J. A., Murphy, S.G., Hennick, L.A. and Wise, H.A. 1980. Active specific immunotherapy of Stage IV renal cell carcinoma with aggregated tumor antigen adjuvant. Cancer. 46:1126.
Nowell, P.C. 1986. Mechanisms of tumor progression. Cancer Res. 46:2203.
Oaks, M. K., Hanson Jr. J.P. and O'Malley, D.P. 1994. Molecular cytogenetic mapping of the human melanoma antigen (MAGE) family to chromosome region Xq27-qter: implications for MAGE immunotherapy. Cancer Res. 54:1627.
Oettgen, H.F. and Old, L.J., 1991. The history of cancer immunotherapy. Biologic Therapy of Cancer. Philadelphia, Lippincott.
Partridge, D.H. 1979. Chemotherapy of Stage III breast carcinoma with BCG and a live allogeneic tumor cell vaccine. Cancer Immunol.Immunother. 5:217.
Patel, P.M., Flemming, C.L., Russell, S.J., McKay, I.A., MacLennan, K.A., Box, G.M., Eccles, S.A. and Collins, M.K.I. 1993. Comparison of the potential therapeutic effects of interleukin-2 or interleukin-4 secretion by tumours. Br.J. Cancer. 68:295.
Patel, P. M., Flemming, C.L., Fisher, C., Porter, C.D., Thomas, J.M., Gore, M.E. and Collins, M.K. 1994. Generation of IL-2 secreting melanoma cell populations from resected metastatic tumours. Hum. Gene Ther. 5:577.
Perlin, E., Oldham, R.K., Weese, J.L., Heim, W., Reid, J., Mills, M., Miller, C., Blom, J., Green, D., Bellinger, Jr. S., Cannon, G.B., Law, I., Connor, R. and Herberman, R.B. 1980. Carcinoma of the lung: immunotherapy with interdermal BCG and allogeneic tumor cells. Int.J.Radiat.Oncol.Biol.Phys. 6:1033.
Porador, A., Tzehoval, E., Katz, A., Vadai, E., Revel, M., Feldham, M. and Eisenbach, L. 1992. Interleukin-6 transfection into Lewis lung carcinoma tumour cells suppresses the malignant phenotype and confers immunotherapeutic competence against parental metastatic cells. Cancer Res. 53:3679.
Prager, M. D., Baechtel, F.S., Peters, P.C., Brown, G.L. and Greene, C.L. 1981. Specific immunotherapy of human metastatic renal cell carcinoma. Proc.Am.Assoc. Cancer Res. 22:163.
Radrizzani, M., Benedetti, B., Castelli, C., Longo, A., Ferrara, G.B., Herlyn, M., Parmiani, G. and Fossati, G. 1991. Human allogeneic melanoma-reactive T helper lymphocyte clones: functional analysis of lymphocyte-melanoma interactions. Int J. Cancer. 49:823.
Ravindranath, M.H. and Irie, R.F. 1988. Gangliosides as antigens of human melanoma. Malignant Melanoma: Biology, Diagnosis and Therapy. Boston, Kluwer Academic Publishers.
Ravindranath, M. H., Morton, D.L. and Irie, R.F. 1989. An epitope common to gangliosides O-acetyl-GD3 and GD3 recognized by antibodies in melanoma patients after active specific immunotherapy. Cancer Res. 49:3891.

Reid, J. W., Perlin, E., Oldham, R.K., Weese, J.L., Heim, W., Mills, M., Miller, C., Blom, J., Green, D., Ballinger, S., Cannon, G.B., Law, I., Connor, R. and Heberman, R.B. 1982. Immunotherapy of carcinoma of the lung with intradermal BCG and allogeneic tumor cells. Immunotherapy of Human Cancer. New York, Excerpta Medica.

Riethmuller, G., Schneider-Gadicke, E., Schlimok, G., Schmiegel, W., Raab, R., Hoffken, K., Gruber, R., Pichlmaier, H., Hirche, H., Pichlmayr, R. 1994 Randomised trial of monoclonal antibody for adjuvant therapy of Duke's C colorectal carcinoma. German Cancer Aid 17-1A study group. 343(8907): 1177.

Risley, E.H. 1911. The Gilman-Coca vaccine emulsion treatment of cancer. Boston Med.Surg.J. 165:784.

Rosenberg, S. A., Lotze, M.T., Yang, J.C., Topalian, S.L., Chang, A.E., Schwartzerntruber, D.J., Aebersold, P., Leitman, S., Linehan, W.M. and Seipp, C.A. 1993. Prospective randomized trial of high-dose interleukin-2 alone or in conjunction with lymphokine-activated killer cells for the treatment of patients with advanced cancer. J. Natl. Cancer Inst. 85:622.

Rosenberg, S. A., Packard, B.S., Aebersold, P.M., Solomon, D., Topalian, S.L., Toy, S.T., Simon, P., Lotze, M.T., Yang, J.C. and Seipp, C.A. 1988. Use of tumor infiltrating lymphocytes and interleukin-2 in the immunotherapy of patients with metastatic melanoma: preliminary report. N.Engl.J.Med. 319:1676.

Sahasrabudhi, D. M., de Kernion, J.B., Pontes, J.E., Ryan, D.M., O'Donnell, R.W., Marquis, D.M., Mudholkar, G.S. and McCune, C.S. 1986. Specific immunotherapy with suppressor function inhibition for metastatic renal cell carcinoma. J.Biol.Resp.Mod. 5:581.

Sato, T., McCue, P., Masuoka, K., Salwen, S., Lattime, E.C., Mastrangelo, M.J. and Berd, D. 1996. Interleukin 10 production by human melanoma. Cl. Cancer Res. 2:1383.

Savage, H. E., Rossen, R.D., Hersh, E.M., Freedman, R.S., Bowen, J.M. and Plager, C. 1986. Antibody development to viral and allogeneic tumor cell-associated antigens in patients with malignant melanoma and ovarian carcinoma treated with lysates of virus infected cells. Cancer Res. 46:2127.

Schulof, R. S., Mai, D., Nelson, M.A., Paxton, H.M., Cox, Jr.J.W., Turner, M.L., Mills, M., Hix, W.R., Nochomovitz, L.E. and Peters, L.C. 1988. Active specific immunotherapy with an autologous tumor cell vaccine in patients with resected non-small cell lung cancer. Mol.Biother. 1:30.

Seiger, H. F., Shingleton, W.W., Metzgar, R.S. and Buckley, C.E. 3rd. 1973. Immunotherapy in patients with melanoma, Annals of Surgery, 178(3):352.

Simmons, R.L. and Rios, A. 1971. Combined use of BCG and neuraminidase in experimental tumor immunotherapy. Surg. Forum. 22:99.

Smith, G.V., Morse, P.A., Deraps, G.D., Raju, S. and Hardy, J.D. 1973. Immunotherapy of patients with cancer. Surgery. 74:59.

Souberbielle, B.E., Knight, B.C., Morrow, W.J.W., Darling, D., Fraziano, M., Marriott, J.B., Cookson, S., Farzaneh, F. and Dalgleish, A.G. 1996 Comparison of IL-2 and IL-4 transfected B16-F10 cells with a novel oil-microemulsion adjuvant for B16-F10 whole cell tumour vaccine. Gene Ther. 3:853.

Sparks, F.C., Wile, A.G., Ramming, K.P., Silver, H.K., Wolk, R.W. and Morton, D.L. 1976. Immunology and adjuvant chemoimmunotherapy of breast cancer. Arch.Surg. 3:1057.

Srivastava, P.K., Udono, H., Blachere, N.E. and Li, Z. 1994. Heat shock protein transfer peptides during antigen processing and CTL priming. Immunogenetics. 39:93.

Stewart, T.H.M., Hollinshead, A.C., Harris, J.A. and Raman, S. 1982. Specific active immunotherapy of Stage II lung cancer patients. Immunotherapy of cancer. New york, Exerpta Medica.

Stone, H.B. 1951. Can resistance to cancer be induced? Ann. Surg. 134:519.

Suto, R. and Srivastava, P.K. 1995. A mechanism for the specific immunogenicity of heat shock protein-haperoned peptides. Science. 269:1585.

Takita, H., Hollionshead, A.C., Bhayana, J.N., Edgerton, F., Conway, D., Moskowitz, R.M., Adler, R.H., Ramundo, M., Han, T., Rao, U., Vincent, R.G., Federico, A., Takita., L. and Smith, R. 1982. Specific active immunotherapy of squamous cell lung carcinoma. In: Immunotherapy of Human Cancer. New York, Excerpta Medica.

Takita, H., Takada, M., Minowada, J., Han, T. and Edgerton, F. 1978. Adjuvant immunotherapy of stage III lung carcinoma. In: Immunotherapy of Cancer: Present status of Trials in Man. New York, Raven Press.

Tallberg, T., Kalimo, T., Halttunen, P., Tykka, H., Mahlberg, K., Matous, B. and Sandell, B. 1986. Post-operative active specific immunotherapy with supportive measures in patients suffering from reccurent metastasized melanoma: Case report of six patients. J.Surg.Oncol. 33: 115.

Taylor, S.G., Bytell, D.E., Sisson, G.A., Nisius, S. and DeWys, W.D. 1977. Methotrexate-leucovorin with immunotherapy as adjuvant to surgery and radiotherapy in Stage III-IV head and neck squamous cancer patients. In: Adjuvant Therapy of Cancer. Amsterdam, Elsevier.

Townsend, C.M., Eilber, F.R. and Morton, D.L. 1976. Skeletal and soft tissue sarcomas. J.A.M.A. 236:2187.

Townsend, S. E. and Allison, J.P. 1993. Tumour rejection after direct costimulation by B7-transfected melanoma cells. Science. 259:368.

Treurniet-Donker, A.D., Meischke-de Jongh, M.L. and van Putten, W.L. 1987. Levamisole as adjuvant immunotherapy in breast cancer. Cancer. 59:1590.

Tykka, H. 1981. Active specific immunotherapy with supportive measures in the treatment of advanced palliatively nephrectomised renal adenocarcinoma. A controlled clinical study. Scand. J. Urol. Nephrol. 63:1.

Udono, H., Levey, D.L. and Srivastava, P.K. 1994. Cellular requirements for tumor-specific immunity elicited by heat shock proteins. Proc.Natl.Acad.Sci. USA., 91:3077.

Van Den Brenk, H.A.S. 1969. Autoimmunization in human malignant melanoma. B.M.J. 4:171.

Van Der Bruggen, P. 1991. A gene encoding an antigen recognised by cytolytic T lymphocytes on a human melanoma. Science. 254:1643.

Vaughan, J.W. 1914. Cancer vaccine and anti-cancer globulin as an aid in the surgical treatment of malignancy. J.A.M.A. 63:1258.

Vogelstein, B., Fearon, E.R., Hamilton, S.R., Kern, S.E., Preisinger, A.C., Leppert, M., Nakamura, Y., White, R., Smits, A.M. and Boss, J.L. 1988. Genetic alterations during colorectal tumor development. N.Engl .J.Med. 319:525.

Volk, B.W. 1975. The gangliosidoses. Hum. Pathol. 6:555.

Von Leyden, V.E. and Blumenthal, F. 1902. Vorlautige Mitteilungen ubber einige Ergebnisse der Krebsforschung auf der 1. medizinischen klinik. Dt. Med. Wschr. 28:637.

Wallack, M.K., McNally, K.R., Leftheriotis, E., Seigler, H., Balch, C., Wanebo, H., Bartolucci, A.A. and Bash, J.A. 1986. A southeastern cancer study group Phase I/II trial with vaccinia melanoma oncolysates. Cancer. 57:649.

Wallack, M. K. and Michaelides, M. 1984. Serologic response to human melanoma lines from patients with melanoma undergoing treatment with vaccinia melanoma oncolysates. Surgery. 96:791.

Wallack, M. K. and Sivanandham, M. 1993. Clinical trials with VMO for melanoma. Ann.N.Y.Acad.Sci. 690:178.

Wallack, M. K., Sivanandham, M., Balch, C.M., Urist, M.M., Bland, K.I., Murray, D., Robinson, W.A., Flaherty, L.E., Richards, J.M. and Bartolucci, A.A. 1995. A Phase III randomised, double blind, multiinstitutional trial of vaccinia melanoma oncolysate -active specific immunotherapy for patients with Stage II melanoma. Cancer. 75:34.

Wallack, M. K., Steplewski, Z., Koprowski, H., Rosato, E., George, J., Hulihan, B. and Johnson, J. 1977. A new approach in specific, active immunotherapy. Cancer. 39:560.

Welt, S., Carswell, E.A., Vogel, C.W., Oettgen, H.F. and Old, L.J. 1987. Immune and non-immune effector functions of IgG3 mouse monoclonal antibody R24 detecting the disialganglioside GD3 on the surface of melanoma cells. Clin.Immunol.Immunopathol. 45:214.

Wollina, U., Kilina, U., Henkel, U., Schaarschmidt, H. and Knopf, B. 1991. The initial steps of tumour progression in melanocytic lineage: a histochemical approach. Anticancer Res. 11:1405.

ISCOMS AS MUCOSAL VACCINE VECTORS

Allan McI. Mowat, Kevin J. Maloy, Rosemary E. Smith
and Anne M. Donachie

Department of Immunology, University of Glasgow, Western Infirmary,
Glasgow, G11 6NT, UK

INTRODUCTION

There is currently a great deal of interest in developing orally active synthetic vaccines containing recombinant proteins as protective antigens. However, purified proteins are poorly immunogenic in general and do not elicit the mucosal immunity essential for protecting against diseases of mucosal surfaces such as the intestine and respiratory tract (McGhee et al 1992). Indeed, the usual result of administering soluble proteins by the oral route is profound immunological tolerance which prevents systemic and local immune responses on subsequent exposure to the antigen (Mowat 1987). Thus there is a need for vectors that will avoid this phenomenon of oral tolerance and prime a full range of immune responses to orally administered protein antigens.

Lipophilic immune-stimulating complexes (ISCOMS) containing the saponin, Quil A are potent adjuvants, inducing powerful humoral and cell-mediated immune responses in vivo (Heeg et al, 1991; Morein et al, 1990; Mowat et al, 1991; Mowat et al, 1993; Takahashi et al, 1990). In addition, ISCOMS based vaccines elicit protective immunity in vivo against a variety of pathogens, including bacteria, viruses and parasites (Araujo and Morein, 1991; Claasen and Osterhaus, 1992; Kersten et al, 1991; Morein et al, 1995) and have the unusual ability to allow exogenous protein antigens to stimulate class I MHC-restricted CTL (Heeg et al, 1991; Mowat et al, 1991; Takahashi et al, 1990; Trudel et al, 1992). Here we describe the use of ISCOMS for inducing a wide range of local and systemic immune responses after oral administration of purified protein antigen and present our preliminary attempts to understand the basis of their potent immunogenicity.

MATERIALS AND METHODS

Mice

C57Bl/6 (B6) and BALB/c mice were purchased from Harlan Olac (Bicester, Oxon, UK).

129/Sv γIFN receptor KO (γIFNRKO) and (B6 x 129)F1 IL4 KO mice were first obtained from Dr H Bluethmann, Hoffmann-La Roche, Basel, before being bred and maintained at the University of Glasgow.

Preparation of ISCOMS Containing OVA

OVA was palmitified and incorporated into ISCOMS containing phosphatidyl choline, cholesterol and Quil A as described previously (Mowat et al 1991; Mowat & Reid 1994). The formation of ISCOMS was confirmed by electron microscopy and OVA content determined by Bradford's stain (Bio-Rad, Hemel Hempstead). The ISCOMS-OVA used in this study were 30-40nm in diameter and contained OVA and Quil A at a ratio of 10:1.

Induction and Measurement of Immunity in vivo

Systemic immune responses were measured in BALB/c mice which had been immunised in the rear footpad with 10μg OVA in ISCOMS, apart from splenic CTL responses which were induced by immunising C57Bl/6 (B6) mice with 10μg ISCOMS-OVA i.p. For oral immunisation, mice received 50-100μg OVA ISCOMS on 6 occasions on days 1,2,3,8,9 and 10.

Measurement of OVA-Specific Immune Responses

As described previously (Maloy et al, 1995; Mowat et al, 1993), systemic DTH was assessed by footpad testing with heat aggregated OVA, while serum IgG and intestinal IgA antibody responses were measured using specific ELISA's. Antigen-specific proliferation and cytokine production were measured in draining popliteal lymph nodes (PLN) or spleens as described previously (Maloy et al, 1995; Garside et al, 1995). OVA-specific CTL activity in the spleen was assayed against OVA transfected EG7.OVA cells after 5 days restimulation with

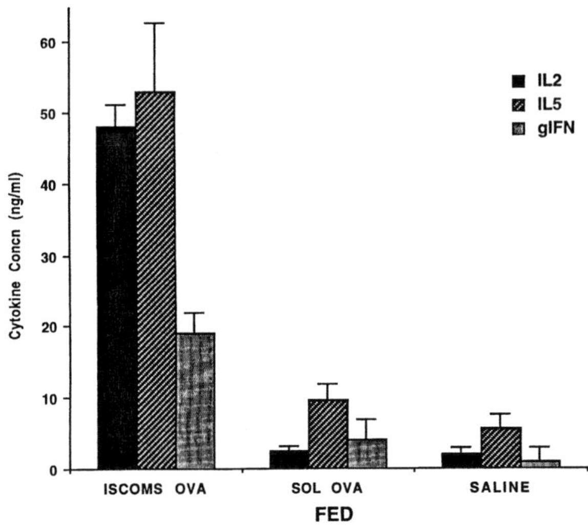

Figure 1. Oral immunisation with OVA ISCOMS primes systemic Th1 and Th2 cells. OVA-specific IL2, IL5 and γIFN production in the spleen of mice immunised on 6 occasions with 100μg OVA in ISCOMS, with 100μg soluble OVA, or with saline. Results are mean levels of cytokine measured by ELISA for triplicate samples restimulated with 1mg/ml OVA in vitro.

EG7.OVA cells in vitro. Intestinal IgA responses were measured by ELISA analysis of small bowel secretions induced by gavage with PEG.

Measurement of Inflammatory Responses in Peritoneal Exudates

Mice were injected ip with 2.5μg ISCOMS OVA and peritoneal exudate cells (PEC) obtained at intervals thereafter by washing out the peritoneal cavity with 10ml cold RPMI 1640. After washing the cells in medium, $2x10^6$ PEC were stimulated in vitro with 10μg/ml LPS, 20ng/ml recombinant mouse γIFN, 10μg/ml ConA, or with 5 x 10^6/ml heat killed Listeria monocytogenes in a final volume of 1ml at 37°C in 5% CO_2 in air. The supernatants were assessed for the production of γIFN, IL6, TNFa and IL12 by sandwich ELISA.

Statistics

Results expressed and means ± 1s.d. were compared by Student's t-test.

RESULTS

Induction of Local and Systemic Immunity by Oral Administration of Quil A

Mice fed 100μg ISCOMS-OVA on a single occasion developed systemic DTH responses equivalent to those found after subcutaneous immunisation with OVA in complete Freund's adjuvant (CFA) (Mowat et al, 1993). Although only low levels of serum IgG antibody were found under these conditions, oral immunisation on 6 occasions induced significant levels of serum IgG antibodies. In addition, mice immunised on repeated occasions had secretory IgA antibodies in the intestine (Mowat et al, 1993).

The immunogenicity of orally administered ISCOMS was confirmed by the fact that spleen and mesenteric lymph node cells proliferated when restimulated in vitro with OVA. In addition, these cells showed antigen-specific production of IL2, IL5 and γIFN in response to OVA (Fig 1).

Induction of Antigen-Specific CTL Following Oral Immunisation with ISCOMS

An unusual feature of parenteral immunisation with ISCOMS is their ability to prime class I MHC restricted CTL in vivo (Mowat et al, 1991; Heeg et al, 1991; Takahashi et al, 1990). This also occurs after oral immunisation and mice immunised orally with 100μg OVA in ISCOMS 6 times developed high levels of OVA-specific CTL in the spleen and MLN (Mowat et al 1993). These CTL are $CD8^+$ T cells which recognise the OVA 257-264 peptide that constitutes the immunodominant epitope recognised with the $H\text{-}2K^b$ class I MHC molecule (data not shown).

Together, these findings underline the potent immunogenicity of ISCOMS when given by the oral route and we have now begun to dissect the mechanisms underlying their adjuvant properties.

ISCOMS Recruit Local Inflammatory Cells and Mediators

One factor which most adjuvants share is an ability to induce inflammation or the production of costimulatory mediators. To examine whether ISCOMS also do this, we injected mice intraperitoneally with ISCOMS containing 2.5μg OVA and assessed the numbers and

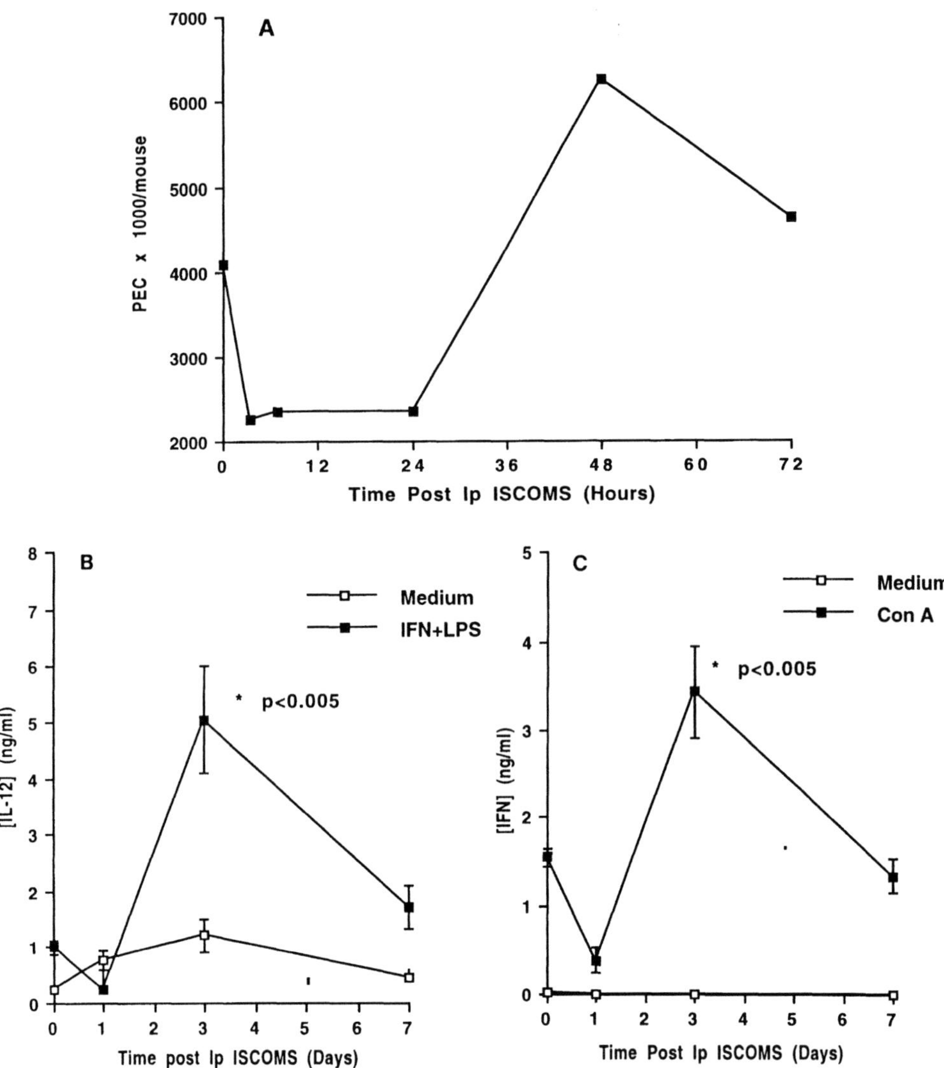

Figure 2. ISCOMS stimulate local infiltrates of inflammatory cells and induce cytokine production. Mice injected ip with ISCOMS have increased numbers of PEC (a) and these cells produce higher levels of IL12 (b) and γIFN (c) when stimulated in vitro with LPS + γIFN, or Con A respectively.

phenotype of peritoneal exudate cells (PEC) and their ability to produce proinflammatory cytokines.

Ip injection of ISCOMS induced a rapid, but transient disappearance of macrophages and other cells from PEC within 6-12 hours, but this was followed by a marked recruitment of cells to the site which peaked 3 days after injection (Fig 2a). These comprised mainly T and B lymphocytes, with lesser numbers of mature macrophages being found. Stimulation of PEC from ISCOMS injected mice in vitro with LPS + γIFN or heat killed Listeria monocytogenes resulted in the production of large amounts of IL12, at levels much higher than equivalently stimulated control PEC (Fig 2b). This was also maximal at 72 hours after injection. ISCOMS induced PEC also showed a moderate enhancement of O_2^- radical production as measured by PMA-stimulated reduction of luminol (data not shown) and there was considerable

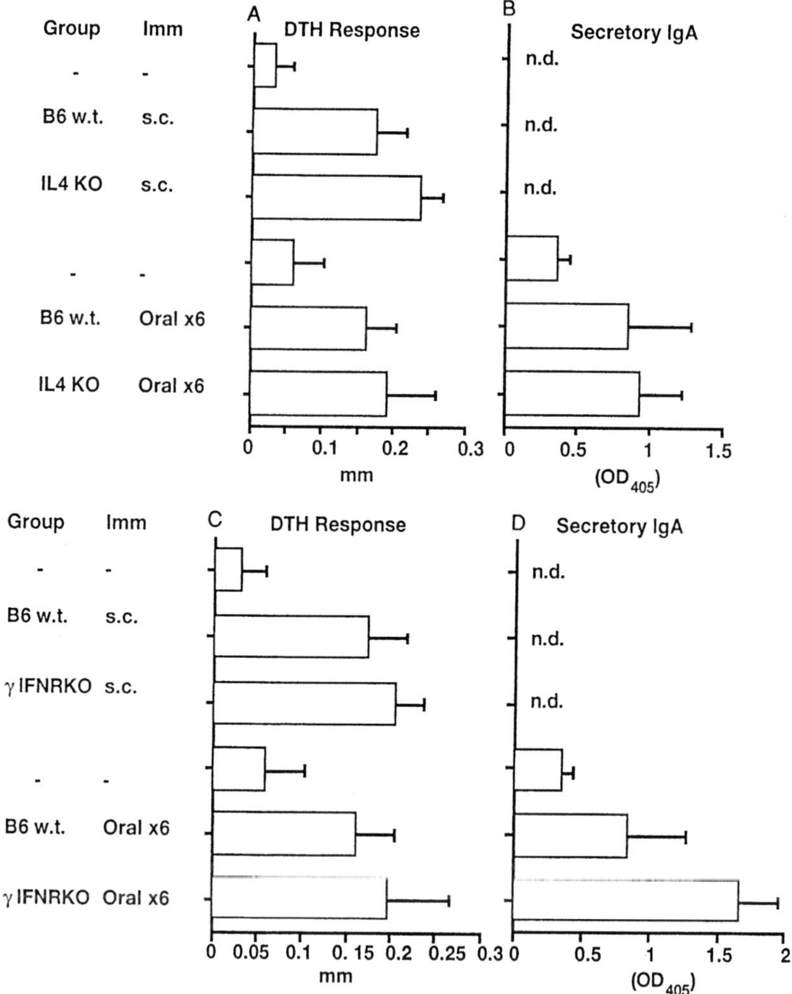

Figure 3. The mucosal immunogenicity of ISCOMS does not require IL4 or γIFN in vivo. Systemic DTH (a & c) and intestinal IgA antibody responses (b & d) in IL4 KO (a & b) or γIFNR KO mice (c & d) immunised orally on 6 occasions with 100μg OVA ISCOMS. Results are means ± 1 standard deviation for 5-6 mice/group.

enhancement of γIFN production (Fig 2c). ISCOMS had no effect on the production of IL4, IL6 or TNFα in response to any of the in vitro stimuli (data not shown).

Immunogenicity of ISCOMS does not Require IL4 or γIFN in vivo

In view of their ability to prime for the production of cytokines, we examined which of these mediators might be required for the immunogenicity of ISCOMS in vivo. Consistent with the lack of IL4 production in ISCOMS immunised mice, but contrary to what is found with cholera toxin as an oral adjuvant (Vajdy et al, 1995), IL4 KO mice developed normal local and systemic immune responses after oral immunisation with OVA ISCOMS (Fig 3a). Similar results were obtained in IL6KO mice (data not shown) and in mice lacking the γIFNR, despite the induction of γIFN after administration of ISCOMS (Fig 3b).

CONCLUSIONS

The results of these studies confirm and extend previous indications that ISCOMS may prove useful vectors for mucosal vaccination. Oral immunisation with the model antigen, ovalbumin, incorporated into ISCOMS primed mice to develop a full range of immune responses in vivo, which included conventional T cell dependent systemic antibody and DTH responses, as well as proliferation, cytokine production and class I MHC-restricted CTL responses. In addition, ISCOMS immunised mice had evidence of local priming, as shown by the presence of secretory IgA antibodies in the intestine and CTL in the MLN. The ability of ISCOMS to prime T cells was also not restricted to a single functional subset of $CD4^+$ Th cell, as we observed production of large amounts of antigen-specific γIFN and IL5, indicators of Th1 and Th2 cell activity respectively. Thus ISCOMS induce a wider range of local and systemic responses than most of the other adjuvants used currently for oral immunisation, such as cholera toxin and recombinant Salmonellae (McGhee et al, 1992).

The basis of the potent immunogenicity of ISCOMS remains to be clarified. Our initial studies using the intraperitoneal route show that administration of ISCOMS recruits inflammatory cells locally and stimulates the production of the inflammatory cytokines γIFN and IL12. However, γIFN was not required in vivo for ISCOMS to prime local or systemic immunity, as γIFNR KO mice developed entirely normal responses after oral or parenteral immunisation. Similar studies are currently underway to explore the requirement for IL12 in mice immunised with ISCOMS. Although IL12 and/or γIFN could help explain the priming of Th1 and $CD8^+$ T cells, the induction of Th2-dependent IgG, IgA and IL5 responses remains to be explained. IL6KO mice were initially reported to have defective mucosal immune responses (Ramsay 1994), while IL4KO mice are resistant to the oral adjuvant effects of CT (Vajdy et al 1995). However, in our experiments, neither of these cytokines was induced after administration of ISCOMS and immune responses to oral or parenteral immunisation were normal in the KO mice. Thus, additional cytokines may be involved in the immunogenicity of oral ISCOMS and these may differ from those required by other mucosal adjuvants. In addition, it will be important to determine the role of other factors known to be important in the induction and regulation of T cell dependent immune responses in vivo, such as costimulatory molecules and adhesion molecules.

It will also be necessary to extend these studies to examine the events occurring locally and systemically in animals given ISCOMS orally, as well as to define the anatomical basis of their mucosal effects. It has been suggested that ISCOMS preferentially target the M cells in Peyer's patches thought to be critical for induction of immune responses via the gut (McGhee et al 1992). However, their effects are clearly more widespread than this and it is not known where T cells are first primed by ISCOMS, nor their subsequent migration routes in vivo. Current studies using T cell receptor transgenic mice should help answer these questions.

In conclusion, our studies indicate that ISCOMS-based adjuvants may provide a useful basis for future orally active recombinant vaccines and that they may also be a flexible model for studying the induction of mucosal immune responses in vivo. Together with evidence that oral and intranasal ISCOMS vaccines can protect against experimental infectious disease, these findings highlight the need for further studies of protective immunisation regimes using ISCOMS given by the oral, or other mucosal routes.

Acknowledgments

This work was supported by the Wellcome Trust.

REFERENCES

Araujo, F.G. and Morein, B.1991, Immunisation with Trypanosoma cruzi epimastigote antigens incorporated into ISCOMS protects against lethal challenge in mice. Infect. Immun., 59:2909.

Claasen, I. and Osterhaus. A., 1992, The ISCOM structure as an immune-enhancing moiety: experience with viral systems. Res. Immunol., 143:531.

Garside, P., M. Steel, E.A. Worthey, A. Satoskar, J. Alexander, H. Bluethmann, F.Y. Liew, and A.McI Mowat. 1995, Th2 cells are subject to high dose oral tolerance and are not essential for its induction. J Immunol., 154:5649.

Heeg, K., Kuon, W. and Wagner, H., 1991, Vaccination of Class I major histocompatibility complex (MHC)-restricted murine CD8+ cytotoxic T lymphocytes toward soluble antigen: immunostimulating complexes enter the Class I MHC-restricted antigen pathway and allow sensitization against the immunodominant peptide. Eur.J.Immunol., 21: 152.

Kersten, G.F.A., Spiekstra, A., Beuvery, E.C. and Crommelin, D.J.A., 1991, On the structure of immune-stimulating saponin-lipid complexes (ISCOMS). Bioch.Bioph.Acta, 1062:165.

Maloy, K.J., Donachie, A.M. and Mowat, A.McI., 1995, Induction of Th1 and Th2 CD4+ T cell responses by oral or parenteral immunization with ISCOMS. Eur J Immunol., 25:2835.

McGhee, J.R., Mestecky, J., Dertzbaugh, M.T., Eldridge, J.H., Hirasawa, M. and Kiyono, H., 1992, The mucosal immune system: from fundamental concepts to vaccine development. Vaccine, 10 :75.

Morein, B., Fossum, C., Lovgren, K. and Hoglund, S., 1990, The ISCOM - a modern approach to vaccines. Semin. Virol., 1:49.

Morein, B., Lövgren, K., Rönnberg, B., Sjölander, A. and Villacres-Eriksson, M., 1995, Immunostimulating complexes. Clinical potential in vaccine development. Clin. Immunother., 3:461.

Mowat, A.McI, 1987, The regulation of immune responses to dietary protein antigens. Immunology Today, 8:93.

Mowat, A.McI., Donachie, A.M., Reid, G. and Jarrett, O., 1991, Immune stimulating complexes containing Quil A and protein antigen prime Class I MHC-restricted T lymphocytes in vivo and are active by the oral route. Immunology, 72 :317.

Mowat, A. McI., Maloy, K.J. and Donachie, A.M., 1993, Immune stimulating complexes as adjuvants for inducing local and systemic immunity after oral immunisation with protein antigens. Immunology, 80:527.

Mowat, A. McI. and Reid, G., 1994, The preparation of immune stimulating complexes (ISCOMS) as adjuvants for local and systemic immunisation with protein antigens. In: "Current Protocols in Immunology", J.E. Coligan Kruisbeek, A.M., Margulies, D , Shevach, E. and Strober, W.v cds., John Wiley and Sons Inc, New York

Ramsay, A. J., Husband, A. J., Ramshaw, I. A., Bao. S., Matthaei, K. I., Koehler, G. and Kopf, M.,1994, The role of interleukin-6 in mucosal IgA antibody responses in vivo. Science, 264:561.

Takahashi, H., T. Takeshita, B. Morein, S. Putney, R.N. Germain, and J. Berzofsky, 1990, Induction of $CD8^+$ cytotoxic T cells by immunisation with purified HIV-1 envelope protein in ISCOMS. Nature, 344: 873-5.

Trudel, M., Nadon, F., Seguin, C., Brault, S., Lusignan, Y. and Lemieux, S., 1992, Initiation of cytotoxic T cell response and protection of BALB/c mice by vaccination with an experimental ISCOMS respiratory syncytial virus subunit vaccine. Vaccine, 10:107.

Vajdy, M., Kosco-Vilbois, M.H., Kopf, M., Kohler, G. and Lycke, N., 1995, Impaired mucosal immune responses in interleukin 4-targeted mice. J. Exp. Med., 181:41.

ADJUVANT DIRECTED IMMUNE SPECIFICITY AT THE EPITOPE LEVEL:

IMPLICATIONS FOR VACCINE DEVELOPMENT

A MODEL STUDY USING SEMLIKI FOREST VIRUS INFECTION OF MICE

H. Snippe, I.M. Fernández and C.A. Kraaijeveld

Eijkman-Winkler Institute for Microbiology, Infectious Diseases and Inflammation, Utrecht University, AZU G04 614, Heidelberglaan 100, 3584 CX Utrecht, The Netherlands

INTRODUCTION

The objective of vaccination is to provide acquired protective immunity against invasive pathogens like viruses, bacteria, protozoa etc. For a number of them there is a vaccine available (against mumps, rubella, poliomyelitis, diphtheria, measles, hepatitis B, tuberculosis...) that shows a variable degree of efficacy and in minor instances unwanted side effects. Socioeconomic status of the population and immunological state of the individual (different for newborns, toddlers, elderly, immunosuppressed) influence the outcome of vaccination to a high extent. Until now no vaccine has been developed for a variety of diseases, malaria and human immunodeficiency virus (HIV) being important examples, and for many others (pneumococcus) an improved version of the current vaccine remains to be prepared.

The majority of the vaccines in use nowadays are based on whole organisms, killed or attenuated in their pathogenic capacity by different methods. An exception to this is the vaccine against hepatitis B which is based on a peptide from the outer glycoprotein envelope of the virus. These conventional vaccines have a number of disadvantages related to degree of efficacy, safety and side effects. Also factors like price, ease of preparation, storage and number of doses needed to reach protective immunity are very important issues and might hamper the introduction of new vaccines in Third-World countries.

The improvements in recent years of techniques in the fields of molecular biology and chemistry like DNA sequence analysis, genetic engineering and automated peptide synthesis might lead to a new generation of vaccines, e.g. based on peptides and recombinant microorganisms, that would be safe, stable, easy to handle and cheap to prepare. In this way the problems of conventional vaccines could be avoided by preparing subunit vaccines based only on those elements from the pathogens that are needed to evoke a protective immune response in the host. An encouraging starting point was the observation that antibodies induced by small peptides could recognize the intact protein (Geysen et al, 1985; Niman et al, 1983). In this manuscript the Semliki Forest virus (SFV) infection of mice was used as an animal model to assess the potential use of synthetic peptide vaccines (Snijders, 1992; Fernández, 1996).

SEMLIKI FOREST VIRUS

This arthropod-borne alphavirus of the Togaviridae family consists of single stranded RNA of positive polarity which is enclosed in an icosahedral nucleocapsid (C-protein), surrounded by a phospholipid bilayer (Simons and Garoff, 1980) in which the viral spikes (maximally 80) are embedded containing trimers of three glycoproteins: E1 (438 aa), E2 (422 aa) and E3 (66 aa) (Vogel et al, 1986). The nucleotide sequence that codes for the glycoproteins is known, which allows peptide synthesis (Garoff et al, 1980). After infection the spikes are inserted in the host cell membrane and once the new virus particle is assembled it is released from the cell by budding (Strauss et al, 1995). The transmembrane protein 6K is involved in this budding process (Lanzrein et al, 1994).

Some strains of the virus produce a lethal encephalitis in mice which makes it possible to assess vaccine efficacy in terms of survival. Specific antibodies (neutralizing or not) are mainly involved in the protection against the virus infection (Boere et al, 1983). Non-neutralizing antibodies bind to the glycoproteins of virus infected cells, providing in that way their protective capacity (Schmaljohn et al, 1982). Virus-neutralizing antibodies are capable of neutralizing the virus in an in-vitro virus neutralization assay. Both types of antibodies can provide protection in mice. Other related viruses are Sindbis virus, Ross River virus and Venezuelan equine encephalitis virus.

PEPTIDE VACCINES

In order to induce a significant, virus specific, antibody response peptide vaccines must contain at least one B- and one T helper (Th)-cell epitope in combination with an adjuvant (Ada, 1990). Once inside the body the antigen will be processed (degraded) by macrophages (an antigen presenting cell) and exposed at the surface of those cells in association with MHC-II molecules. The Th cells recognize the peptide-MHC-II complex through their T cell receptor and, as a consequence of that, T cells will become activated. The antigen is also recognized by B cells through the immunoglobulin receptor located at their surface. The B cells can also function as antigen presenting cells especially in secondary immune responses. After internalization and processing the peptide-MHC-II complex will appear at the cell surface. Recognition of this complex by an already macrophage-activated Th cell will lead to activation of the B cells, resulting in proliferation and antibody production.

Two subsets of antigen specific Th cells have been defined, Th1 and Th2, that differ in their cytokine profiles and the functions they perform (Mosmann et al, 1986; Noelle and Snow, 1992; Stevens et al, 1988; Valensi et al, 1994). Cytokines are proteins secreted by T cells and many other types of cells that exert regulatory functions during an immune response. Cells called Th1 secrete among others gamma interferon that will induce the production of antibodies of the IgG2a subclass, whereas Th2 cells will induce IgG1 antibodies through the secretion of interleukin-4. It is alleged that murine IgG2a antibodies are most effective in activating complement, promoting phagocytosis and inducing antibody-dependent cellular cytotoxic mechanisms, leading finally to a better protective capacity. Only Th2 cells can stimulate resting B cells (Boom et al, 1988) whereas Th1 cells help already activated B cells. The latter cells are involved in cell-mediated immune responses, such as delayed hypersensitivity.

Peptides containing a B- and a Th-cell epitope alone do not elicit a high antibody response after immunization. High immune responses are only achieved after addition of an appropriate adjuvant. The term adjuvant comprises a wide range of substances which are able to specifically enhance the immune response to a given antigen (in this case peptides) being themselves ideally not immunogenic. The mode of action of adjuvants is not completely understood but they are supposed to interact with macrophages during the processing of the peptides (Allison and Byars, 1986). A complex, strongly regulated interaction between different cells and their secreted cytokines takes place during this process (Finkelman et al, 1988; Paul, 1992; Schrader, 1991; Staruch and Wood, 1983). Different factors like type of antigen and its configuration (Cox et al, 1988; Francis et al, 1987; Levely et al, 1990), dose, route of administration and adjuvant used (Kalish et al, 1991; Karagouni and Hadjipetrou-Kouronakis, 1990; Kenney et al, 1989; Robinson et al, 1995) will influence this interaction and as a consequence the type of immune response that is generated. The search for less (or non-) toxic effective adjuvants has been very intense during the last years and still continues. Some new adjuvant formulations are very promising, even for application in humans (Scalzo et al, 1995).

The main drawback in the development of peptide vaccines is that B-cell epitopes can be discontinuous, e.g. the essential amino acid sequences forming the epitope are located far apart when one looks at the primary structure of the protein. In the native antigen they are brought together by folding. A number of strategies have been designed to overcome this problem:

1. In the multiple antigen peptide system (MAP) (Clarke et al, 1987; Francis et al, 1987; Brown et al, 1991;) the epitopes of interest are presented to the immune system in a multimeric form that can resemble the conformation in the original antigen;
2. In the immunostimulating complex (ISCOM) multiple copies of the antigen or peptide are incorporated in a matrix of the adjuvant Quil A and cholesterol (Lovgren and Morein, 1991);
3. In liposomes; the antigen or peptides are chemically linked to the surface of multimeric lipid bilayers with or without concomittant incorporation of adjuvants (Alving, 1991; Thérien et al, 1991);
4. In solid matrix-antibody-antigen complexes (SMAA) (Randall, 1989, Randall and Young, 1989) with an intrinsic adjuvant activity;
5. On the tip of loops of viral envelopes (Durda et al, 1990; Javaherian et al, 1990; Langedijk et al; 1991, Langeveld et al, 1994; Robinson et al, 1995).

Another problem to be solved concerns the MHC restriction of the T-cell epitopes. In other words, T cells recognize the processed peptides only in association with one or a few of the many different MHC molecules that are normally found in a given population. However, a number of promiscuous T-cell epitopes has been described (Kilgus et al, 1991; Panina-Bordignon et al, 1989; Sinigaglia et al, 1988) able to react with different MHC haplotypes; another possiblity is to use a cocktail of peptides for vaccination containing different T cell epitopes with different MHC specificities.

SCOPE OF THIS MANUSCRIPT

The efficacy of a vaccine depends on the amount, the (sub)isotype distribution, avidity and epitope specificity of the induced antibodies. This holds true for both protein-, peptide- and carbohydrate vaccines. This manuscript focuses on the effects of epitope polarity e.g. T-B or B-T orientation, and addition of adjuvants on the immune response to synthetic peptide vaccines.

The first part of this manuscript deals with the immunogenicity and efficacy of synthetic peptide vaccines against Semliki Forest virus (SFV). Antibody titers, subclass distribution and reactivity to SFV-infected L-cells in relation to protective efficacy in BALB/c mice will be presented. **In the second part** the fine specificity of the humoral response to these synthetic peptide vaccines in relation to the adjuvant used will be discussed. This fine specificity of the humoral immune response was studied by the **PEPSCAN** technique.

PEPTIDES

The peptide vaccines consisted of amino acid sequences 240-255 (B) and 137-151 (T) of the E2 membrane protein of SFVcolinearly synthetized in orientation T-B and B-T. The identification of the linear B-cell epitope was based on the binding of SFV-specific antibodies to a set of overlapping synthetic hexapeptides representing the complete E2 amino acid sequence as determined by **PEPSCAN** (Snijders et al. 1991). The mapping of the T- helper cell epitope on the stuctural protein of SFV was performed by measuring the ability of recombinant SFV protein fragments to induce SFV-specific delayed type hyper-sensitivity **DTH**, (Snijders et al. 1991, 1992) .

Peptide B CGG-------^{240}PFVPRADEPARKGKVH^{255}
Peptide T ^{137}GREKFTIRPHYGKEI^{151}---C
Peptide T-B ^{137}GREKFTIRPHYGKEI^{151}------- ^{240}PFVPRADEPARKGKVH^{255}
Peptide B-T ^{240}PFVPRADEPARKGKVH^{255}------ ^{137}GREKFTIRPHYGKEI^{151}

ADJUVANTS

The nonionic block copolymer surfactant L 180.5 alone and L 180.5 in a squalane-in-water emulsion (water-oil-water [W/O/W] L 180.5) with the antigen in the aqueous phase was kindly donated by R. Hunter, Emory University, Atlanta.The saponins Quil A and Q-VAC, extracted from the bark of the tree Quillaia saponaria were obtained from Superfos (Vedbaek, Denmark) and NOR-VET (Hvidovre, Denmark), respectively. The water -in-oil emulsion Montanide ISA 740 is manufactured by SEPPIC, Paris, France. The latter adjuvant is used in a proportion 70/30 with the antigen solution. Freund's complete adjuvant was purchased from Difco, Detroit, Mich.

RESULTS

Effects of epitope polarity and adjuvants on the sfv-specific response

The B-cell epitope alone was unable to elicit a humoral antibody response in BALB/c mice. The T-helper cell epitope, however, evoked a strong antibody response to the peptide but not a significant antibody response against SFV. In contrast, the combination of the T-helper cell epitope and the B-cell epitope in the T-B orientation evoked high serum levels of SFV-reactive antibodies (data not shown). In the next experiments, the effects of epitope polarity and adjuvants on the serum antibody responses to peptides and SFV were investigated. Groups of male BALB/c mice were immunized subcutaneously with synthetic SFV peptides of either the T-B or B-T polarity combined with the adjuvants L 180.5, W/O/W L180.5, Montanide, and Q VAC. Eight weeks after the primary immunization, the mice received an booster immunization with the same formulations as used for the primary injection. Two weeks later, blood was obtained for determination of both antipeptide and SFV-reactive antibodies. Therafter, mice were intraperitoneally challenged with 10 LD_{50} of SFV. The combined results of two separate experiments are presented in Table 1. Except with adjuvant L 180.5, the mean antipeptide

Table 1. Effect of epitope polarity of synthetic peptide vaccines on induction of protective immunity against SFV using different adjuvants[a]

Epitope polarity of peptide	Adjuvants used for immunization	Log_{10} antibody titres (± SD) against			Survival ratio[b]
		homologous peptide	SFV infected L cells		
		(EXP.1)	(EXP.1)	(EXP.2)	(EXP.2)
None	L 180.5	NT[c] 0/4	NT	NT	
B-T	L 180.5	3.2 ± 1.0	1.6 ± 0.2	1.7 ± 0.3	0/6
T-B	L 180.5	5.0 ± 0.5	1.9 ± 0.6	2.2 ± 0.8	1/6
None	W/O/W L 180.5	NT	NT	NT	0/4
B-T	W/O/W L 180.5	5.5	<1.5	<1.5	0/6
T-B	W/O/W L 180.5	5.5	4.1 ± 0.4	4.2 ± 0.3	5/6
None	Montanide	NT	NT	NT	0/4
B-T	Montanide	5.5	2.6 ± 1.0	2.7 ± 1.0	2/6
T-B	Montanide	>5.5	3.1 ± 0.9	3.2 ± 0.6	4/6
None	Q VAC	NT	NT	NT	0/4
B-T	Q VAC	>5.5	<1.5	<1.5	1/6
T-B	Q VAC	>5.5	4.4 ± 0.2	>4.5	4/5

[a] Male mice were immunized subcutaneously with 50 μg peptide combined with adjuvant. After 8 weeks an identical booster immunization was given. Control mice for the protection experiment received adjuvant only. Two weeks later blood was obtained by retro-orbital puncture from ether-anesthetized mice for determination of antibody titres in serum. Three sera were tested for anti-peptide antibodies (log_{10} serum dilutions: 2.0 - 5.5) and six mice for SFV-reactive antibodies (log_{10} serum dilutions: 1.5 - 4.5) (Fernández et al,1993).

[b] Mice were intraperitoneally challenged with 10 LD_{50} of virulent SFV two weeks after booster immunization.

[c] NT, not tested.

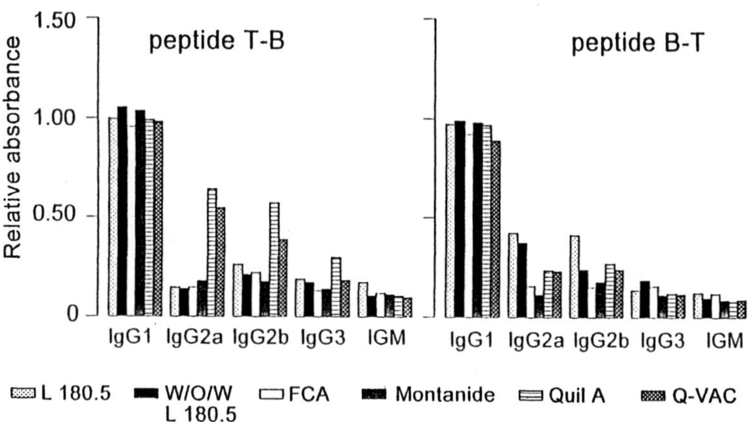

Figure 1. Distribution of IgG isotypes in antipeptide sera. Pooled sera were obtained from groups ($n = 5$) of mice immunized twice with either the T-B or B-T peptide, using adjuvants as indicated. Absorbance values of the individual mouse sera were determined by indirect ELISA on either peptide, using enzyme-labeled isotype-specific antibodies. To make the results comparable for both peptides, the relative absorbance was calculated as the absorbance value obtained for a particular isotype divided by the absorbance value observed for total IgG with the same antipeptide serum at the same dilution. Serum dilutions were chosen to give an A_{450} of about 1.0, using a pool of enzyme-labeled isotype-specific sera. Normal mouse serum at the same dilution gave an absorbance of less than 0.15 for all isotypes. Each bar represents the mean relative absorbance for the indicated subclass (Fernández et al, 1993)

antibody titer did not differ greatly between sera of mice immunized with either the B-T or the T-B peptide. In contrast to the antipeptide response, the SFV-specific response differed greatly with the adjuvants W/O/W L180.5 and Q VAC. The B-T peptide induced no SFV-specific antibody response, but with the T-B peptide, the titers were more than 10,000. This difference in antibody response against glutaraldehyde-fixed SFV-infected L cells was matched by the difference of the number of mice surviving a lethal challenge. With use of the adjuvant Montanide, an SFV-specific response was observed in both the T-B and B-T peptides. L 180.5 alone was not effective as an adjuvant. Although the SFV-specific response could be quite high, only nonneutralizing antibodies were detected (in vitro assay). However, as shown in Table 1, the serum levels of SFV-nonneutralizing antibodies correlate quite well with protective immunity. The mechanism by which these nonneutralizing antibodies provide protection to a lethal challenge of SFV has been discussed previously (Boere et al. 1983): enhanced uptake and clearance by macrophages thereby limiting viremia.

Effect of epitope polarity and adjuvant on induction of igg subclasses

Both the T-B and B-T peptides induced antibodies of all IgG subclasses, as measured by indirect ELISA on plastic-absorbed peptides (Fig.1). When Q-VAC and Quil A were used as adjuvants for the T-B peptide, higher levels of IgG2a and IgG2b antibodies were induced than with the other adjuvants. With the B-T peptide, the enhancing effect of Q-VAC on IgG2a and IgG2b development was not observed.

Table 2. PEPSCAN for the T-B peptide GREKFTIRPHYGKEI-PFVPRADEPARKGKVH

	Montanide	Quil-A
Dodecapeptide tested	Reactivity	Reactivity
GREKFTIRPHYG	-	-
REKFTIRPHYGK	-	-
EKFTIRPHYGKE	+/-	+/-
KFTIR***PHYGKEI***	-	+/-
FTIR***PHYGKEI***P	+/-	+
TIR***PHYGKEI***PF	+/-	+
IR***PHYGKEI***PFV	+/-	+
R***PHYGKEI***PFVP	+/-	+
PHYGKEIPFVPR	+/-	+
HYGKEIPFVPRA	+/-	+/-
YGKEIPFVPRAD	-	+/-
GKEIP***FVPRAD***E	++	++
KEIP***FVPRAD***EP	+	++
EIP***FVPRAD***EPA	+	+
IP***FVPRAD***EPAR	++	+++
P***FVPRAD***EPARK	++	++
FVPRADEPARKG	++	++
VPRADEPARKGK	+/-	-
PRADEPARKGKV	+/-	+/-
RADEPARKGKVH	+/-	-

Extinction between 0.0 - 0.5: -
0.5 - 1.0: +/-
1.0 - 1.5: +
1.5 - 2.0: ++
2.0 - 2.5: +++

Identification of epitopes on sfv-specific peptide vaccines by PEPSCAN

Twenty overlapping, 12 amino acid long peptides, were made accordingly to the amino acid sequences of peptides T-B and B-T. For example the 12-mer peptides GREKFTIRPHYG and REKFTIRPHYGK are the first two of the panel of peptide T-B. Different polyclonal immune sera were tested against the overlapping peptides. The reactivity of a serum was measured as absorbance value in indirect ELISA. The results of two relevant sera (anti T-B with Quil A or montanide as adjuvant) are presented in Table 2 and the results of all experiments combined are summarized in Table 3.

Serum from mice immunized with the B-cell amino acid sequence PFVPRADEPARKGKVH coupled to the protein carrier keyhole limpet haemocyanin (KLH) in combination with the adjuvant Quil A, showed a reactivity with the whole sequence and most probably with PFVP and KGKVH as minimal reactivity determining sequences (Table 2).

With serum from mice immunized with the peptide T-B and using Quil A as an adjuvant, FVPRAD and PHYGKEI were identified as epitopes. With Montanide as an adjuvant, the antibodies were directed against the same epitopes and in addition a third epitope was revealed (EPARKGKVH) (Table 2, data not shown).

A panel of 9 MAbs, induced by peptide immunization and selected for reactivity against SFV-infected L cells, were also applied in Pepscan analysis. Most SFV-reactive MAbs bind to

Table 3. Distinct amino acid sequences determining immune serum reactivity in the Pepscan using pooled sera from mice immunized with different peptides

Immunogens	Adjuvant	Amino acid sequences determining reactivity[a]			Protective efficacy of synthetic peptide vaccines[b]
KLH-B	Quil A	PFVPRAD	EPARKGKVH		90% (15)
T-B	Quil A	FVPRAD		PHYGKEI	74% (47)
T-B	Montanide	FVPRAD	EPARKGKVH	PHYGKEI	NT[c]
B-T	Quil A	PFVPRADE		PHYGKEI	NT
B-T	Montanide	PFVPRADE	EPARKGKVH	PHYGKEI	NT

[a] Minimal epitopes are underlined.
[b] Results derived from previous studies (Snijders, 1992, Fernández, 1993, 1994). Survival of nonimmunized mice 8% (73). Number of mice between parentheses.
[c] NT, not tested.

amino acid sequence FVPRAD of the E2 membrane protein of SFV. The only exception was MAb 23 which reacts against the peptide T within the peptide T-B. Pepscan reactivity was located between dodecapeptide number 2 (REKFTIRPHYGK) and 11 (YGKEIPFVPRAD) of peptide T-B (data not shown) and the minimal reactive sequence was identified as PHYGKEI. This MAb is not reactive against SFV-infected L cells and very likely not protective. So the results obtained with MAbs and polyclonal immune sera as well suggest that the protection inducing sequence is FVPRAD.

DISCUSSION

This manuscript deals with the detailed analysis of previously developed peptide vaccines using the Semliki Forest virus (SFV) infection of mice as a model. The advantages of using this model have been described earlier (Snijders, 1992). In short, SFV is a rather simple, extensively studied virus that produces a lethal encephalitis in mice making it possible to perform protection experiments. This is of importance when developing vaccines because it allows the vaccine efficacy to be monitored.

Peptides are quite simple antigens due to their small size. That is why the SFV peptide vaccines, containing a virus specific B- and a T helper (Th)-cell epitope in combination with an adjuvant, proved to be excellent tools to address our objectives. Those objectives were: first, modulation of the immune response against peptides using different epitope polarity and/or different adjuvants and secondly, a study of the variability of the humoral immune response against an SFV protective linear epitope, including a study of the antibody specificity using the Pepscan. The B-cell epitope was identified at the amino acid sequence 240-255 of the E2 membrane protein of SFV and the Th-cell epitope at 137-151 of the same protein.

A colinearly synthesised peptide, designated T-B, that had proved its vaccine efficacy in previous studies (Snijders, 1992) is compared with the peptide in the opposite orientation, B-T. In addition, different adjuvants were used and hence the immune responses were compared. It was found that both epitope polarity and adjuvants profoundly influence the immunogenicity and vaccine efficacy of SFV peptide vaccines. Peptide T-B showed a much higher vaccine (protective) efficacy than the peptide in the orientation B-T. The protective antipeptide antibodies did not neutralize SFV directly but were highly reactive with SFV-infected cells. The epitopes located in both peptides are probably seen by B-cells in a different manner depending on the epitope orientation. Other factors, like adjuvants and peptide polymerization, can also influence the antigen degradation and presentation by antigen presenting B-cells (APCs).

Different adjuvants have different modes of action (Allison and Byars, 1986; Karagouni and Hadjipetrou-Kourounakis, 1990; Kenney et al, 1989). For example adjuvants can release the antigen slowly in the body, in such a way that the antigen is localized in a lot of different sites resulting in an increased antigen interaction with T lymphocytes and macrophages; the adjuvant Montanide is supposed to interact accordingly (Steward-Tull, 1983). Other adjuvants activate the complement system, or they intervene with the activity of phagocytic cells thereby influencing the antigen processing. Adjuvants that belong to the group of the nonionic block polymer surfactants (L180.5 among them) are thought to act by this principle (Zigterman et al, 1988). But L180.5 applied in a different emulsion, like in the adjuvant W/O/W, behaved quite differently and an additional mechanism remains to be described. It has been extensively studied that nonionic block polymer surfactants show a wide spectrum of adjuvant activities depending on their different structures (Hunter et al., 1984 and 1991; Hunter and Bennett, 1984 and 1986). In many studies, Quil A has widely proved its excellent adjuvant activity (Bomford, 1984; Scott et al., 1985) but due to its haemolytic effect it can only be used subcutaneously. Its mode of action is probably related to the presence in the skin of a high concentration of Langerhans cells (an APC) which in turn activate T cells (Braathen et al., 1984, Streilein and Bergstresser, 1984).

To assess the alleged superiority of murine IgG2a antibodies providing protection a panel of antipeptide monoclonal antibodies (MAbs) of different subclasses was generated and tested. It was found that no particular antibody isotype was superior to the others (Stevens et al., 1988). We think that the experiment should be repeated, using several antipeptide monoclonal antibodies of every subclass to obtain a more definitive conclusion. In another panel of neutralizing MAbs generated against SFV the IgG2a subclass seemed to be indeed superior to other subclasses, in vitro and in vivo.

An exhaustive analysis of the humoral response against the linear, protective B-cell epitope of SFV ^{241}FVPRAD^{246} was carried out with the help of the Pepscan technique. Different sera of peptides containing an SFV specific B- and a Th-cell epitope in different orientations with two different adjuvants were tested. Using Quil A as adjuvant, the Pepscan revealed one immunodominant epitope at the B-cell epitope, ^{241}FVPRAD^{246}, and one at the Th-cell epitope, ^{145}PHYGKEI^{151} (Cease et al., 1987; Marx, 1988). An extra one was found at the B-cell sequence using Montanide as adjuvant, ^{247}EPARKGKVH^{255} (data not shown). A switch in immunodominancy was detected when peptides T-B and B-T were tested. The sequence ^{241}FVPRAD^{246} was immunodominant in the peptide T-B while sequence ^{145}PHYGKEI^{151} was in the peptide B-T. Specific virus antiserum recognized one epitope at the B-cell amino acid sequence and one at the Th-cell amino acid sequence. Antibodies that are reactive with the epitope located in the Th-cell sequence are not reactive with virus infected cells and are not protective. It was concluded that the epitope ^{241}FVPRAD^{246} located at the B-cell epitope and recognized by virus antibodies was the protective one. The same sequence was found to be reactive with a set of protective monoclonal antibodies.

CONCLUSIONS

A broader humoral immune response seems to be evoked by peptides in a water-in-oil emulsion (Montanide ISA 740) compared to saponin.

Interactions of peptides with adjuvant and thereby exposure of potential epitopes might be different for each adjuvant and each synthetic peptide vaccine. Therefore we recommend **PEPSCAN** analysis of the humoral response for each immunization protocol that includes a peptide to assess the specificity and quantity of the humoral response to each B-cell epitope detected by solid phase ELISA.

The affinity and isotype profiles of the evoked antibodies after immunization with peptide based vaccines should preferably be determined because these profiles are also influenced by adjuvants. It is alleged that IgG isotypes 2a and 2b are more effective against viral infections than the other isotypes.

Acknowledgements

We would like to thank R.H. Meloen and J.P.M. Langedijk from the ID-DLO, Lelystad, The Netherlands for performing the PEPSCAN analyses and A.F.M. Verheul for carefully reading the manuscript.

REFERENCES

Ada, G.L., 1990, Modern vaccines. The immunological principles of vaccination, The Lancet, 335:523.

Allison, A.C. and Byars, NE, 1986, An adjuvant formulation that selectively elicits the formation of antibodies of protective isotypes and cell-mediated immunity, J. Immunol. Meth., 95:157.

Alving, C.R., 1991, Liposomes as carriers of antigens and adjuvants. J. Immunol. Meth., 140:1.

Boere, W.A.M., Benaissa-Trouw, B.J., Harmsen, M., Kraaijeveld, C.A. and Snippe, H., 1983, Neutralizing and non-neutralizing monoclonal antibodies to the E2 glycoprotein of Semliki Forest virus can protect mice from lethal encephalitis, J. Gen. Virol., 64:1405.

Bomford, R, 1984, Relative adjuvant efficacy of $Al(OH)_3$ and saponin is related to the immuno genicity of the antigen, Int. Archs. Allergy Appl. Immun., 75:280

Boom, W.H., Liano, D. and Abbas, A.K., 1988, Heterogeneity of helper/inducer T lymphocytes II. Effects of interleukin 4- and interleukin 2-producing T cell clones on resting B lymphocytes, J. Exp. Med., 167:1350.

Braathen, L.R., Bjercke, S. and Thorsby, E., 1984, The antigen-presenting function of human Langerhans cells, Immunobiol., 168:301.

Brown, A.L., Francis,M.J., Hastings, G.Z., Parry, N.R., Barnett, P.V.,. Rowlands, D.J. and Clarke, B.E., 1991, Foreign epitopes in immunodominant regions of hepatitis B core particles are highly immunogenic and conformationally restricted, Vaccine, 9:595.

Cease, K.B., Margalit, H., Cornette, J.L., Putney, S.D., Robey, W.G., Ouyang, C., Streicher, H.Z., Fischinger, P.J., Gallo, R.C., Delisi, C. and Berzofsky, J.A., 1987, Helper T-cell antigenic site identification in the acquired immunodeficiency syndrome virus gp120 envelope protein and induction of immunity in mice to the native protein using a 16-residue synthetic peptide, Proc. Natl. Acad. Sci. USA, 84:4249.

Clarke, B.E., Newton, S.E., Carroll, A.R., Francis, M.J., Appleyard, G., Syred, A.D., Highfield, P.E., Rowlands, D.J. and Brown, F. 1987, Improved immunogenicity of a peptide epitope after fusion to hepatitis B core protein, Nature, 330:381.

Cox, J.H., Ivanyi, J., Young, D.B., Lamb, J.R., Syred, A.D. and. Francis, M.J., 1988, Orientation of epitopes influences the immunogenicity of synthetic peptide dimers, Eur. J. Immunol., 18:2015.

Durda, P.J., Bacheler, L., Clapham, P., Jenoski, A.M., Leece, B., Matthews, T.J., McKnight, A., Pomerantz, R., Rayner, M. and Weinhold, K.J., 1990. HIV-1 neutralizing monoclonal antibodies induced by a synthetic peptide, AIDS Res. Hum. Retrov., 6:1115.

Fernández, I.M., Snijders, A., Benaissa-Trouw, B.J., Harmsen, M., Snippe, H. and Kraaijeveld, C.A., 1993, Influence of epitope polarity and adjuvants on the immunogenicity and efficacy of a synthetic peptide vaccine against Semliki Forest virus, J. Virol., 67:5843.

Fernández, I.M., Ovaa, W., Harmsen, M., Benaissa-Trouw, B.J., Bos, N.A., Kraaijeveld, C.A. and Snippe, H., 1994, A shared idiotope among antibodies against Semliki Forest virus. Viral Immunol., 7:71.

Fernández, I.M., 1996, Diversity of the humoral response against peptide and anti-idiotypic vaccines in the Semliki Forest virus model, Academic Thesis, Utrecht.

Finkelman, F.D., Katona, I.M., Mosmann, T.R. and Coffman, R.L., 1988, IFN-gamma regulates the isotypes of Ig secreted during in vivo humoral immune responses, J. Immunol., 140:1022.

Francis, M.J., Fry, C.M., Rowlands, D.J., Bittle, J.L., Houghten, R.A. Lerner, R.A. and Brown, F., 1987, Immune response to uncoupled peptides of foot-and-mouth disease virus, Immunology, 61:1.

Garoff, H., Frischauf, A.-M. Simons, K., Lerach, H. and Delius, H., 1980, Nucleotide sequence of cDNA coding for Semliki Forest virus membrane glycoproteins, Nature , 288:236.

Geysen, H.M., Barteling, S.J. and Meloen, R.H., 1985, Small peptides induce antibodies with a sequence and structural requirement for binding antigen comparable to antibodies raised against the native protein, Proc. Natl. Acad. Sci. USA, 82:178.

Hunter, R.L. and Bennett,B., 1984, The adjuvant activity of nonionic block polymer surfactants. II. Antibody formation and inflammation related to the structure of triblock and octablock copolymers, J. Immunol., 133:3167.

Hunter, R.L. and Bennett, B., 1986, The adjuvant activity of nonionic block polymer surfactants. III. Characterization of selected biologically active surfaces, Scand. J. Immunol., 23:287.

Hunter, R., Olsen, M., and Buynitzky, S., 1991, Adjuvant activity of non-ionic block copolymers. IV. Effect of molecular weight and formulation on titre and isotype of antibody, Vaccine, 9:251.

Javaherian, K., Langlois, A.J., LaRosa, G.J., Profy, A.T., Bolognesi, D.P., Herlihy, W.C., Putney, S.D. and Matthews, T.J., 1990, Broadly neutralizing antibodies elicited by the hypervariable neutralizing determinant of HIV-, Science, 250:1590.

Kalish, M.L., Check, I.J., and Hunter, R.L. 1991, Murine IgG isotype responses to the Plasmodium cynomolgi circumsporozoite peptide $(NAGG)_5$, J. Immunol., 146:3583.

Karagouni, E.E. and Hadjipetrou-Kourounakis, L., 1990. Regulation of isotype immunoglobulin production by adjuvants in viv,. Scand. J. Immunol., 31:745.

Kenney, J.S., Hughes, B.W., Masada, M.P. and Allison, A.C., 1989. Influences of adjuvants on the quantity, affinity, isotype and epitope specificity of murine antibodies, J. Immunol. Meth., 121:157.

Kilgus, J., Jardetzky, T., Gorga, J.C., Trzeciak, A., Gillessen, D. and Sinigaglia, F., 1991, Analysis of the permissive association of a malaria T cell epitope with DR molecules, J. Immunol., 146:307.

Langedijk, J.P.M., Back, N.K.T., Durda, P.J., Goudsmit, J. and Meloen, R.H., 1991, Neutralizing activity of anti-peptide antibodies against the principal neutralization domain of human immunodeficiency virus type 1, J. Gen. Virol., 72:2519.

Langeveld, J.P.M., Casal, J.I., Osterhaus, A.D.M.E., Cortés, E., Swart, R. De, Vela, C., Dalsgaard, K., Puijk, W.C., Schaaper, W.M.M. and Meloen, R.H., 1994, First peptide vaccine providing protection against viral infection in the target animal: studies of canine parvovirus in dogs, J. Virol., 68:4506.

Lanzrein, M., Schlegel, A. and Kempf, C., 1994, Entry and uncoating of enveloped viruses, Biochem. J., 302:313.

Levely, M.E., Mitchell, M.A. and Nicholas, J.A., 1990, Synthetic immunogens constructed from T-cell and B-cell stimulating peptides (T:B chimeras): preferential stimulation of unique T- and B-cell specificities is influenced by immunogen configuration, Cell. Immunol., 125:65.

Lovgren, K., and Morein, B., 1991, The iscom: an antigen delivery system with built-in adjuvant, Mol. Immunol., 28:285.

Marx, J.L., 1988, What T cells see and how they see it, Science, 242:863.

Mosmann, T.R., Cherwinsky, H., Bond, M.W., Giedlin, M.A. and Coffman, R.L., 1986, Two types of murine helper T cell clone. I. Definition according to profiles of lymphokine activities and secreted proteins, J. Immunol., 136:2348.

Niman, H.L., Houghten, R.A., Walker, L.E., Reisfeld, R.A.,. Wilson, I.A., Hogle, J.M. and Lerner, R.A., 1983, Generation of protein-reactive antibodies by short peptides is an event of high frequency: implications for the structural basis of immune recognition, Proc. Natl. Acad. Sci. USA, 80: 4949.

Noelle, R. and Snow, E.C., 1992, T helper cells, Curr. Opin. Immunol., 4:333.

Panina-Bordignon, P., Tan, A., Termijtelen, A., Demotz, S., Corradin, G. and Lanzavecchia, A., 1989, Universal ly immunogenic T cell epitopes: promiscuous binding to human MHC class II and promiscuous recognition by T cells. Eur. J. Immunol., 19:2237.

Paul, W.E., 1992, Poking holes in the network, Nature, 357:16.

Randall, R.E., 1989, Solid matrix-antibody-antigen (SMAA) complexes for constructing multivalent subunit vaccines, Immunol. Today, 10:336.

Randall, R.E. and Young, D.F., 1989, Immunization against multiple viruses by using solid-matrix-antibody-antigen complexes, J. Virol., 63:1808.

Robinson, K., Mostratos, A., and Grencis, R.K., 1995, Generation of rubella virus-neutralising antibodies by vaccination with synthetic peptides, FEMS Immunol. and Med. Microbiol., 10:191.

Scalzo, A.A., Elliott, S.L., Cox, J., Gardner, J., Moss, D.J. and Suhrbier, A., 1995, Induction of protective cytotoxic T cells to murine cytomegalovirus by using a nonapeptide and a human-compatible adjuvant (Montanide ISA 720) J. Virol., 69:1306.

Schmaljohn, A.L., Johnson, E.D., Dalrymple, J.M. and Cole, G.A., 1982, Non-neutralizing monoclonal antibodies can prevent lethal alphavirus encephalitis, Nature, 297:70.

Schrader, J.W., 1991, Peptide regulatory factors and optimization of vaccines, Mol. Immunol., 28:295.

Scott, M.T., Goss-Sampson, M. and Bomford, R., 1985. Adjuvant activity of saponin: antigen localization studies, Int. Archs. Allergy appl. Immun., 77:409.

Simons, K. and Garoff, H., 1980 The budding mechanisms of enveloped animal viruses, J. Gen. Virol., 50:1.

Sinigaglia, F., Guttinger, M., Kilgus, J., Doran, D.M., Matile, H., Etlinger, H., Trzeciak, A., Gillesen, D. and Pink, J.R.L., 1988. A malaria T-cell epitope recognized in association with most mouse and human MHC class II molecules, Nature, 336:778.

Snijders, A., Benaissa-Trouw, B.J., Oosterlaken, T.A.M., Puijk, W.C., Posthumus, W.P.A., Meloen, R.H., Boere, W.A., Oosting, J.D., Kraaijeveld, C.A. and Snippe, H., 1991, Identification of linear epitopes on Semliki Forest virus and their efficacy as synthetic peptide vaccine, J. Gen. Virology, 72: 557.

Snijders, A., Benaissa-Trouw, B.J., Snippe, H. and Kraaijeveld, C.A., 1992, Immunogenicity and vaccine efficacy of synthetic peptides containing Semliki Forest virus B and T cell epitopes, J Gen Virology, 73 :2267.

Snijders, A., 1992, Vaccine efficacy of synthetic peptides. A model study using Semliki Forest virus infection of mice. Academic Thesis, Utrecht.

Staruch, M.J. and Wood, D.D., 1983 The adjuvanticity of interleukin 1 in vivo, J. Immunol., 130:2191.

Stevens, T.L., Bossie, A., Sanders, V.M., Fernandez-Botran, R,. Coffman, R.L., Mosmann, T.R. and Vitetta, E.S., 1988, Regulation of antibody isotype secretion by subsets of antigen-specific helper T cells, Nature, 334:255.

Steward-Tull, D.E.S., ed., 1983. in: "Biology of Microbacteria"; vol. 2, Academic Press, London.

Strauss, J.H., Strauss, E.G., and Kuhn, R.J., 1995, Budding of alphaviruses, Trends in Microbiol., 3:346.

Streilein, J.W. and Bergstresser, P.R., 1984, Langerhans cells: antigen presenting cells of the epidermis. Immunobiol., 168:285.

Thérien, H.-M., Shahum, E. and Fortin, A., 1991, Liposome adjuvanticity: influence of dose and protein:lipid ratio on the humoral response to encapsulated and surface-linked antigen, Cell. Immunol., 136:402.

Valensi, J.-M. M., Carlson, J.R. and Van Nest, G.A., 1994, Systemic cytokine profiles in BALB/c mice immunized with trivalent influenza vaccine containing MF59 oil emulsion and other advanced adjuvants, J. Immunol., 153:4029.

Vogel, R.H., Provencher, S.W.,Bonsdorff, C.-H. von, Adrian, M., and Dubochet, J 1986, Envelope structure of Semliki Forest virus reconstructed from cryo-electron micrographs, Nature, 320:533.

Zigterman, G.J.W.J., Snippe, H., Jansze, M. and Willers, J.M.N., 1988, Adjuvant effects of nonionic block polymer surfactants on liposome-induced humoral immune response. II. Mode of action. Chapter 3, Academic Thesis, Utrecht

INTERLEUKIN 1 AND ITS SYNTHETIC PEPTIDE 163-171 AS VACCINE ADJUVANTS

Aldo Tagliabue and Diana Boraschi

Dompé Research Center- 67100 L'Aquila, Italy

INTRODUCTION

Interleukin 1 (IL-1) is a family of cytokines of key importance in the mechanisms of host defense, being involved in the onset and development of both immune and inflammatory reactions (Dinarello, 1991; Boraschi and Tagliabue, 1989). The IL-1 family includes IL-1α and IL-1β, which have similar structures and overlapping biological activities, and IL-1ra, which is a pure receptor antagonist, able to occupy the activating IL-1 receptor (IL-1R_I) without exerting any agonistic effect. IL-1 binds to two types of receptors on the cell surface. IL-1R_I (CDw121a) is an 80 kDa monomeric transmembrane glycoprotein of the immunoglobulin superfamily which is responsible for initiating the cell activation mechanism upon IL-1 binding. Both agonist IL-1α and IL-1β and antagonist IL-1ra bind equally well to IL-1R_I. Conversely, IL-1R_{II} (CDw121b) is a 68 kDa receptor very similar to IL-1R_I in its extracellular domain, but apparently unable to initiate cell activation. The extracellular IL-1 binding domain of IL-1R_{II} can be naturally released from the cell surface and can capture IL-1β (Fig. 1).

Several reports have suggested that within the IL-1β molecule it is possible to identify active domains responsible for biological effects. In particular we found that the region 163-171 of IL-1β is essential for immunomodulation and does not elicit the proinflammatory effects of the parental molecule (Nencioni et al., 1987; Boraschi et al, 1988) (Table 1). In fact, synthetic peptides encompassing this area could selectively mimic the immunomodulating activities of the entire IL-1β in vivo.

The direct proof that this sequence is of great importance for IL-1β activities is provided by mutant SMIL-3, where the IL-1β amino acid stretch QGEESNDKIP (in position 164-173) has been replaced with the corresponding sequence present in the IL-1ra protein (EPHA) (Boraschi et al., 1995). In fact, the substitution of the active fragment 164-173 resulted in a profound loss of IL-1R_I-binding capacity and in a dramatic reduction of IL-1 agonist capacity both in vitro and in vivo (Table 2). On the other hand, introduction of the sequence QGEESN of IL-1β at the corresponding region of the biologically inactive IL-1ra results in aquisition of agonist activity (Greenfeder, 1995). Thus all together these results demonstrate beyond any

Vaccine Design: The Role of Cytokine Networks
Edited by Gregoriadis *et al.*, Plenum Press, New York, 1997

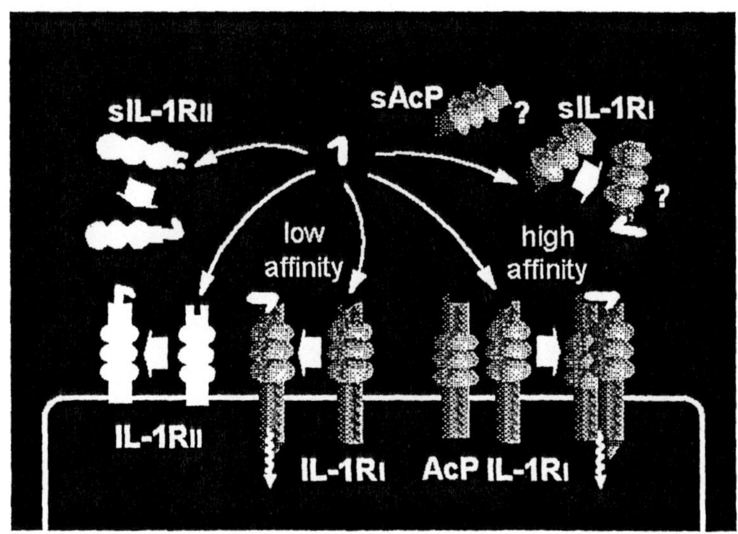

Figure 1. The IL-1 system. Schematic representation of the IL-1 system, where the number 1 represents IL-1 agonists IL-2α and IL-1β, IL-1R_I, and IL-1R_{II} are the membrane forms of the two receptors, AcP is the IL-1R accessory protein, sIL-1R_I, sIL-1R_{II} and sAcP are the soluble forms of the corresponding chains

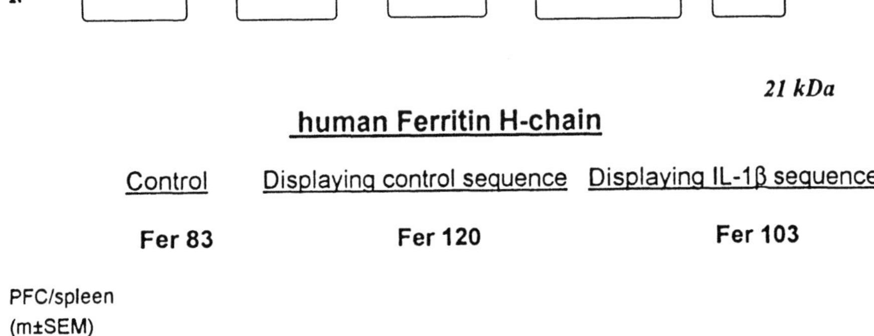

Figure 2. Schematic representation of protein construct. The H chain of human ferritin showing the five helices (A-E) and the site of insertion of the nonapeptide 163-171 of IL-1β. Biological activity is reported as described by Beckers et al., 1993.

doubt that the region of the β-bulge which includes peptide 163-171 is of extreme importance in the expression of biological activity for the members of the IL-1 family.

On the basis of the above mentioned results, the synthetic peptide 163-171 was tested to assess its efficacy as vaccine adjuvant. Encouraging results were obtained by us using T-dependent as well as T-independent antigens in experimental systems, including a recombinant hepatitis B virus antigen (Table 3). Moreover, the fragment of IL-1 was an effective adjuvant in an antitumor vaccine of irradiated tumor cells (McCune and Marquis, 1990) and it can provoke rejection of poorly immunogenic syngeneic tumors by stimulating the host effector cells (Forni et al, 1989).

The adjuvant effect of the synthetic fragment has been also compared to that of other known adjuvants. As summarized in Table 4, in the stimulation of the immune response to SRBC the 163-171 peptide proved as effective as muramyl dipeptide (MDP), an immunostimulatory component of bacterial cell wall, in terms of maximal immunostimulation attained, but it was several orders of magnitude more effective in terms of dose necessary to

Table 1. In vivo IL-1-like effects of the IL-1 synthetic fragment 163-171

In vivo activities	**IL-1β**	**163-171 peptide**
Inflammation-related effects		
Fever	↑↑↑	=
Food intake	↓↓	=
Circulating PMN	↑↑	=
Platelets	↑↑↑	=
Glycemia	↓↓↓	=
Triglyceridemia	↑↑	=
Insulinemia	↑↑↑	=
Corticosterone	↑↑↑	=
SAA	↑↑↑	=
Serum fibrinogen	↑↑	=
Plasmatic Fe^{++}	↓↓	=
Circulating PLA_2	↑↑↑	=
Metastatization	↑↑	=
Systemic effects		
Shock and death	↑↑↑	=
Radioprotection	↑↑↑	↑
Desensitization		
From shock & death	↑↑↑	↑
Adjuvanticity		
Protein antigens	↑↑↑	↑↑
Peptides	↑↑↑	↑↑
Polysaccharides	↑↑↑	↑↑
Bacterial antigens	↑↑↑	↑↑
Viral antigens	↑↑↑	↑↑
Entire cells	↑↑↑	↑↑

Table 2. Biological effects of the IL-1β mutant SMIL-3

Activity	IL-1β	SMIL-3	Ratio IL-1β/SMIL-3
In vitro			
Binding to IL-1R_I (K_D; M)	3.60×10^{-11}	4.00×10^{-8}	900
Binding to IL-1R_{II} (K_D; M)	1.11×10^{-10}	1.27×10^{-10}	1.1
Thymocyte proliferation (U/mg)	2.50×10^{7}	1.67×10^{4}	1,500
D10.G4.1 proliferation (U/mg)	5.34×10^{9}	5.26×10^{5}	10,152
IL-6 production (U/mg)	4.75×10^{7}	4.33×10^{4}	1,332
IL-8 production (U/mg)	2.94×10^{7}	3.45×10^{4}	852
MMP9 induction (U/mg)	1.92×10^{6}	1.59×10^{3}	1,208
Inhibition Ca^{++} flux (U/mg)	1.34×10^{6}	1.33×10^{3}	1,075
Bone resorption (U/mg)	5.00×10^{6}	5.56×10^{2}	8,993
In vivo			
Anorexia (U/kg)	3.13×10^{3}	3.85×10^{0}	813
Hypoglycemia (U/kg)	8.33×10^{3}	7.69×10^{0}	1,083
Neutrophilia (U/kg)	5.26×10^{3}	3.08×10^{0}	1,708

reach maximal effect. In another system, *i.e.* induction of circulating antibodies to HBsAg, the 163-171 fragment proved to be even more active than alum (aluminum hydroxide, presently one of the choice adjuvants for human use) in inducing specific antibodies. Taken all together these results clearly demonstrated that IL-1β and, more importantly, its noninflammatory peptide 163-171 possess in vivo immunostimulatory activity that can be exploited for use as adjuvants in vaccination.

Our results were further confirmed by other groups with the use of viral and bacterial antigens administered either with the peptide as adjuvant or in chimeric constructs containing both the antigen and the adjuvant peptide in sequence. In fact, Rao and Nayak (1990) coupled

Table 3. Adjuvant characteristics of the IL-1β peptide 163-171

Antigen	Route[(1)]	Isotype	T-cells	Reference
Proteins:				
viral HBsAg	iv/ip	total	NI	Tagliabue et al., 1992
Polysaccharides:				
bacterial SIII	iv/ip	M	NI	Nencioni et al., 1987 Boraschi et al., 1988
Cells:				
SRBC	iv/ip/sc/oral	M,G	Th	Nencioni et al., 1987 Boraschi et al., 1988
Tumor L1/C2	id	-	rejection	McCune & Marquis, 1990
Tumor CE-2	sc	-	Th (reject.)	Forni et al., 1989

[(1)] Route of antigen immunization
NI = not investigated

Table 4. Adjuvanticity of 163-171 peptide compared with classical adjuvants

Assay	Antigen	Adjuvant	Dose/mouse	Response
Specific PFC/spleen[(1)]	SRBC iv (10^8 cells)	Saline	---	36,898
		163-171	20 μg iv	81,846
		MDP	25 mg iv	81,283
Antibody to viral HBsAg[(2)]	HBsAg ip (4 mg)	Saline	--- iv/ip	206
		163-171	20 μg ip	10,595
			200 pg iv	6,489
		Alum	0.5 mg iv	6,784

[(1)] Measured 4 days after immunization
([2]) Specific serum Ab anti-HBsAg measured by RIA 4 weeks after immunization in mU/ml

the peptide 163-171 to a 21-amino acid sequence spanning positions 12-32 of the large protein of hepatitis B surface antigen, with a spacer of two glycine residues (Table 5), and showed that the new peptide S1-(12-32)-IL-(163-171) could elicit a much stronger immune response than the antigen alone (Rao and Nayak, 1990). Indeed the new peptide is able to elicit an increased primary and secondary response anti-S1-(12-32), measurable in terms of increased number of responders to the primary immunization and of specific antibody titers. These results clearly indicate that it is possible to obtain by synthetic ways a peptide with built-in adiuvanticity through insertion of the IL-1 163-171 sequence. This concept of including the adjuvant 163-171 moiety together with the antigen within the same construct was further confirmed with recombinant chimeric peptides. The sequence of peptide 163-171 was inserted into the loop between helices D and E of recombinant human ferritin H chain (Figure 2) and into the hypervariable region of recombinant flagellin from Salmonella muenchen (Beckers et al, 1993). The chimeric proteins were injected into mice and the level of humoral immune response developed against the native protein was assessed by measuring the number of antigen-specific plaque forming cells/spleen or as the level of serum IgG response. The response was compared to that of mice receiving injections with control chimeric proteins containing unrelated foreign peptide sequences of the same length. A significantly higher immune response was observed in mice immunized with chimeric constructs containing the 163-171 sequence (Beckers et al,

Table 5. Adjuvanticity of peptide 163-171 with a hepatitis B surface peptide

PEPTIDE	SEQUENCE	SPECIFIC ANTIBODY TITER
S1 (12-32)	MGTNLSVPNPLGFLPDHQLDP	15[1]
IL (163-171)	VQGEESNDK	--
S1 (12-32)-IL (163-171)	MGTNLSVPNPLGFLPDHQLDPGGVQGEESNDK	63

[(1)] Secondary response in terms of specific antibody titers (1/dilution) in C3H/CH mice against S1(12-32) peptide assessed by ELISA after immunization with peptides (Rao and Nayak, 1990).

1993), proving that the insertion of the peptide sequence increases immune response against poorly immunogenic recombinant proteins.

In a very recent paper (Hakim et al, 1996), the adjuvanticity of the nonapeptide was also demonstrated for naked DNA vaccine. In fact, Levy and co-workers at Stanford University have described in the last few years a generation of idiotype vaccines that were tested in animal tumor models such as the 38C13 mouse cell lymphoma. Initially, they have shown that effective anti-tumor immunity could be elicited by immunization with a syngeneic idiotype when conjugated to a carrier protein and mixed with an adjuvant. The subsequent generation of idiotype vaccines eliminated the need for a carrier protein and for an adjuvant by incorporating cytokines into fusion proteins containing the idiotype. A third generation vaccine consisting of naked DNA encoding the idiotype-GM-CSF fusion protein was equally effective in inducing anti-tumor immunity. Then it was attempted to determine whether Ig variable regions, in the absence of constant regions, could be immunotherapeutic in the 38C13 model employing single-chain Fv (scFv). When scFv protein produced in bacteria and naked DNA encoding scFv were used with GM-CSF as adjuvant, it was observed that the scFv-GM-CSF construct was effective only when injected as a protein and not as a DNA vaccine. In contrast, the construct including the peptide 163-171 from IL-1β and scFv could induce protection against the tumor challenge either as a protein or as a DNA vaccine (Table 6) (Hakim et al, 1996).

It can be concluded that the peptide 163-171 from IL-1β is a fully safe, non immunogenic, potent adjuvant that can be used to enhance the immune response in a variety of experimental situations including naked DNA vaccines.

Table 6. Effect of 163-171 peptide in a DNA vaccine

DNA Vaccine	Expression System	% Survivors
pBCL1	Plasmid DNA encoding unrelated tumor id	0
pscFv	Plasmid DNA encoding scFv of 38C13 tumor id	0
pscFv-IL-1β peptide	Plasmid DNA encoding scFv of 38C13 tumor id plus IL-1β peptide	40

from Hakim et al., 1996.

REFERENCES

Beckers, W., Villa, L., Gonfloni, S., Castagnoli, L., Newton, S.M.C., Cesareni, G. and Ghiara, P., 1993, Increasing the immunogenicity of protein antigens through the genetic insertion of VQGEESNDK sequence of human IL-1β into their sequence, J.Immunol., 151:1757.

Boraschi, D. and Tagliabue, A., 1989, Structure-function relationship of interleukin-1 giving new insights for its therapeutic potential. Biotherapy, 1:377.

Boraschi, D., Nencioni, L., Villa, L., Censini, S., Bossù, P., Ghiara, P., Presentini, R., Perin, F., Frasca, D., Doria, G., Forni, G., Musso, T., Giovarelli, M., Ghezzi, P., Bertini, R., Besedovsky, H.O., del Rey, A., Sipe, J.D., Antoni, G., Silvestri S. and Tagliabue, A., 1988, In vivo stimulation and restoration of the immune response by the noninflammatory fragment 163-171 of human interleukin 1β, J.Exp.Med., 168:675.

Boraschi, D., Bossù, P., Ruggiero, P., Tagliabue, A., Bertini, R., Macchia, G., Gasbarro, C., Pellegrini, L., Melillo, G., Ulisse, E., Visconti, U., Bizzarri , C., Del Grosso, E., Mackay, A.R., Frascotti, G., Frigerio, F., Grifantini, R. and Grandi, G., 1995, Mapping of receptor binding sites on IL-1β by reconstruction of IL-1ra-like domains, J.Immunol., 155:4719.

Dinarello, C.A., 1991, Interleukin-1 and interleukin-1 antagonism, Blood, 77:1627.

Forni, G., Musso, T., Jemma, C., Boraschi, D., Tagliabue, A. and Giovarelli, M., 1989, Lymphokine activated tumor inhibition (LATI) in mice. Ability of a nonapeptide of the human IL-1β to recruit anti-tumor reactivity in recipient mice, J.Immunol., 142:712.

Greenfeder, S.A., Varnell, T., Powers, G., Lombard-Gillooly, K., Shuster, D., McIntyre, K.W., Ryan, D.E., Levin, W., Madison, V. and Ju, G., 1995, Insertion of a structural domain of interleukin (IL)-1β confers agonist activity to the IL-1 receptor antagonist, J.Biol.Chem., 270:22460.

Hakim, I., Levy, S. and Levy, R., 1996, A nine-amino acid peptide from IL-1β augments antitumor immune response induced by protein and DNA vaccines. J. Immunol., 157: 5503.

McCune, C.S. and Marquis, D.M., 1990, Interleukin 1 as an adjuvant for active specific immunotherapy in a murine tumor model. Cancer Res., 50:1212.

Nencioni, L., Villa, L., Tagliabue, A., Antoni, G., Presentini, R., Perin, F., Silvestri, S. and Boraschi, D., 1987, In vivo immunostimulating activity of 163-171 peptide of human IL-1β, J.Immunol., 139:800.

Rao, K.V.S. and Nayak, A.R., 1990, Enhanced immunogenicity of a sequence derived from hepatitis B virus surface antigen in a composite peptide that includes the immunostimulatory region from human interleukin 1, Proc.Natl.Acad.Sci. USA, 87:5519.

Tagliabue, A., Ghiara, P. and Boraschi, D., 1992, Non-inflammatory peptide fragments of IL1 as safe new-generation adjuvants, Res.Immunol.,143:563.

THE IMMUNOLOGICAL CO-ADJUVANT ACTION OF LIPOSOMAL INTERLEUKIN-15

Mayda Gursel and Gregory Gregoriadis

Centre for Drug Delivery Research, The School of Pharmacy, University of London, Brunswick Square, London, UK

INTRODUCTION

It is well known that the immunological adjuvant property of liposomes established in the early 70's (Gregoriadis, 1990) can be further enhanced by interleukin-2 (IL-2) (Tan and Gregoriadis, 1989; Ho et al, 1992; Abraham and Shah, 1992; Sencer et al, 1991; Mbawuike et al, 1990; Anderson et al, 1994; Gursel and Gregoriadis, 1997a). It has been suggested (Meuer et al, 1989) that the co-adjuvant activity of liposomal IL-2 could prove useful in the vaccination of certain individuals who are low or non-responders (eg. immunosuppressed patients). Such findings with liposomal IL-2 have raised the question as to whether the recently discovered (Grabstein et al, 1994) interleukin-15 (IL-15) exhibits a similar action: IL-15 interacts with components of the IL-2 receptor and, as with IL-2, promotes T cell growth (Giri et al, 1994; Matthews et al, 1995; Carson et al, 1994), serves as a chemoattractant for human blood T-cells (Wilkinson and Liew, 1995) and induces B-cell proliferation and differentiation in the presence of stimuli (Armitage et al, 1995). Here we have studied IL-15 behaviour in vivo by entrapping the cytokine together with a model antigen (tetanus toxoid) into liposomes in a variety of formulations and monitoring its co-adjuvant activity in mice. Data indicate that IL-15 augments immune responses against the toxoid to levels well above those achieved with liposomal toxoid alone, but only when both the cytokine and the antigen are associated with the same vesicles.

METHODOLOGY

Sources of materials used in the present study have been described elsewhere (Gregoriadis et al, 1987; Gursel and Gregoriadis, 1997b).

Vaccine Design: The Role of Cytokine Networks
Edited by Gregoriadis *et al.*, Plenum Press, New York, 1997

Entrapment of interleukin-15 and tetanus toxoid into liposomes

The proteins were entrapped into liposomes according to the procedure of Kirby and Gregoriadis (1984). In short, small unilamellar vesicles (SUV) composed of 16 μmoles egg phosphatidylcholine (PC) and equimolar cholesterol and prepared (Kirby et al, 1980) by probe sonication were mixed with tetanus toxoid (supplemented with ^{125}I-labelled tracer toxoid) and/or IL-15 (for amounts of proteins used see Table 1). The mixtures were dehydrated by freeze-drying and rehydrated under controlled conditions (Kirby and Gregoriadis, 1984) to generate dehydration-rehydration vesicles (DRV liposomes). DRV were then diluted with 0.05 M sodium phosphate buffer containing 0.9 % NaCl, pH 7.4 (PBS) and centrifuged at 27,300 xg for 20 min. The pellet consisting of multilamellar (Gregoriadis et al, 1993) DRV was washed in PBS by centrifugation as above and resuspended in the same buffer. Percent solute entrapment was estimated on the basis of ^{125}I radioactivity recovered in the washed pellet (toxoid) and by the CTLL-2 proliferation assay (IL-15).

Covalent coupling of interleukin-15 and/or tetanus toxoid to the surface of liposomes

The toxoid and IL-15 were coupled to the surface of liposomes as described elsewhere (Garçon et al, 1986): DRV generated from SUV composed of 16 μmoles PC, 16 μmoles cholesterol and 0.75 μmoles aminophenyl stearylamine (APSA) were activated by the sequential addition of cold (4°C) 0.2 M $NaNO_2$ and 0.2 M HC1/NaCl solutions. They were then separated from the reagents by centrifugation as above and the pellet obtained was suspended in 0.05 M borate buffer (pH 10) containing ^{125}I-labelled toxoid alone or together with IL-15 (for amounts of toxoid and IL-15 used, see Table 1). Samples were placed in an ice-bath and allowed to reach 20° C overnight. DRV with covalently coupled material were separated from free materials by centrifugation and washing as above. Estimation of the amount of coupled toxoid was carried out on the basis of ^{125}I radioactivity values in the pellet

Table 1. Incorporation of tetanus toxoid and interleukin-15 into DRV liposomes

Preparation	Entrapped or coupled toxoid (% of used[a])	Entrapped or coupled IL-15 (% of used[a])
Entrapped toxoid	32.5	
Linked toxoid	21.0	
Separately entrapped toxoid and IL-15	32.5	44.7
Co-entrapped toxoid and IL-15	28.6	31.8
	31.7	32.3
Surface-co-linked toxoid and IL-15	23.6	20.7
	21.8	21.6

a, Amounts of toxoid (8-50μg) and IL-15 used (6.2×10^3 - 2.5×10^5) were adjusted (on the basis of entrapment and coupling values anticipated from preliminary work) to give, after appropriate dilutions, final preparations containing 0.1 μg antigen and the appropriate units of IL-15 per 0.1 ml injected volume. (Modified from Gursel and Gregoriadis, 1997b).

suspended in PBS (1ml final volume) and wash solutions. The CTTL-2 proliferation assay was used for the estimation of IL-15 coupling.

CTLL-2 proliferation assay

CTLL-2 cells (10^4/ml) were maintained in complete medium composed of RPMI 1640, 5% foetal calf serum and 30 units interleukin-2/ml. Following 3 days of incubation at 37° C in a humidified chamber in the presence of 5 % CO_2, the cells were washed three times by centrifugation and resuspended (10^5 cells/ml) in RPMI 1640 in the absence of IL-2. Samples for the quantitation of the cytokine and a IL-15 standard were distributed in 96 well tissue culture plates, 50 μl cell suspension was added in each well and the plates were incubated for 48 h at 37°C. Assessment of cell proliferation was carried by the mitochondrial stain MTT method (Roehm et al, 1991).

Immunization protocol

CD-1 mice in groups of four were injected intramuscularly with 0.1μg each of free toxoid mixed with free IL-15 (and "empty" DRV in one case) or toxoid with or without IL-15 in a variety of liposomal formulations (for details see legend to Table 2). The same preparations were used for boosting the animals 29 days later. Blood sera samples on days 28

Table 2. The effect of interleukin-15 on immune responses against liposomal tetanus toxoid

Liposomal preparation	IgG ($\log_{10}$ reciprocal end point dilution)		
	IgG_1	IgG_{2a}	IgG_{2b}
A Entrapped toxoid	2.5±0.0	1.3±0.0	1.9±0.0
B Surface-linked toxoid	2.6±0.1	1.3±0.0	2.0±0.1
C1 Separately entrapped toxoid and IL-15[a]	3.1±0.2	1.5±0.0	2.0±0.1
C2 Separately entrapped toxoid and IL-15[b]	2.8±0.4	1.8±0.3	2.0±0.3
D1 Entrapped toxoid + free IL-15[a]	4.2±0.1	1.4±0.1[c]	2.4±0.2
D2 Entrapped toxoid + free IL-15[b]	2.8±0.2[c]	1.4±0.1[c]	2.0±0.3[c]
E1 Co-entrapped toxoid and IL-15[a]	3.7±0.1	1.4±0.2[c]	2.0±0.1[c]
E2 Co-entrapped toxoid and IL-15[b]	3.6±0.2	1.3±0.0[c]	2.0±0.1[c]
F1 Surface co-linked toxoid and IL-15[a]	3.7±0.2	1.4±0.1[c]	2.6±0.3
F2 Surface co-linked toxoid and IL-15[b]	3.7±0.4	2.0±0.3	2.5±0.2

Mice were immunized twice with 0.1μg tetanus toxoid in a variety of preparations in the absence or presence of a low (a) or high (b) dose of interleukin-15. IL-15 units injected were: C1, 246; C2, 2461; D1, 150; D2, 1500; E1, 139; E2, 1269; F1, 734; F2, 7049.
Injected mixtures of 0.1μg free toxoid and free IL-15 (150 and 1500 units) or of 0.1μg free toxoid, free IL-2 (150 and 1500 units) and "empty" liposomes led to IgG responses which were similar to those for entrapped toxoid. c, Denotes IgG values which were not significantly (Student's test) different from those obtained with entrapped and surface-linked toxoid or with separately entrapped toxoid and IL-15. (Modified from Gursel and Gregoriadis, 1997b).

(primary response) and 39 (secondary response) were kept at -20°C until they were tested for anti-toxoid IgG_1, IgG_{2a} and IgG_{2b} by ELISA as described elsewhere (Gursel and Gregoriadis, 1997b). ELISA values were statistically analyzed by the Student's test.

RESULTS AND DISCUSSION

Antigen and interleukin-15 content of liposomes

Results of tetanus toxoid and IL-15 entrapment or coupling are shown in Table 1. As expected from previous work (Gregoriadis et al, 1987; Gregoriadis et al, 1993; McCormack and Gregoriadis, 1994; Gregoriadis et al, 1997) in which the same method was used for the entrapment of a variety of solutes, entrapment of the toxoid was considerable (29.7-32.5 %) even when the protein was co-entrapped with IL-15. Values of IL-15 entrapment (31.8-44.7% of the two different amounts used) were also high and similar to those obtained previously with IL-2 (Tan and Gregoriadis, 1989; Gursel and Gregoriadis, 1997a). Values of covalent coupling for the toxoid (21.8 and 23%) and IL-15 (20.7 and 21.6 % for two different amounts used) were also considerable (Table 1). In addition, as the values obtained for IL-15 were based on the CTLL-2 proliferation assay, covalent coupling to the liposomal surface did not appear to affect the biological activity of the cytokine.

The effect of interleukin-15 on immune responses against liposomal tetanus toxoid

The immunological co-adjuvant activity of "low" (150-734 units) and "high" (1270-7049 units) doses of IL-15 was monitored in experiments where animals were immunized with 0.1 μg free toxoid alone or in the presence of the two different doses of free IL-15 as such or in mixture with preformed empty liposomes, or with 0.1 μg toxoid in a variety of liposomal formulations in the absence or presence of IL-15 (see legend to Table 2). These included separately entrapped IL-15 and toxoid (mixed before injection), and IL-15 and toxoid either co-entrapped in or covalently linked to the same liposomes (Table 2). Antibody responses obtained with these formulations were compared with responses observed in animals injected with liposome-entrapped or coupled toxoid alone. As established in preliminary work, immune responses obtained with 0.1μg liposomal toxoid were low (Table 2) and similar to those obtained with the same amount of free toxoid (see legend to Table 2).

A modest but significant ($P<0.02-0.05$) rise in primary IgG_1 response was observed against the toxoid from a $\log_{10}$ value of 2.0 (liposomal toxoid alone) to values of 2.5-3.0 when IL-15 was present together with the antigen in the same liposomes, or where toxoid-containing DRV were mixed with free cytokine ($\log_{10}$ 2.7). However, there was no change in responses for liposomes with separately entrapped antigen and cytokine (results not shown). As expected, the co-adjuvant effect of IL-15 was greater for secondary responses (Table 2). For instance, there was a ten-fold increase (to $\log_{10}$ values of about 3.7) in immune responses (IgG_1) for formulations with co-entrapped or surface co-linked toxoid and IL-15 (both doses) compared to liposomal toxoid alone, liposomal toxoid mixed with separately entrapped IL-15 or free toxoid mixed with free IL-15 (Table 2 and legend).

As with the primary response, entrapped toxoid mixed with free IL-15 (low dose) also gave a significantly higher anti-toxoid IgG_1 response (Table 2) suggesting a physical association of IL-15 with the liposomal surface. Indeed, such association was confirmed in experiments (Gursel and Gregoriadis, 1997b) where DRV liposomes composed of equimolar PC and cholesterol were mixed with IL-15 and stored at 4°C for one week which is the period of time elapsed between the preparation of co-entrapped or surface co-linked toxoid and IL-15 and use in the immunization studies. After centrifugation of the stored mixture and assay of

IL-15 in the supernatant, 46% of the cytokine was estimated to be adsorbed onto the liposomal surface. This same preparation as well as those with co-linked antigen and cytokine (both doses) also boosted the secondary anti-toxoid IgG_{2b} titers significantly more when compared with liposomal toxoid alone or even with co-entrapped toxoid and IL-15 (Table 2). However, only the co-linked antigen and cytokine (high dose) preparation was effective in significantly increasing the IgG_{2a} subclass titers (Table 2). The effectiveness of the latter preparation may be due to an interaction of the surface linked antigen with B-cells by which it is eventually presented. In contrast, there appears to be only one possible route of processing and presentation for the liposome-entrapped antigen, namely via the macrophages (Shahum and Therien, 1994). It is also conceivable that IL-15 linked to the surface of liposomes interacts directly, and thus more effectively, with its receptor on B cells (Armitage et al, 1995), leading to their proliferation and differentiation. The mechanism through which entrapped IL-15 exerts its co-adjuvant action is not clear at present but it is likely to result, at least to some extent, from cytokine molecules adsorbed to the liposomal surface during the process of their entrapment.

CONCLUSIONS

The present immunization studies (Gursel and Gregoriadis, 1997b) strongly suggest that IL-15 acts similarly to IL-2 (Gursel and Gregoriadis, 1997a) as an immunological co-adjuvant in conjunction with liposomes. It appears that the spatial distribution of the liposomal antigen and cytokine in the vesicles may influence the extent and subclass of IgG production. For instance, for IL-15 to act as a co-adjuvant, its presence together with the antigen in the same liposomes is required, either as co-entrapped, co-linked or adsorbed. The observation that IL-15 fails to potentiate immune responses against the toxoid when entrapped separately from it, or in the presence of a mixture of free toxoid and empty liposomes, suggests a need for the cytokine and the antigen to contact the same antigen-presenting cells. This is supported by data (Heath and Playfair, 1990) showing increased adjuvanticity for IFN-γ conjugated to the antigen.

Acknowledgements

This work was part of M.G.'s Ph.D. Thesis. We thank the Turkish Government for a scholarship to M. G. and Mrs Concha Perring for excellent secretarial assistance.

REFERENCES

Abraham, E. and Shah, S., 1992, Intranasal immunization with liposomes containing IL-2 enhances bacterial polysaccharide antigen-specific pulmonary secretory antibody responses, J.Immunol., 149:3719.

Anderson, P.M., Hanson, D.C., Hasz, M.R., Halet, Blazar, B.R. and Ochoa, A.C., 1994, Cytokines in liposomes: preliminary studies with IL-1, IL-2, IL-6, GM-CSF and interferon-γ, Cytokine, 6:92

Armitage, R.J., Macduff, B.M., Eisenman, J., Paxton, R. and Grabstein, K.H., 1995, IL-15 has stimulatory activity for the induction of B cell proliferation and differentiation, J. Immunol., 154:483

Carson, W.E., Giri, J.G., Lindermann, M.J., Linett, M.L., Ahdieh, M., Paxton, R., Anderson, D., Eisenmann, J., Grabstein, K. and Caliguri, M.A., 1994, Interleukin (IL) 15 is a novel cytokine that activates human natural killer cells via components of the IL-2 receptor, J.Exp. Med., 180:1395

Garçon, N., Senior, J. and Gregoriadis, G., 1986, Coupling of ligands to liposomes before entrapment of agents sensitive to coupling procedures, Biochem.Soc.Trans., 14:1038

Giri, J.G., Ahdieh, M., Eisenmann, J., Shanebeck, K., Grabstein, K., Kumaki, S., Name, A., Park, L.S., Cosman, D. and Anderson, D., 1994, Utilization of the β and γ chains of the IL-2 receptor by the novel cytokine IL-15, EMBO J., 13:2822

Grabstein, K.H., Eisenmann, J., Shanebeck, K., Rauch, C., Srinivasan, S., Fung, V., Beers, C., Richardson, J., Schoenborn, M.A., Ahdieh, M., Johnson, L., Alderson, M.R., Watson, J.D., Anderson, D.M. and Giri, J.G., 1994, Cloning of a T cell growth factor that interacts with the β chain of the interleukin-2 receptor, Science, 264:965

Gregoriadis, G., 1990, Immunological adjuvants: A role for liposomes (Review) Immunol.Today, 11:89

Gregoriadis, G., Davis, D. and Davies, A., 1987, Liposomes as immunological adjuvants: Antigen incorporation studies, Vaccine, 5:145

Gregoriadis, G., Saffie, R. and de Souza, B., 1997, Liposome-mediated DNA vaccination, FEBS Lett, 402:107.

Gregoriadis, G., Garçon, N., da Silva, H. and Sternberg, B., 1993, Coupling of ligands to liposomes independently of solute entrapment: Observations on the formed vesicles, Biochim.Biophys.Acta, 1147:185

Gursel, M. and Gregoriadis, G., 1997a, Interleukin-2 as a co-adjuvant for liposomal tetanus toxoid: The effect of cytokine and antigen mode of localization in the vesicles, J.Drug Targeting, in press

Gürsel, M. and Gregoriadis, G., 1997b, Interleukin-15 acts as an immunological co-adjuvant for liposomal antigen in vivo, Immunology Letters, 55:161

Heath, A.W. and Playfair, J.H.L., 1990, Conjugation of interferon-γ to antigen enhances its adjuvanticity, Immunology, 71:454

Ho, R.J.Y., Burke, R.L. and Merigan, T.C., 1992, Liposome-formulated interleukin-2 as an adjuvant of recombinant HSV glycoprotein gD for the treatment of recurrent genital HSV-2 in guinea-pigs, Vaccine, 10:209

Kirby, C. and Gregoriadis, G., 1984, Dehydration-rehydration vesicles (DRV): A new method for high yield drug entrapment in liposomes, Biotechnology, 2:979

Kirby, C., Clarke, J. and Gregoriadis, G., 1980, Effect of the cholesterol content of small unilamellar liposomes on their stability in vivo and in vitro, Biochem.J., 186:591

Matthews, D.J., Clark, P.A., Herbert, J., Morgan, G., Armitage, R.J., Kinnon, C., Minty, A., Grabstein, K.H., Caput, C., Ferrara, P. and Callard, R., 1995, Function of the interleukin-2 (IL-2) receptor γ-chain in biologic responses of X-linked severe combined immunodeficient B cells to IL-2, IL-4, IL-13 and IL-15, Blood, 85:38

Mbawuike, I.N., Wyde, P.R. and Anderson, P.M., 1990, Enhancement of the protective efficacy of inactivated influenza A virus vaccine in aged mice by IL-2 liposomes, Vaccine, 8:347

McCormack, B. and Gregoriadis, G., 1994, Drugs-in-cyclodextrins-in liposomes: A novel concept in drug delivery, Int.J.Pharm., 112:249

Meuer, S.C., Dumann, H., Zum-Buschenfelde, K.H.M. and Kohler, H., 1989, Low-dose interleukin-2 induces systemic immune responses against HbsAg in immunodeficient non-responders to hepatitis B vaccination, The Lancet, 1:15

Roehm, N.W., Rodgers, G.H., Hatfield, S.M. and Glasebrook, A.L., 1991, An improved colorimetric assay for cell proliferation and viability utilizing the tetrazolium salt XTT, J.Immunol.Meth., 142:257

Sencer, S.F., Rich, M.L., Katsanis, E., Ochoa, A.C. and Anderson, P.M., 1991, Anti-tumor vaccine adjuvant effects of IL-2 liposomes in mice immunized against MCA-102 sarcoma, Eur.Cytokine Netw., 2:311

Shahum, E. and Therien, H.-M., 1994, Correlation between in vitro and in vivo behaviour of liposomal antigens, Vaccine, 12:1125

Snyder, S.L. and Vannier, W.E., 1984, Immunologic response to protein immobilized on the surface of liposomes via covalent azo-bonding, Biochim.Biophys.Acta, 772:288

Tan, L. and Gregoriadis, G., 1989, Dehydration-rehydration vesicles (DRV): A new method for high yield drug entrapment in liposomes, Biochem.Soc.Trans., 17:693

Wilkinson, P.C. and Liew, F.Y., 1995, Chemoattraction of human blood T lymphocytes by interleukin-15, J Exp Med., 181:1255

PROTECTION AGAINST TUBERCULOSIS BY PLASMID DNA

R.E. Tascon, M.J. Colston, E. Stavropoulos, S. Ragno, D. Gregory and D.B. Lowrie

Division of Mycobacterial Research, National Institute for Medical Research, London, UK

INTRODUCTION

The availability of cloned mycobacterial genes and suitable vectors for expression in mammalian cells has now opened a new avenue in which individual mycobacterial protein antigens can be tested for their ability to confer protective immunity. Expression of protection against mycobacteria is largely a function of antigen specific CD4 and cytotoxic CD8 T cells. We have found that intramuscular injection of plasmid DNA expressing several mycobacterial immunodominant genes can induce both T cell populations and confer protection equivalent to BCG, suggesting that this approach may lead to a new vaccine.

RESULTS AND DISCUSSION

Tuberculosis continues to be a major health problem particulary in developing countries, this is despite the existence of highly effective chemotherapeutic drugs and widespread use of BCG vaccine. Part of the explanation for the modest impact of BCG vaccination on the global problem is that it gives little or no protection in some parts of the world, although it is highly effective in others.

Major steps forward are now being made as a result of recombinant DNA technology; by expressing mycobacterial genes directly within mammalian cells we have found that individual mycobacterial protein antigens can protect as effectively as the living, antigenically complex BCG vaccine; the key appears to be the development of an intense antigen specific CD4 and CD8 cytotoxic T cell response following endogenous expression of the antigen as a transgene.

Previous work using a retroviral vector to express the Mycobacterium leprae gene encoding the 65 kDa heat shock protein (MLhsp65) in the macrophage-like cell line J774 established that the transfected cells (J774-hsp65) presented the antigen for recognition by MHC class I- and MHC class II-restricted T cells and when they were injected into syngeneic Balb/c mice the mice were protected against subsequent challenge with virulent Mycobacterium tuberculosis H37Rv (Silva and Lowrie, 1994). Listeria monocytogenes or immunization with the protein with adjuvant showed no protection.

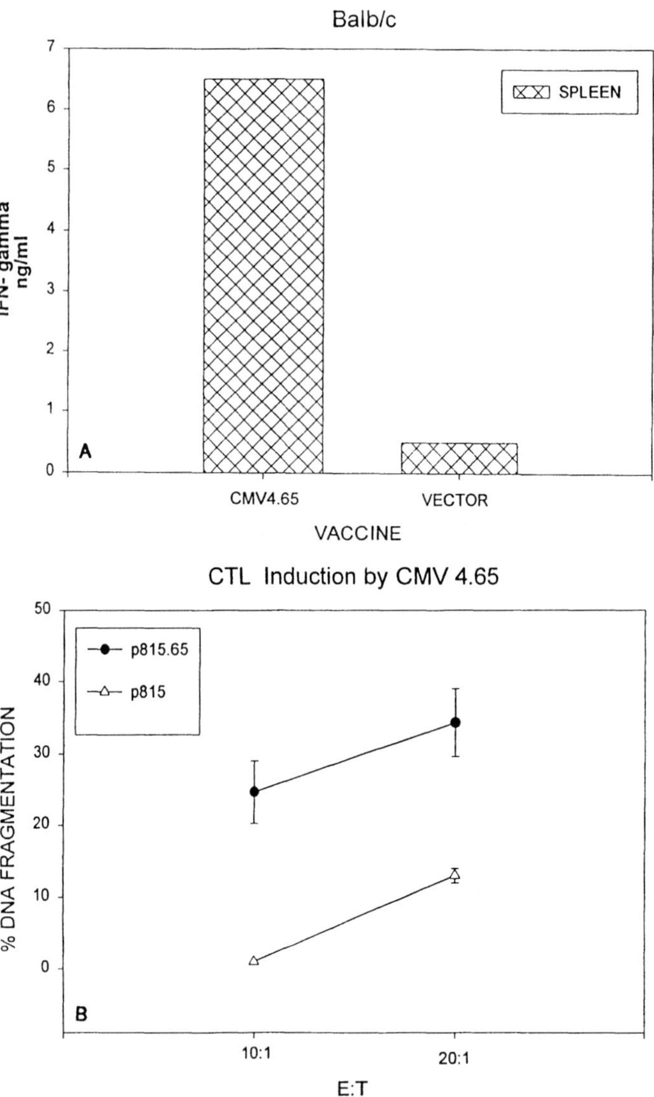

Figure 1. Cellular immune responses induced by vaccination with plasmid pCMV4.65. (A) IFN-gamma production by spleen cells of pCMV4.65 or vector (pCDNA3) vaccinated mice in response to hsp65 stimulation. (B) CTL responses against P815 or P815 cells transfected with the hsp65 gene (p815-65) by T cell effector cells of pCMV4.65 vaccinated mice. Plasmid pCMV4.65 was obtained by cloning the CMV intron A as a Hind III 0.9kb DNA fragment in the unique Hind III site of the vector pCMV3.65 (Tascon et al, 1996). Mice received the plasmid pCMV4.65 or pCDNA3 on four occasions at 3-4 weeks intervals, 4-6 weeks after the the last DNA injection the mice were sacrificed and the spleen cells collected; for the IFN-gamma experiments the spleen cells were stimulated with the recombinant hsp65 antigen for 72-96h and the supernatants were analized by ELISA (Genzime). For the CTL determinations the CMV4.65 immune spleen cells were reestimulated in vitro for 5 days in the presence of P815-65 irradiated cells and IL-2(20 U.I/ml) and then used in a standard JAM (Matzinger P, 1991) assay, using P815 or P815-65 target labeled cells.

Limiting dilution analysis (Tasswell, 1981), of hsp65-reactive T cells with $CD4^+CD8^-$ and $CD4^-CD8^+$ phenotypes in spleens of J774-hsp65 vaccinated mice showed that both types were present at very high frequency, whereas immunization with the hsp65 protein mixed with J774 cells or in Freund's incomplete adjuvant preferentially increased cells with $CD4^+CD8^-$ phenotype

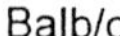

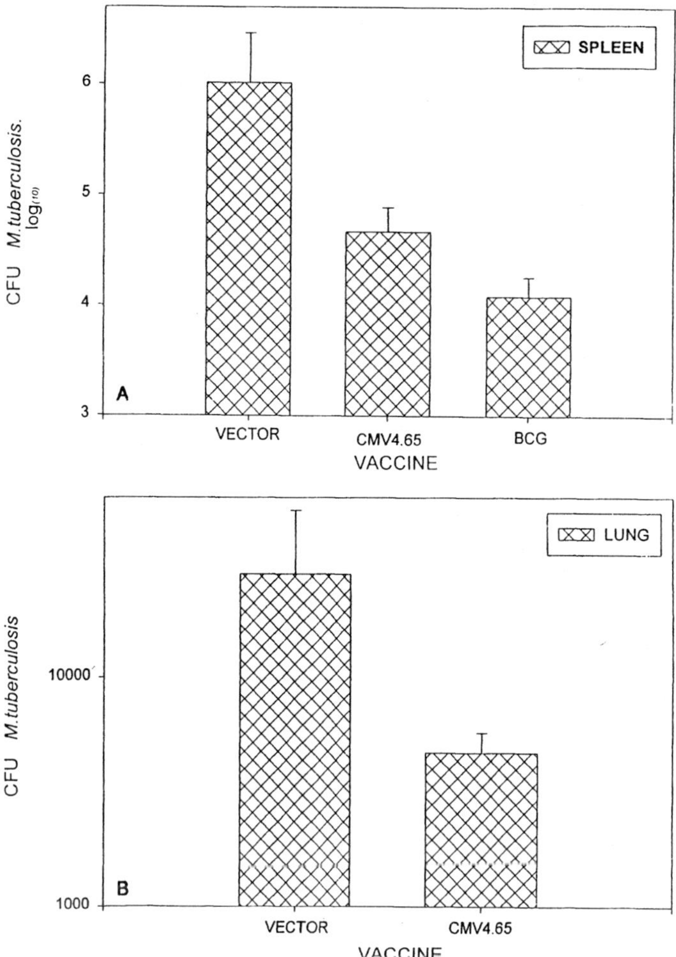

Figure 2. Protection against tuberculosis by immunisation with DNA encoding the mycobacterial hsp65 (A) or hsp70 (B) proteins. Mice were immunised on four occasions at 3-4 wk intervals by injections of 50-75 mg plasmid DNA into each quadriceps muscle. Mice received the plasmids pCMV4.65, pCMV70, or vector without the antigen-encoding sequences; a positive control group in each experiment, received a single intradermal injection of live BCG vaccine at the time of the first DNA dose. Four weeks after the last DNA dose they were infected by intraperitoneal injection with M. tuberculosis and 6 wk later the numbers of live bacteria (mean ± SD) were assessed in spleens and lungs.

suggesting that the $CD8^{+}$ T cells contributed to the protective response, an inference that was substantiated by passive transfer of immunity with such T cells (Silva et al, 1994).

Hence, a key requirement for a protective effect of vaccination against tuberculosis seems to be the ability of the vaccine to prime a large population of antigen specific CD4 and cytotoxic CD8 T cells. Vaccination by endogenous antigen arising from a transgene apparently establishes this state, whereas injection of exogenous antigen does not or does it very inefficiently.

For DNA vaccination we have introduced the hsp65 gene into suitable plasmids downstream of either the CMV immediate early gene promoter (pCMV) or the promoter of the murine 'housekeeping' gene for hydroxymethylglutaryl-CoA-reductase (pHMG) (Tascon et al, 1996, Gautier et al, 1989). Both promoters effectively drive expression of mycobacterial genes in mammalian cells. In our standard protocol we injected the DNA into the quadriceps muscles of groups of 4-6 mice, 50-75μg into the left leg and 50-75μg into the right leg, four times at 3-4 wk intervals (400-600 μg/mouse). Control mice received empty plasmid DNA, hsp65 protein in saline or in Freund's incomplete adjuvant, or a single intradermal dose of BCG.

High antibody levels and strong cellular immune responses against the mycobacterial antigen were found in the hsp65 plasmid vaccinated mice (Tascon et al, 1994), these responses were not obtained following immunization with plasmids that did not contain the inserted mycobacterial DNA; further, spleen cells from hsp65 treated mice specifically reacted to the hsp65 antigen in vitro producing high levels of IFN-gamma (Figure 1a) and low levels of IL-4 (Tascon et al, 1996), indicating a predominantly Th1 type of response.

Splenocytes from hsp65 DNA vaccinated mice also displayed antigen specific cytotoxicity against P-815 target cells that had been either transfected with the hsp65 gene (Figure 1b) or that had been loaded with synthetic peptides representing predicted MHC class I restricted T cell epitopes (Tascon et al, 1996).

This standard protocol of vaccination with hsp65 DNA protected against tuberculosis challenge (Figure 2a). The level of protection differed between strains of mice but was high in outbred Parkes mice and in CBA/B10 strain (Tascon et al, 1996). Hsp65 is not unique in having this capacity to induce protective immune response when given as a DNA vaccine. We have now tested several mycobacterial protein antigens individually as DNA vaccines using CMV based constructs in Balb/c mice. High specific cellular immune responses have been found and preliminary results

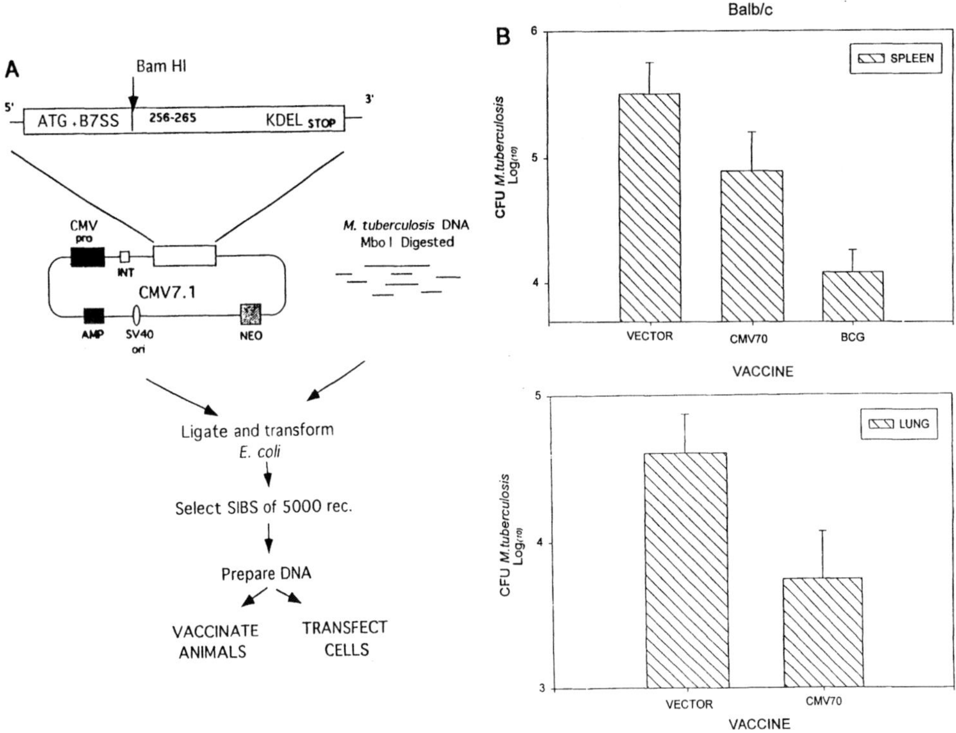

Figure 3. Schematic representation of the vector pCMV7.1 used to construct partial genomic DNA libraries of Mycobacterium tuberculosis. The vector contain the CMV promoter, intron A, an ATG codon and a signal peptide encoding region; derived from the murine B7-1 molecule (Freeman et al, 1991); followed by a unique Bam HI restriction site. A mini gene encoding the peptide: MALSTLVVNKIKDEL, has been cloned 'in frame' to the signal peptide coding region, to target expression to the endoplasmic reticulum.

suggest that vaccination with plasmid DNA constructs encoding the hsp70 (Figure 2b) and the 6 kDa antigen (ESAT-6) (Sorensen et al, 1995), also elicit significant protection. Comparisons in outbred mice, and in other experimental models of tuberculosis will be needed before conclusions can be drawn as to which antigens are the best candidates for inclusion in a practical vaccine. However, the best antigens may yet remain to be discovered and it would be surprising if new candidates are not revealed by this approach; in fact, a new interesting alternative for the identification and characterization of protective antigens is the vaccination with cDNA or genomic DNA libraries constructed in optimised plasmid expression vectors. We have vaccinated mice with partial DNA libraries of M. tuberculosis H37Rv, cloned in our CMV 7.1 expression vector (Figure 3) and found that the immune spleen cells were able to produce significant levels of IFN-gamma, in response to mycobacterial antigen in vitro, suggesting that even very low doses of DNA are sufficient for effective priming of naive T cells. Recently (Barry et al, 1995) reported that immunisation with partial DNA expression libraries from Mycoplasma pulmonis provided protection against challenge from the pathogen, further indicating that this approach holds great promise for vaccinology.

A vaccine that gives protection better than BCG by endogenous expression of only a few proteins will leave the majority of the species specific antigens available for diagnostic tests in vaccinated populations. Furthermore, and of potentially far greater significance, there is the prospect that such a vaccine might function in those populations in wich BCG does not. However, special safety issues have to be addressed before clinical evaluation in humans can be contemplated; the possibility of promoting oncogenesis or autoimmunity have to be seriously studied; Such issues will have a high priority as DNA vaccines are optimized.

Acknowledgements

This work received financial support from the WHO Global Programme for Vaccines. We thank Colin Anderson for his technical assistence.

REFERENCES

Barry M. A., Lai W. C., Johnston S.A., 1995, Protection against mycoplasma infection using expression library immunization. Nature, 377:632.

Freeman, G. J., Gray, G. S., Gimmi, C. D., Lombard, D. B., Zou, L. White, M., Fingeroth, J. D., Gribben, J. G., and Nadler, L. M., 1991, Structure, expression, and T cell costimulatory activity of the murine homologue of the human B lymphocyte activation antigen B7. J. Exp. Med., 174:625.

Gautier, C., Mehtali, M. and Lathe, R., 1989, A ubiquitous mammalian expression vector, pHMG based on a housekeeping gene promoter. Nucleic Acids Res., 17:8389.

Matzinger-P., 1991, The JAM test a simple assay for DNA fragmentation and cell death. J.Immunol.Methods., 145:185.

Silva, C.L. and Lowrie, D.B., 1994, A single mycobacterial protein (hsp65) expressed by a transgenic antigen-resenting cell vaccinates mice against tuberculosis. Immunol., 82:244.

Silva, C.L., Silva, M.F., Pietro, R.C.L.R. and Lowrie, D.B. 1994, Protection against tuberculosis by passive transfer with T-cell clones recognizing mycobacterial heat-shock protein 65. Immunol., 83:341.

Sorensen, A.L., Nagai, S., Houen, G., Andersen, P. and Andersen, A.B., 1995, Purification and characterization of a low-molecular-mass T-cell antigen secreted by Mycobacterium tuberculosis. Infect. Immun., 63:1710.

Tascon, R.E., Colston, M. J., Ragno S., Stavropoulos, E., Gregory D., Lowrie D.B., 1996, Vaccination against tuberculosis by DNA injection. Nature Medicine, 2:888.

Taswell, C., 1981, Limiting dilution assays for the determination of immunocompetent cell frequencies. I. Data analysis. J. Immunol., 126:1614.

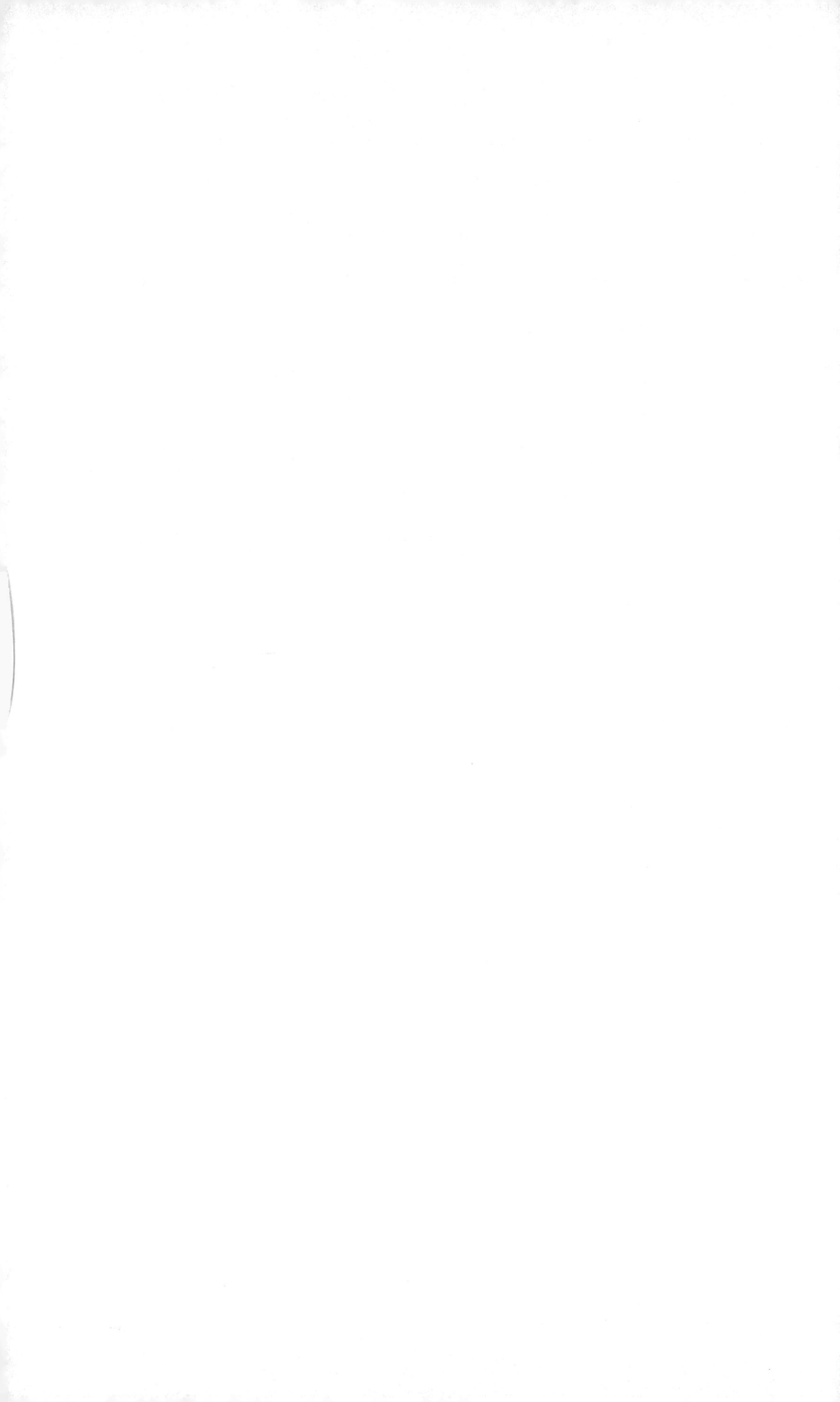

FROM SCIENTIFIC DISCOVERY TO CLINICAL TRIAL:

OVERCOMING THE REGULATORY HURDLES -

A GUIDE FOR ACADEMIC RESEARCHERS

Jillian K. Bennet

Research & Development Division, CSL Ltd,
45 Poplar Road Parkville, Victoria 3052, Australia

INTRODUCTION

Vaccines have a distinguished history originating from the demonstration by Jenner in 1796 that cowpox could protect against the development of smallpox. Historically, the objective of vaccination was to provide effective immunity to the target disease, and with the introduction earlier this century of widespread immunisation for diseases such as diphtheria, tetanus, polio, smallpox and pertussis, the occurrence of these diseases has been significantly reduced if not eliminated. However, the acceptance of immunisation programs in the community could have been jeopardised by the rare events which occurred as a result of poor vaccine manufacture.

Over the past thirty years the objective of vaccination has been refined to additionally incorporate safety and quality considerations into the manufacture and supply of vaccines. The control of human vaccine development and manufacture is governed by regulatory bodies such as the European Medicines Evaluation Agency (EMEA) in Europe, the Food and Drug Administration (FDA) in the USA, the Ministry of Health and Welfare (MHW) in Japan, the Health Protection Branch (HPB) in Canada, and the Therapeutic Goods Administration (TGA) in Australia. Their role is to ensure the consistency, safety, quality and efficacy of vaccines.

In order to progress the development of a vaccine from discovery through to a marketed product, a range of investigational studies need to be undertaken. These studies can be divided into the non-clinical and clinical development stages (refer to Figure 1).

Non-clinical development studies are directed towards defining the characteristics of the product, including the parameters which determine product quality, the demonstration of safety, and assessment of action or potency in appropriate animal models.

Clinical development is undertaken in three phases with increasing numbers of participants at each phase. Initial Phase I studies are designed to demonstrate safety in small numbers of individuals, these are followed by safety and efficacy studies to establish the treatment regimen and then large, statistically-significant studies in the target population to demonstrate safety and efficacy.

The Phase I studies are usually undertaken in normal healthy volunteers (n = 20-80 subjects) and offer no therapeutic benefit to the participants. The studies are designed to demonstrate tolerance and safety, and to provide some pharmacokinetic data. However, sometimes these studies are undertaken in individuals who are affected by life threatening disease (eg HIV and oncology patients).

Phase II studies can only proceed once a review of adverse events reported in Phase I has been undertaken. Phase II studies are undertaken in a limited defined patient population (n = several hundred). The major objectives are to establish comparative evidence of the product's effectiveness and safety in controlled trials. At the completion of these studies and prior to proceeding to Phase III studies the effective dose and maximum safe dose will have been established.

Phase III studies are undertaken to provide substantial confirmatory evidence of effectiveness and safety as established at Phase II. Larger, controlled trials are undertaken during Phase III and are designed to provide pivotal clinical data to support marketing approval of a new product. These studies are designed to incorporate statistical power to support the findings of effectiveness and safety of the product.

All clinical studies should be undertaken in compliance with Good Clinical Practice, have Ethics Committee Approval and in accordance with the principles of the Declaration of Helsinki. Formal approval to undertake a clinical development program varies considerably between countries. The documentation requirements to initiate a clinical trial ranges from no regulatory agency notification or approval, through to notification with no approval or no objection, and notification and approval from the agency. Thus, although the principles governing clinical research leading to product registration are identical, the procedures for initiating clinical trials differ.

At the completion of the clinical development phase an application for approval to market the product is submitted for regulatory agency review. Regulatory agencies review the product application in terms of product quality and purity, safety and efficacy. Upon a favourable review by the regulatory agency, the product is registered for marketing within the country/countries of responsibility of the agency.

In certain life threatening diseases such as HIV and cancer it is possible to accelerate the product development process. The rationale for this is based on a risk versus benefit analysis. The requirements for a product such as a vaccine intended for use in normal healthy children will be such that the risk must be perceived to be negligible relative to the benefit.

Discovery	Non-clinical Development	Clinical Development	Registration	Post Marketing
Research Investigation	Characterisation Purification Formulation Optimisation Animal Models Safety Testing	Phase I → Phase II → Phase III →	Regulatory Agency Review and Evaluation, Registration	Phase IV

Figure 1. Stages of product development.

The purpose of this paper is to address some of the regulatory issues that academic researchers should consider when initiating a development program which may lead to the clinical development of a new biological product such as a vaccine. It is unlikely that many academic researchers will have sufficient funding to undertake a full product development program alone, therefore it is the intention of this paper to address the basic regulatory requirements that will provide a sound basis for attracting a commercial sponsor or partner.

There are many regulatory issues to consider in the early stages of development of a new biological product. These issues relate to documentation, quality and purity, safety and efficacy. The resources used in the preparation of this paper are listed at the end.

DOCUMENTATION

Good documentation practices form the basis of the principles of Good Laboratory Practice (GLP). Thorough documentation of experimental protocols, observations, outcomes and conclusions provides evidence of the conduct of studies, and validity and integrity of the scientific data generated. The inclusion of appropriate standards and/or controls in the experiment ensures future reproducibility of the experimental findings (OECD 1992).

To ensure that laboratory and pre-clinical findings can be reproduced it is essential that good records are maintained. This would involve the daily recording of materials and methods used as well as the results and/or observations of experiments. Additionally, materials used during the course of any study should be clearly and unambiguously labelled.

Good documentation practices enable a researcher to back-track ,or trace exactly what was done, why something was done, and what was used during an experiment. As a consequence, unexpected or ambiguous results can be investigated to determine a causality, experimental findings can be reproduced, and records can be produced to support intellectual property claims.

Records should be maintained in a workbook which has pre-numbered secured pages and not on loose or scrap pieces of paper, it provides an assurance that critical details are not lost or misplaced. Such events could jeopardise the timely completion of a work program, and prove costly in terms of resources, and perhaps could result in the loss of a competitive edge.

QUALITY AND PURITY, SAFETY AND EFFICACY

It is difficult to give a comprehensive account of the all of the requirements for the demonstration of quality and purity, safety and efficacy for biological products. In an attempt to illustrate the requirements, examples will be used that may be familiar to many of you in your current fields of research.

Quality and purity

For the purposes of this paper I will define product quality as the attributes which are unique to that product. These attributes will specify the product profile in terms of how we will ultimately characterise the product to enable it to be reliably and reproducibly manufactured, thus enabling consistency of performance of the product in the target species. Therefore every aspect that may affect the product quality must be assessed, this ranges from the origin and quality of the starting materials, through to the method and equipment by which the product is made, the identification of impurities, and the development and validation of tests to demonstrate of reliability of performance or potency.

By establishing a specification for the product, this means that a product of consistent purity and quality can be consistently and reliably produced, thus claims for therapeutic action/benefit and safety may be made. If the product is of inconsistent quality, the safety and efficacy data may be invalidated.

Origin and history of starting materials

One of the basic requirements for the development of a biological product is knowledge of the origin and history of the biological starting material. If it is a virus, bacteria or parasite it is important to record where it was isolated, how it was isolated and the history of passage in the laboratory. Additionally, if the biological product is a gene product it is important to document how the gene was isolated, the origin and construction of the expression vector including promoters and flanking sequences used and the origin and maintenance of the host cell line. Once the cell line or microorganism has been optimised for growth and/or expression of the gene product a seed lot system should be established to ensure a stable genetic composition of the inoculum or cell line, each time culture of the product is required. A summary of the requirements for characterisation of starting materials including expression constructs, seedlots and strains is shown in Figure 2.

2.1 Characterisation of expression construct

Origin of the source/gene sequence
Construction of the expression construct:
- promoter sequence
- flanking sequences
- origins of replication
- antibiotic resistance genes
- expression as a fusion protein

Restriction endonuclease maps
Complete nucleotide sequence

2.2 Characterisation of host cell line

Description of :-
source
phenotype
genotype
Amplification methods
Method of transfer of construct into host cell
Stability of the clone

2.3 Characterisation /preparation of seedlot

Selection of single clone
Document methods and history of propagation
Dispense aliquots
Preserve by cryopreservation/lyophilisation
Test for :-
viability
identity
purity
presence of gene product

Figure 2. Characterisation of biological starting material/host.

Product characterisation

It is important to establish a set of criteria or measured parameters which is known as the specification, which will reliably ensure the quality of the product. This should include validated methods to ensure product purity, stability, activity or potency, yield, and identity. Validation is the characterisation of assay performance that enables the understanding of the significance of the results obtained in an assay. What is required from an assay is accuracy, reproducibility of performance, specificity and to establish a range. It is essential that this be done, because this will enable you to reproduce your experiments consistently, and hence reliably establish your claims for the product. If the product is of inconsistent quality leading to significant batch to batch variation, the safety and efficacy data for the product may be invalidated.

If you are intending to test your product in the clinic it is essential that you have stability data to support the product shelf life for the duration of the clinical trial. This stability data should be generated for product stored in identical containers under identical conditions to those which are proposed for clinical use. Some of the methods used to characterise vaccine products are shown in Figure 3.

3.1 Stability

- Appearance
- Temperature
- Light
- Humidity

3.2 Potency/Activity

- Bioassays:
    - *in vitro*
    - *in vivo*

- Selection of reference standards

3.3 Purity

- Characterisation of degradation products
- Freedom from adventitious agents
- Removal of host cell protein
- Removal of endotoxin
- Quantitation of excipients
- Quantitation/characterisation of impurities
- Quantitation/characterisation of DNA

3.4 Identity and Yield

- NH_2 - terminal sequence
- Amino acid composition
- Peptide mapping
- Appearance
- Western blot/EIA
- SDS-PAGE
- HPLC
- Chromatographic procedures
- Mass Spectroscopy

Figure 3. Characterisation of product.

Safety

Characterisation and safety testing of mammalian cell lines

In general we think of safety in terms of the product itself. However it is advisable to consider safety issues early in the development of a product associated with a biological compound grown or expressed in mammalian cell lines.

Potential viral contamination of product may arise from the host cell lines, or from adventitious introduction of virus during production processes. To overcome contamination in mammalian cell lines it is recommended that you source your cell line from a recognised culture collection where documentation on the history of that cell line can be provided.

A range of tests are recommended for characterisation of the master cell bank and working cell bank, these are shown in Figure 4. However, this battery of tests may be cost prohibitive to many research programs. In the first instance I would recommend testing to ensure:

- freedom from mycoplasma contamination
- sterility
- electron microscopy for retroviruses

as the minimal requirement for preliminary research investigations.

Safety of the product

Safety testing of biological products is an important consideration. The objectives of animal safety studies are to predict the toxicity in humans, to identify target organs which may be affected, to provide an estimation of risk for humans and to establish the potential effects of an overdose. Many of the safety testing requirements have been developed for new chemical entities and are not applicable to some categories of biological products. Such comprehensive safety testing includes pharmacokinetics, pharmacodynamic, immunotoxicity, reproductive toxicity, acute toxicity, chronic toxicity, mutagenicity, tumorigenicity and local tolerance studies.

In general, the safety testing requirements for polypeptides and proteins which are shown to be identical to naturally occurring human polypeptides or proteins are minimal and may only require pharmacodynamic data. Closely related polypeptides/proteins that have known differences in amino acid sequences or post-translational modifications that may affect biological activity and/or immunogenicity may additionally require pharmacokinetic and acute and chronic toxicity data (James,1994).

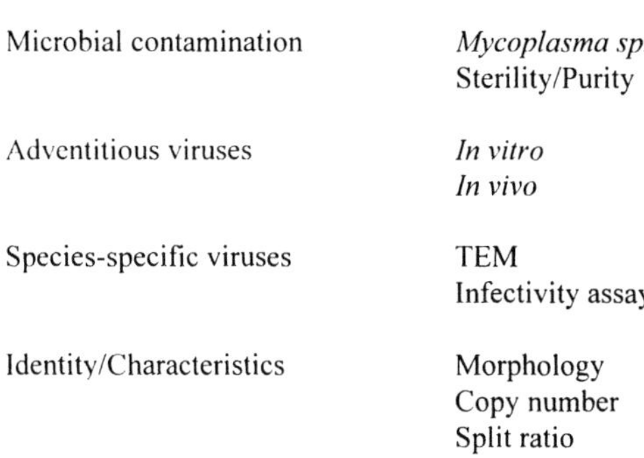

Microbial contamination	*Mycoplasma sp.* Sterility/Purity
Adventitious viruses	*In vitro* *In vivo*
Species-specific viruses	TEM Infectivity assay
Identity/Characteristics	Morphology Copy number Split ratio

Figure 4. Master cell bank characterisation.

Pharmacodynamic studies investigate the mode of action of the test substance on an organism and include:

- dose-effect relationships
- mechanisms of side effects
- duration of response

however, in the context of a vaccine this may be related to the type of immune response and the duration of the immune response.

Pharmacokinetic studies investigate the influence of the organism on the test substance and include the mode of :

- adsorption
- distribution
- metabolism
- elimination of the product

these studies help establish the dosage regime.

Pharmacokinetic studies are not generally applicable to vaccines, but may involve studies looking at the retention of the dosage form at the injection site.

Acute toxicity - (single dose toxicity) (rodents)

Acute toxicity studies involve a single application of high doses of the test substance and establish a dose response relationship. These studies are used to identify the "approximate lethal dose" of the substance and are useful to predict the events associated with an accidental overdosage. The application route for acute toxicity testing should reflect the proposed clinical application route and should also ensure systemic exposure.

Chronic toxicity - (Repeat dose toxicity) (Rodent and non-rodent)

Chronic toxicity studies involve administration of the test substance by the proposed clinical route daily at least three dose levels for at least four weeks. Slight toxicity should be observed at the highest dose level, the intermediate dose should correspond to the therapeutic dose.

Since vaccines are administered only a few times these studies are generally not applicable.

Local tolerance - Assessed at the application site

Local tolerance testing investigates the effect of the vaccine at the administration site. It is recommended that vaccine components be tested separately and together.

Local tolerance testing is the only absolutely essential safety/toxicity test recommended routinely for vaccines. The test is simple in principle and practice, and can be done by researchers providing good laboratory practice is observed. Careful documentation of any observations made at the administration site in terms of reactions such as swelling (firmness, size and duration of the swelling), redness, tenderness and abscess formation should be undertaken.

It is fair to say that in general, extensive safety toxicity testing of vaccines is not required. The standard test procedures described have been established to assess the pharmacological and safety features of chemical compounds or pharmacologically active biopharmaceuticals that are applied frequently (eg. clotting factors). However if a new adjuvant or excipient is proposed for inclusion in the product, the full battery of safety tests may need to be applied.

The costs of safety testing are high and it is for this reason that many researchers and vaccine manufacturers have chosen to use vaccine components with a well established quality and safety profile (excipients and adjuvants).

I would like to focus briefly on nucleic acid immunisation which is an example of a new technology which is currently being trialed for application in new and improved vaccines. The first major regulatory hurdle for a new technology is a lack of precedents, and initially the most challenging issues for nucleic acid vaccines were related to safety because there were already precedents in terms of methods for characterising recombinant DNA products. Issues pertaining to safety may affect society's willingness to accept these new vaccines.

The safety issues initially mooted were:

- integration or insertion of the DNA into the host genome leading to inactivation of an essential gene, or a transformation event as a result of insertion into a tumour suppressor gene,
- unexpected and undesirable sequelae which may develop as a result of persistent expression of foreign antigens,
- the formation of anti-DNA antibodies
- the nature of the immune response generated (sufficient antigen expressed to overcome maternal antibody and antibody dependent immune suppression, tolerisation, adverse consequences of an unnecessary CTL response).

To date these safety issues appear to be theoretical, however, there is still a greater understanding required from long term toxicological studies before we can absolutely discount the theoretical safety issues raised.

Efficacy

Ultimately true efficacy can only be established in the target species and during clinical development this is usually at Phase III. However, the predictive value of a good animal model for the disease should not be overlooked, it is a useful and worthwhile substitute for establishing the criteria to measure the safety and efficacy of the product in clinical development. However, many diseases do not have predictive animal models and it is not until phase II or III trials that the certainty of success of a new product can be gauged after a costly development program.

CONCLUSION

In closing I would like to briefly address the issues of the new vaccine technologies including new adjuvants, vaccine vectors, naked DNA immunisation and the incorporation of cytokines.

It is exciting to participate in the development of new vaccines using "cutting-edge" technologies, however you must ask yourself :

- can we clearly define/characterise our product?
- do we understand its mode of action?
- is the desired effect reproducible?
- has it been evaluated for safety and toxicity?

Ultimately it is the issue of safety that the regulatory agencies and ethics committees must address when considering an application to undertake a clinical trial of a vaccine.

I hope that this paper has provided a basic introduction to some of the data required at the research phase to demonstrate the quality, purity and safety of a product. It is unlikely that many of you will have sufficient funding to carry out the extensive testing that is required to take a product to trial alone. However, with good documentation supporting the demonstration of sound preliminary quality and safety data you will have the basis of a potential biological product development program.

REFERENCES

James, R.W., 1994, Toxicity Testing Strategies for Biotechnology-Derived and High Technology Products, BIRA Journal, 12:10.

OECD, 1992, The OECD Principles of Good Laboratory Practice, Environment Monograph No.45. Organisation For Economic Co-operation and Development, OCDE/GD(92)32, Paris

RESOURCES

Food and Drug Administration, Bethesda Maryland, USA

Points to Consider in the Production and Testing of New Drugs and Biologicals Produced by Recombinant DNA Technology, 1985, Office of Biologics Research and Review, Center for Drugs and Biologics, FDA

Points to Consider in the Characterization of Cell Lines Used to Produce Biologicals, 1987, Office of Biologics Research and Review, FDA

Points to Consider in Human Somatic Cell Therapy and Gene Therapy, 1992 Center for Biologics Evaluation and Research, Food and Drug Administration Pharmaceutical Engineering, 12:28

Supplement to the Points to Consider in the Production and testing of New Drugs and Biologicals Produced by Recombinant DNA Technology: Nucleic Acid Characterization and Genetic Stability, 1992, Center for Biologics Evaluation and Research, FDA

Points to Consider in the Characterization of Cell Lines Used to Produce Biologicals, 1993, Center for Biologics Evaluation and Research, FDA

Draft Points to Consider in the Manufacture and testing of Monoclonal Antibody Products for Human Use, 1994, Center for Biologics Evaluation and Research, FDA

Committee for Proprietary Medicinal Products, Commission of the European Communities

Stability testing of new drug substances and products, December 1993, CPMP Note for Guidance III/3335/92 Final

Stability Testing of Biotechnological/Biological Products, 1995, Annex to the Tripartite ICH Guideline for the Stability testing of New Drug Substances and Products

Production and Quality Control of Medicinal Products Derived by Recombinant DNA Technology (Revision 1994), CPMP Note for Guidance III/3477/92 Draft 7

Analysis of the Expression Construct in Cell Lines Used for the Production of r-DNA Derived Protein Products, November 1995, Note for Guidance on Quality of Biotechnological Products, CPMP/ICH/139/95

Gene Therapy Products: Quality, Safety and Efficacy Aspects in the Production of Vectors and Genetically Modified Somatic Cells, December 1994, CPMP III/5863/93

Viral Safety Evaluation of Biotechnology Products Derived from Cell Lines of Human or Animal Origin, December 1995, Draft 2, Note for Guidance on Quality of Biotechnological Products, CPMP/ICH/295/95

Validation of Analytical Methods: Methodology, November 1995, Note for Guidance on Validation of Analytical Methods, CPMP/ICH/281/95

Safety Testing of Biotechnological Products, November 1995, Draft 5 in the Development of Recommendations on "Internationally Accepted Principles for the Safety Evaluation of Biotechnologically-Derived Products"background paper for ICH3

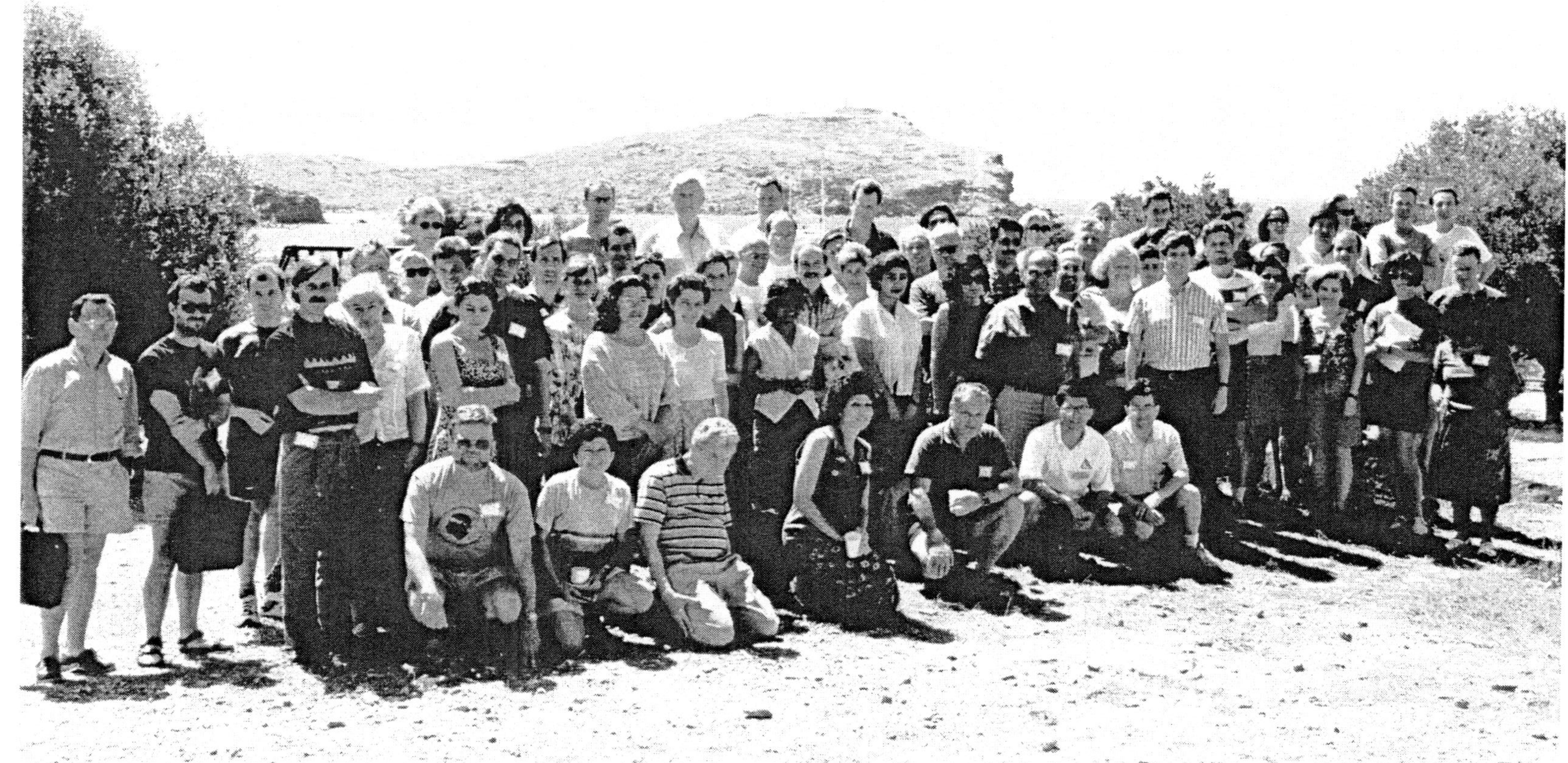

Participants of the NATO Advanced Studies Institute "Vaccine Design: The Role of Cytokine Networks" held at Cape Sounion Beach, Greece, during 24 June - 5 July 1996. The Organizing Committee included G. Gregoriadis (ASI Director and Chairman), A.C. Allison (ASI Co-Director), G. Kollias, B. McCormack and J.-L. Virelizier.

CONTRIBUTORS

A.C. Allison, Dawa Corporation, 2513 Hastings Drive, Belmont, CA 94002, U.S.A.

A. Amara, Unité d'Immunologie Virale, Institut Pasteur, 75724 Paris Cedex 15, FRANCE

J.M. Austyn, The Nuffield Dept of Surgery, John Radcliffe Hospital, Headington, Oxford OX3 9DU, UK

J. Bates, Commonwealth Serum Laboratories Ltd., 45 Poplar Road, Parkville, Victoria 3052, AUSTRALIA

L. Beezum, Commonwealth Serum Laboratories Ltd., 45 Poplar Road, Parkville, Victoria 3052, AUSTRALIA

S. Behboudi, Swedish University of Agricultural Sciences, Section of Virology, Biomedical Centre, Uppsala, SWEDEN

J.K. Bennet, Commonwealth Serum Laboratories Ltd., 45 Poplar Road, Parkville Victoria 3052, AUSTRALIA

D. Boraschi, Biotechnology Department, Dompe SpA, 67100 L'Aquila, ITALY

A. Capron, CIBP, INSERM U167, Institut Pasteur, 1, rue du Professeur Calmette, 59019 Lille, FRANCE

G. Cates, Connaught Laboratories Ltd, 1755 Steeles Avenue West, North York, Ontario, CANADA M2R 3T4

N. Challanáin, Dept of Medical Microbiology, The University of Sheffield Medical School, Beech Hill Rd, Sheffield S10 2RX, UK

M.J. Colston, Leprosy Unit, National Institute for Medical Research, The Ridgeway, Mill Hill, London NW7 1AA, UK

E. Comoy, CIBP, INSERM U167, Institut Pasteur, 1, rue du Professeur Calmette, 59019 Lille, FRANCE

A. Coulter, Commonwealth Serum Laboratories Ltd., 45 Poplar Road, Parkville, Victoria 3052, AUSTRALIA

J. Cox, Commonwealth Serum Laboratories Ltd., 45 Poplar Road, Parkville, Victoria 3052, AUSTRALIA

A. Gus Dagleish, Dept of Oncology, St Georges Medical School, Crammer Terrace, London SW17 0RE, UK

A.M. Donachie, Department of Immunology, University of Glasgow, Western Infirmary, Glasgow, Scotland G11 6NT, UK

D. Drane, Commonwealth Serum Laboratories Ltd., 45 Poplar Road, Parkville, Victoria 3052, AUSTRALIA

R.P. Du, Connaught Laboratories Ltd, 1755 Steeles Avenue West, North York, Ontario, CANADA M2R 3T4

M. Ewasyshyn, Connaught Laboratories Ltd, 1755 Steeles Avenue West, North York, Ontario, CANADA M2R 3T4

I.M. Fernández, Utrecht Univ., Eijkman-Winkler Laboratory, of Medical Microbiol., Medical School AZU, rm G04.614 Heidelberglaan 100, 3584 CX Utrecht, THE NETHERLANDS

H.O. Ghazi, Dept of Medical Microbiology, The University of Sheffield Medical School, Beech Hill Rd, Sheffield S10 2RX, UK

P. Ghiara, Istituto Ricerche Immunobiologiche Siena s.r.l., via Fiorentina 1, 53100 Siena, ITALY

B. Golding, Center for Biologics Evaluation and Res, Plasma Derivatives Bldg 29, Room 309 HFM 345, 8800 Rockville Pike Bethesda, MD 20892, USA

H. Golding, Chief, Retrovirology, Div of Viral Products, CBER USFDA HFM 445 Bldg 29A, Rm 1A-21, 8800 Rockville Pike, Bethesda, MD 20892, USA

G. Gregoriadis, Centre for Drug Delivery Research, The School of Pharmacy, University of London, 29-39 Brunswick Square, London WC1N 1AX, UK

D. Gregory, Leprosy Unit, National Institute for Medical Research, The Ridgeway, Mill Hill, London NW7 1AA, UK

M. Gursel, Centre for Drug Delivery Research, The School of Pharmacy, University of London, 29-39 Brunswick Square, London WC1N 1AX, UK

G. Jackson, Connaught Product Development Centre, Pasteur Mérieux Connaught Canada, 1755 Steeles Avenue West, North York, Ontario, CANADA M2R 3T4

R. Jennings, Dept of Medical Microbiology, The University of Sheffield Medical School, Beech Hill Rd, Sheffield S10 2RX, UK

M. Klein, Connaught Centre for Biotechnology Research, 1755 Steeles Avenue West, North York, Ontario, CANADA M2R 3T4

G. Kollias , Hellenic Pateur Institute, Dept of Molecular Genetics, 127 Vas Sofias Avenue, Athens 115 21, GREECE

C.A. Kraaijeveld, Utrecht Univ., Eijkman-Winkler Laboratory, of Medical Microbiol., Medical School AZU, rm G04.614 Heidelberglaan 100, 3584 CX Utrecht, THE NETHERLANDS

M. Kroll, Unité d'Immunologie Virale, Institut Pasteur, 75724 Paris Cedex 15, FRANCE

C.K. Lapham, Laboratory of Retrovirology Research, Div of Viral Products, CBER USFDA HFM 445, 8800 Rockville Pike, Bethesda, MD 20892, USA

D.B. Lowrie, Leprosy Unit, National Institute for Medical Research, The Ridgeway, Mill Hill, London NW7 1AA, UK

R. Macfarlan, Commonwealth Serum Laboratories Ltd., 45 Poplar Road, Parkville, Victoria 3052, AUSTRALIA

K.J. Maloy, Department of Immunology, University of Glasgow, Western Infirmary, Glasgow, Scotland G11 6NT, UK

A. Maraveyas, Dept of Oncology, St Georges Medical School, Crammer Terrace, London SW17 0RE, UK

C.S. McLean, Dept of Medical Microbiology, The University of Sheffield Medical School, Beech Hill Rd, Sheffield S10 2RX, UK

K. Lövgren-Bengtsson, Swedish University of Agricultural Sciences, Section of Virology, Biomedical Centre, Uppsala, SWEDEN

B. Morein, Swedish University of Agricultural Sciences, Section of Virology, Biomedical Centre, Uppsala, SWEDEN

A. Mowat, Department of Immunology, University of Glasgow, Western Infirmary, Glasgow, Scotland G11 6NT, UK

E. Oberlin, Unité d'Immunologie Virale, Institut Pasteur, 75724 Paris Cedex 15, FRANCE

S. Ragno, Leprosy Unit, National Institute for Medical Research, The Ridgeway, Mill Hill, London NW7 1AA, UK

M. Rodriguez, Unité d'Immunologie Virale, Institut Pastcur, 75724 Paris Cedex 15, FRANCE

D. Rousset, Unité d'Immunologie Virale, Institut Pasteur, 75724 Paris Cedex 15, FRANCE

N. Scollard, Connaught Laboratories Ltd, 1755 Steeles Avenue West, North York, Ontario, CANADA M2R 3T4

D.E. Scott, Center for Biologics Evaluation and Res, Plasma Derivatives Bldg 29, Room 309 HFM 345, 8800 Rockville Pike Bethesda, MD 20892, USA

R.E. Smith, Department of Immunology, University of Glasgow, Western Infirmary, Glasgow, Scotland G11 6NT, UK

H. Snippe, Utrecht Univ., Eijkman-Winkler Laboratory, of Medical Microbiol., Medical School AZU, rm G04.614 Heidelberglaan 100, 3584 CX Utrecht, THE NETHERLANDS

E. Stavropoulos, Leprosy Unit, National Institute for Medical Research, The Ridgeway, Mill Hill, London NW7 1AA, UK

A. Symington, Connaught Product Development Centre, Pasteur Mérieux Connaught Canada, 1755 Steeles Avenue West, North York, Ontario, CANADA M2R 3T4

A. Tagliabue, Biotechnology Department, Dompe SpA, 67100 L'Aquila, ITALY

R. Tascon, Leprosy Unit, National Institute for Medical Research, The Ridgeway, Mill Hill, London NW7 1AA, UK

G. Thyphronitis, CIBP, INSERM U167, Institut Pasteur, 1, rue du Professeur Calmette, 59019 Lille, FRANCE

M. Villacres-Ericksson, Swedish University of Agricultural Sciences, Section of Virology, Biomedical Centre, Uppsala, SWEDEN

J.-L. Virelizier, Unité d'Immunologie Virale, Institut Pasteur, 75724 Paris Cedex 15, FRANCE

Tuen-Yee Wong, Commonwealth Serum Laboratories Ltd., 45 Poplar Road, Parkville, Victoria 3052, AUSTRALIA

M.B. Zaitseva, Laboratory of Retrovirology Research, Div of Viral Products, CBER USFDA HFM 445, 8800 Rockville Pike, Bethesda, MD 20892, USA

INDEX